UROLOGIC ENDOSCOPY

UROLOGIC ENDOSCOPY
A Manual and Atlas

Demetrius H. Bagley, M.D.

Associate Professor of Urology and Radiology, Jefferson Medical College of Thomas Jefferson University; Attending Urologist, Thomas Jefferson University Hospital, Philadelphia

Jeffry L. Huffman, M.D.

Fellow in Urologic Oncology, Memorial Sloan-Kettering Cancer Center, New York

Edward S. Lyon, M.D.

Associate Professor of Urology, Department of Surgery, University of Chicago/The Pritzker School of Medicine; Section of Urology, University of Chicago Medical Center, Chicago

Little, Brown and Company

Boston / Toronto

Contents

Contributors

Donald W. Benson, M.D., Ph.D.

Professor and Chairman, Department of Anesthesiology, University of Chicago/The Pritzker School of Medicine; University of Chicago Hospitals and Clinics, Chicago

W. B. Gill, M.D., Ph.D.

Associate Professor of Surgery, University of Chicago/The Pritzker School of Medicine; Section of Urology, University of Chicago Medical Center, Chicago

Elizabeth M. Hickey

Illustrator

R. Lawrence Kroovand, M.D.

Associate Professor of Surgery (Pediatric Urology) and Pediatrics, and Director of Pediatric and Re-constructive Urology, Bowman Gray School of Medicine of Wake Forest University, Winston-Salem, North Carolina, and Former Associate Professor of Urology, Wayne State University School of Medicine, Detroit; Former Associate Chief of Pediatric Urology, Children's Hospital of Michigan, Detroit

Preface

There has been a definite need for a work describing urologic endoscopic techniques and findings that serves both as a training manual for residents and as a basic reference for practicing urologists on some of the less common procedures. As the writing of UROLOGIC ENDOSCOPY: *A Manual and Atlas* progressed, however, an exciting explosion in urologic endoscopy appeared with the extension of endoscopic techniques throughout the urinary tract. The need for such a book became overwhelming.

This volume in its final form describes endoscopic anatomic appearance and techniques throughout the urinary tract, grouped by anatomic areas. Normal and abnormal anatomy are presented initially with an emphasis on endoscopic or intraluminal anatomy and the relationship of other structures to the urinary lumen. The authors' color photographs illustrate the actual endoscopic appearance within the urinary tract. These illustrations demonstrate the normal and abnormal structures and the techniques discussed.

Every urologist will find specific subjects of interest. Although the younger resident may benefit most from a chapter such as that on cystourethroscopy, many advanced residents and practitioners will refer to the discussions of visual internal urethrotomy in the treatment of urethral strictures, transurethral resection of the prostate, and the endoscopic treatment of bladder calculi, which summarize newer techniques and the results with these procedures. The chapters on pediatric cystourethroscopy, ureteral catheterization, retrograde ureteropyelography, and self-retaining ureteral stents, and brush biopsy of the upper urinary tract review the state of the art in each area and summarize and compare the results of different techniques, while those on chromocystoscopy and microscopic cystoscopy, ureteropyeloscopy, percutaneous and operative nephroscopy, and endoscopic photography provide a unique collection of new techniques and color illustrations of endoscopic findings. These discussions summarize the pioneer efforts that have resulted in practical techniques applicable throughout the world today. In addition, other chapters describe supporting procedures, such as anesthesia, irrigation, and the care and sterilization of endoscopic instruments, without which the endoscopic techniques themselves would be impossible.

UROLOGIC ENDOSCOPY: *A Manual and Atlas* will provide a ready resource for the techniques and results of endoscopic procedures and serve as a focal point for the future development of urinary endoscopy. The entire urinary collecting system has now been opened to endoscopic inspection and manipulation. Every urologist should be familiar with these techniques and the endoscopic appearance throughout the urinary tract.

D. H. B.
J. L. H.
E. S. L.

I
NORMAL
ENDOSCOPIC
ANATOMY

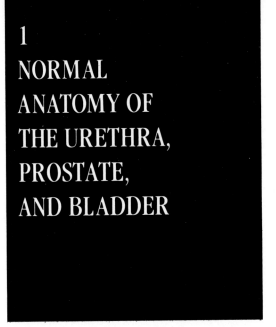

1

NORMAL ANATOMY OF THE URETHRA, PROSTATE, AND BLADDER

Demetrius H. Bagley

Jeffry L. Huffman

Edward S. Lyon

The urethra and bladder, along with the prostate in the male, constitute what is generally considered the lower urinary tract. These structures have been accessible to endoscopic inspection and manipulation since the earliest experience with endoscopic instruments. The greater length of the urethra in the male provides a greater expanse of the lumen for inspection as well as a greater potential for disorder. The prostate itself can be considered an additional region subject to anatomic variation and disease. The bladder in the normal male differs from that in the normal female; the range of abnormality may also differ. Familiarity with the normal anatomic variations and the anatomic relationships will enable the urologist to recognize the presence of significant disorders and minimize the complications from endoscopic procedures.

MALE URETHRA. The normal male urethra can be thought of as being divided into two portions, the anterior and the posterior urethra, separated by the urogenital diaphragm (Fig. 1-1). The course of the male urethra extends from the vesical neck to the external meatus and is approximately 20 to 24 cm in total length. It lies along the ventral penile shaft.

The external meatus is normally approximately 8 mm in diameter (24 Fr.) in the adult male, and appears as a slit in the distal, ventral portion of the glans. Congenital variations can be seen in the specific placement of the meatus. These result from variations in closure of the urethral groove and are recognized clinically as *hypospadius.*

The anterior or more distal portion of the urethra can be further subdivided into three distinct areas: the glandular, the penile, and the bulbous portions of the urethra. The *glandular urethra,* which is the most distal portion of the anterior urethra, terminates at the urethral meatus and is approached first with any instrument passed through the meatus. The more proximal portion of the glanular urethra includes the *fossa navicularis,* which is a dilated portion of the urethra extending from the meatus to the level of the corona. The diameter within this portion often reaches 10 to 11 mm. Congenital anomalies, seen as redundancies in the mucous membrane, often form short pseudodiverticula in this area. In the proximal portion of the fossa, the lumen of the urethra continues from the ventral aspect of the fossa. A ridge is often formed at this level, known as the *valve of the fossa navicularis* or *valve of Guerrin.* This configuration of the urethra must be considered before passing any instrument, which could lodge within the fossa if passed along the dorsal aspect. To continue within the urethra, the instrument should be passed along the ventral aspect at the fossa navicularis. The proximal junction of the fossa navicularis with the penile urethra is often quite narrow and, in fact, may require dilation for passage of the urethroscope. The distal portion of the fossa navicularis is lined with squamous epithelium while the more proximal portions of the urethra are lined with stratified or pseudostratified columnar epithelium.

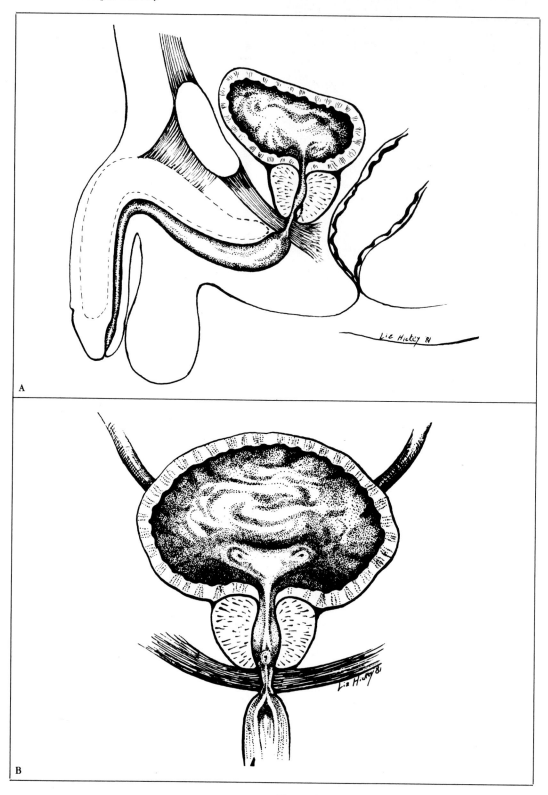

Figure 1-1. *Midline sagittal section (A) and coronal section (B) of the male lower urinary tract.*

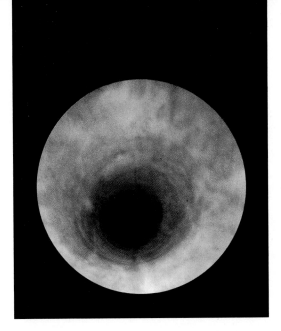

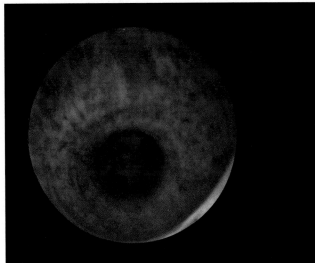

Figure 1-2. *The pendulous urethra in the male has a cylindrical lumen with a pink gray, mottled mucosa. The caliber and the mucosa remain uniform in this portion of the urethra.*

Figure 1-3. *In the bulbous urethra, the lumen becomes larger and the mucosa is often slightly more erythematous with a distinctly linear vascular pattern.*

The next most proximal anatomic division of the urethra is the *penile* or *pendulous urethra,* which extends from the proximal aspect of the fossa navicularis at the level of the corona of the glans penis to the point of attachment of the suspensory ligament of the penis at the penoscrotal junction. It is a cylinder of uniform caliber, usually 9 to 10 mm in diameter (27–30 Fr.). The mucosa in this portion of the urethra appears mottled pink gray. The major endoscopic characteristic, however, is the cylindrical appearance of the lumen (Fig. 1-2).

The *glands of Littré* are mucous glands and follicles within the submucosal tissue of the urethra, predominantly located anteriorly and laterally in the pendulous portion. There are also small pitlike openings or lacunae of varying sizes, the orifices of which open distally.

The *bulbous urethra* is that portion of the anterior urethra extending from the penoscrotal junction proximally to the urogenital diaphragm. The lumen is larger in this area, ranging from 11 to 12 mm in diameter. Proximally, within this portion of the urethra are the openings of the ducts of the bulbous urethral, or Cowper's, glands. The glands themselves lie more proximally in the area of the external sphincter.

There is a more linear vascular pattern in the mucosa in the bulbous urethra, which is oriented distally and proximally toward the membranous urethra (Fig. 1-3). The proximal portion of the bulbous urethra is somewhat redundant and may provide a depression or partial obstruction to the passage of instruments through this portion of the urethra. Careful attention, therefore, must be paid when passing instruments through this portion, and the beak of an endoscope or the curve of a sound should be utilized to negotiate the curve of the bulbous urethra toward the membranous urethra at the urogenital diaphragm (Fig. 1-4). This is a frequent site of perforation when stiff catheters or rigid instruments are passed into the urethra by inexperienced personnel.

Throughout the anterior portion of the urethra, the mucosa lies surrounded by a thin submucosal layer, adjacent to which is the erectile tissue of the *corpus spongiosum.* Proximally, the corpus spongiosum is applied only to the ventral surface of the bulbous urethra but is distributed circumferentially along the distal bulbous and entire pendulous urethra. Distally, the corpus spongiosum is continuous with the erectile tissue of the glans penis.

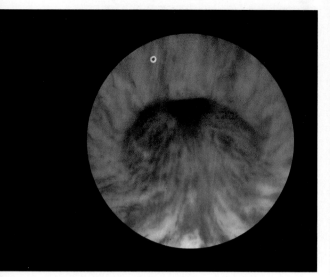

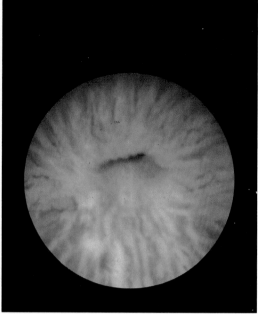

Figure 1-4. *Proximally within the bulbous urethra, the lumen turns cephalad and the posterior wall can be seen directly in the field of view. The lumen narrows abruptly as it approaches the membranous urethra.*

Figure 1-5. *The sphincteric area in the membranous urethra has a shutterlike appearance with a vascular mucosal pattern converging toward the lumen. In an anesthetized patient, the lumen may open under the pressure of the irrigation fluid.*

The membranous urethra is the shortest (only 1–2 cm in length) and, except for the urethral meatus, the narrowest portion of the urethra. It extends from the bulbous urethra proximally to the apex of the prostate and includes the portion traversing the urogenital diaphragm. The length of the membranous urethra may vary with relaxation of the pelvic floor. Endoscopically, there is a sharp demarcation as the instrument passes from the proximal bulbous urethra toward the membranous urethra (see Fig. 7-9). The mucosa in the membranous urethra is characterized by the concentric closure of the musculature forming the sphincterlike mechanism. There are a few mucosal glands but considerably less than in the anterior urethra. The membranous urethra will distend with the pressure of the irrigating fluid during endoscopy, particularly in the anesthetized patient.

The *external sphincter* is not a specific circular muscle but rather represents the combination of several muscle fibers in the area adjacent to the membranous urethra (Fig. 1-5). There is a concentration of spiral muscle fibers at the lower border of the prostate. This thickening of the muscle bands is most apparent endoscopically in the adult male; no comparable collection or mass of muscle fibers is present in the female.

The external sphincter has been defined anatomically as a layer of striated muscle limited above by the superior fascial layer and below by the inferior fascial layer of the urogenital diaphragm. Voluntary contraction of this muscle compresses the membranous urethra within the urogenital diaphragm and obstructs the flow of urine. Hutch[2] has postulated that the external sphincter also includes the *periurethral striated muscle,* which exerts its action by constricting the lower half of the urethra lying above the urogenital diaphragm. It is this area that Hutch postulates can be damaged, resulting in incontinence postprostatectomy.

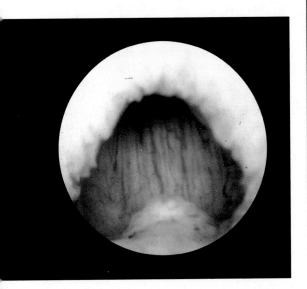

Figure 1-6. *The verumontanum marks the distal prostatic urethra. The inverted V of the anterior distal prostate is evident at the 12 o'clock position, and the posterior lip of the bladder neck, with its parallel vascular pattern, is visible in the distance.*

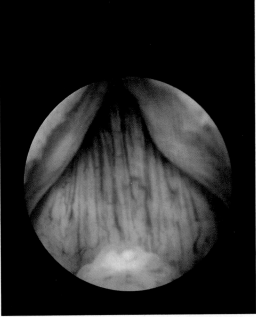

Figure 1-7. *As the urethroscope is advanced proximally, the verumontanum remains in view but the minimally enlarged lateral lobes of the prostate become visible. The high posterior bladder neck remains in view obscuring the lumen of the bladder.*

As the endoscope is passed proximally through the membranous urethra, the distal margin or the apex of the prostate is identified by the presence of the *verumontanum,* also called the *colliculus seminalis* (Fig. 1-6). Mucosal folds of varying prominence can also be identified. In the proximal membranous urethra two folds of mucosa (the inframontanal folds) course laterally and distally from the verumontanum and merge into the urethral wall. Extending proximally from the verumontanum, the urethral crest is a longitudinal ridge on the posterior floor within the prostatic urethra. On either side of this ridge lies the area of the prostatic sinus, which contains the orifices of the prostatic ducts from the lateral lobes. The verumontanum represents the elevation of urethral mucosa by the ejaculatory ducts and the utricle. The utricle itself is only a few (approximately 6) millimeters long, running posteriorly within the substance of the prostate. It has been labeled the *uterus masculinus* since it is a remnant of the paramesonephric, or müllerian, ducts in the male and is homologous with the uterus and upper portion of the vagina in the female.

The prostatic portion of the urethra runs proximally from the verumontanum to the bladder neck through the substance of the prostate gland (Figs. 1-7, 1-8). It is located more anteriorly than posteriorly within the gland. The lumen is indented by the lateral lobes of the prostate and is subject to obstruction in the presence of prostatic hypertrophy.

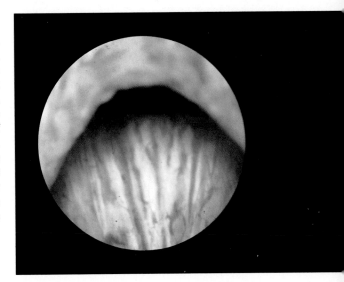

Figure 1-8. *As the beak of the endoscope is elevated (anteriorly), the lip of the bladder neck and the lumen of the bladder come into view. The inverted V formed by the lateral lobes meeting the anterior portion of the prostate remains.*

PROSTATE

Anatomic Relationship. The prostate lies on the urogenital diaphragm inferiorly and is juxtaposed to the bladder superiorly. The urethra traverses the prostate. It is because of this intimate relationship of the prostate to the bladder and urethra that many of the abnormalities of the prostate are manifest by voiding symptoms.

The prostate itself is somewhat conical, with the base adjacent to the bladder and the apex directed inferiorly toward the urogenital diaphragm. The anteroposterior dimension is shorter than the lateral diameter. Although the prostate may vary widely in size, the normal gland is approximately 3 to 4 cm long, 4 cm wide, and 2 to 3 cm thick.

Posteriorly, the prostate is adjacent to the rectum, separated by the rectovesical (Denonvilliers') fascia. Anteriorly, the prostate is approximately 2 cm posterior to the symphysis pubis. It is surrounded by adipose tissue and a venous plexus and is connected to the pubic bone by the puboprostatic ligaments. Laterally, the prostate is associated with the levator ani. The ejaculatory ducts pass through the posterior portion of the prostate and open into the urethra at the level of the verumontanum.

The prostate is surrounded by a thin, tough, fibrous capsule, which is densely adherent and continuous with the stroma of the gland. Smooth muscular tissue is arranged as a dense layer immediately within the fibrous capsule. Another prominent layer of circular fibers is seen around the urethra within the substance of the prostate. This layer is continuous with the muscular layer of the bladder and distally blends into the fibers around the membranous urethra. Smooth muscle fibers also course as a meshwork through the substance of the gland. Anteriorly, the smooth muscle is denser with minimal glandular tissue.

Structure of the Prostate. The glands of the prostate consist of numerous follicles with papillary linings. Some of these open into canals, which join to form 12 to 20 secretory ducts. The prostatic ducts open into the floor of the prostatic urethra and have been described as lacking sphincters. These are considered the *external glands* of the prostate.

The *internal* or *periurethral glands* include the mucosal and submucosal glands. The mucosal glands are located mainly on the roof of the urethra and are similar to the glands of Littré in the anterior urethra. The submucosal glands are located at the bladder neck and laterally within the prostate adjacent to the urethra. These glands can hypertrophy and then become recognizable clinically, although anatomically they remain indistinguishable. They form the posterior and median lobes as well as the lateral and anterior lobes of the prostate. When located beneath the neck of the bladder, they can develop into the clinically recognized subcervical lobe of Albarran, or the sixth lobe. In the subtrigonal position, they can form the subtrigonal lobe of Home, or the seventh lobe.

Vascular Supply of the Prostate. The blood supply of the prostate is derived from a branch of the inferior vesical artery, which arises from the anterior division of the internal iliac artery. The inferior vesical artery courses medially along the levator muscles to the neck of the bladder where it arborizes to supply the lower ureter, seminal vesicles, vas deferens, and prostate. The prostatic artery divides into two branches, the ascending and descending. The former enters the prostate posterolaterally at the base and supplies the glandular tissue as it courses through the prostate at that level. This branch appears in the substance of the prostate posterolateral to the urethra and must be controlled during resection of the prostate[1]. The accessory arteries from the middle hemorrhoidal and internal pudendal arteries supply only the inferior (apical) portion of the prostate.

The veins of the prostate form a plexus, particularly in the lateral prostatic ligaments, and also join the dorsal vein of the penis anteriorly to form the plexus of Santorini, which ultimately enters the internal iliac veins. There is also a minor portion of drainage through the hemorrhoidal veins.

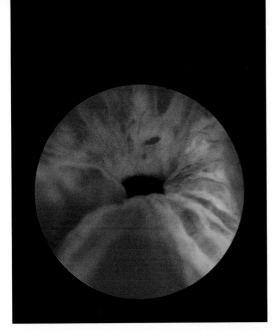

Figure 1-9. *The female urethra is a short structure that is not well distended by irrigation. There is a linear vascular and mucosal pattern. The bladder neck merges less distinctly with the urethra in the female than in the male.*

FEMALE URETHRA. The female urethra is a much shorter structure, approximately 4 cm in length, extending from the bladder to the urethral meatus in the vaginal vestibule. The urethra is located dorsal to the symphysis pubis and courses along the anterior wall of the vagina and through the fascia of the urogenital diaphragm as it descends to the meatus. It is approximately 8 mm in diameter. Endoscopically, the urethral membrane is gathered in longitudinal folds with a comparable vascular pattern (Fig. 1-9). One of these folds, called the *urethral crest,* is more prominent than the others and is located along the floor of the canal. The periurethral glands (of Skene) open through ducts just within the urethral meatus. The distal portion of the urethra is lined by a stratified squamous epithelium and the proximal portion by a transitional epithelium.

THE BLADDER. The bladder is the major reservoir of the urinary system and constitutes the largest surface area in contact with the urine. This entire surface is accessible to the endoscopic approach.

Anatomic Relationship. The bladder is supported on the pelvic floor. It is fixed by the prostate at the level of the neck of the bladder in the male, as well as by the visceral pelvic fascia, the pubovesical ligaments, and the urachal or umbilical ligaments. The bladder is also attached by the ureters, the vascular supply, the obliterated umbilical vessels, and the peritoneal surface.

In the adult, the bladder, when empty, is located entirely within the pelvis. As it fills, the superior surface of the bladder rises into the abdominal cavity. The bladder itself lies posterior to the symphysis pubis, superior to the prostate, and anterior to the seminal vesicals and the rectum in the male. In the female, the bladder is immediately anterior to the uterus and the upper portion of the vagina. The superior surface of the bladder is roughly triangular in shape and is covered by peritoneum. It is directly related to the sigmoid colon and small bowel. The inferior and lateral surfaces are not covered by peritoneum. The surfaces are bound together in the relationships described above with an areolar tissue.

Structure of the Bladder. The bladder is composed of two major layers, the muscular coat and the mucosal lining, which are separated by a small submucosal layer. The muscle is arranged in a meshwork that is continuous to the level of the bladder neck and into the urethra[3]. The most external coat of the muscular layer is longitudinal and courses from the dome posteriorly into the urethra. The muscles are arranged to contract the bladder for emptying and to open the bladder neck and posterior urethra in the process.

The mucosa is formed of transitional epithelial cells that flatten and form a single epithelial layer during bladder distention. In the distensible portions of the bladder, the mucosa is only loosely attached to the submucosa but is more firmly attached directly to the muscular layer over the trigone. It remains smooth in this area regardless of the state of distention since the trigonal area does not distend. In the distensible areas, the mucosal pattern can be related to the degree of filling. The mucosa appears flat when the bladder is filled but can appear redundant or wrinkled when the bladder contains a lesser volume.

The thickness of the musculature of the bladder is related to its activity and hypertrophy. In the younger patient, particularly the female, the bladder may be only a few millimeters thick. There may be only a minimal appearance of the underlying musculature endoscopically.

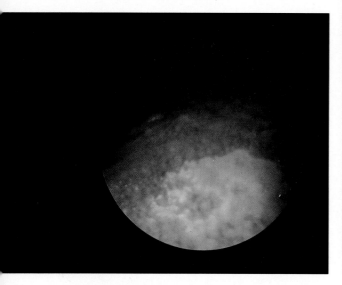

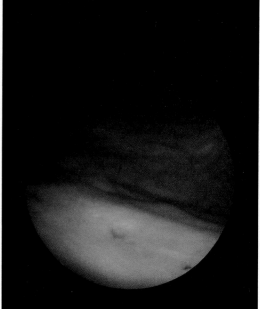

Figure 1-10. *Squamous metaplasia is prominent on the trigone of this 42-year-old female. The right ureteral orifice is evident in the left midfield (70-degree lens).*

Figure 1-11. *The right ureteral orifice is seen with the 12-degree lens in the lower center of the field. The interureteric ridge extends entirely across the lower center of the field.*

Within the bladder, the surface can be divided into several regions. The *vesical neck,* which limits the bladder inferiorly and distally, appears as a funnel-shaped opening of the urethra into the bladder. Endoscopically, the vesical neck is seen when the instrument passes proximally into the bladder. From that point, the vesical neck appears as a concentric muscular ring. If the bladder neck is viewed from the superior aspect, either with the bladder opened or with an endoscope placed through a suprapubic tract, the vesical neck remains the major landmark and reference point in the anatomy of the bladder.

The *trigone* is that area limited by the ureteral orifices and the intravesical urethral opening at the bladder neck. It is formed by musculature thought to be an expansion of the muscle fibers surrounding the ureters, in addition to the normal bladder muscle. The trigone is less prominent in the female than in the male. In the female, squamous metaplasia may be seen on the trigone extending to the bladder neck (Fig. 1-10). It appears in the form of white, slightly raised patches that cannot be scraped from the surface with an instrument. Squamous metaplasia is a normal variation in the female and does not represent an inflammatory process. The presence of squamous epithelium in the bladder has been thought to result from developmental variations, migration of vaginal epithelium, or, less commonly, true metaplasia of the trigonal mucosa.

The elevation extending between the ureteral orifices is known as the *interureteric ridge.* It is more prominent in males than females, in whom it may be poorly defined. It is rare, however, that some prominence identified as the interureteric ridge cannot be located. The ureteral orifices are located along the interureteric ridge symmetrically, usually 1 to 2 cm from the midline (Figs. 1-11 to 1-14). Various anomalies may develop with the orifices placed along the interureteric ridge or its lateral extension, inferiorly to the bladder neck, or even in the urethra (see Chap. 18).

There is great variation in the appearance of the normal ureteral orifice. In the adult, a normal, nonrefluxing orifice may have the configuration described as a volcano, a horseshoe, or some other variation. The orifice may either be quite prominent and obvious on endoscopic examination or appear as an inconspicuous slit distinguishable from the surrounding mucosa only through careful inspection.

The ureteral orifice is often surrounded by a characteristic mucosal vascular pattern. Prominent mucosal vessels course in an arc medial, inferior, and lateral to the orifice (see Figs. 1-11, 1-13). This pattern is often obscured in the presence of generalized mucosal inflammation.

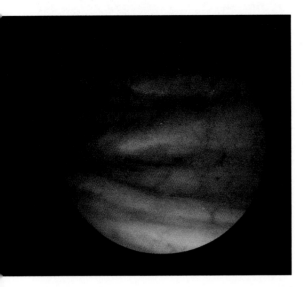

Figure 1-12. *The interureteric ridge continues in this view with the 12-degree lens located at the bladder neck.*

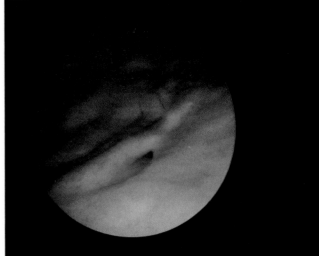

Figure 1-13. *As the 12-degree lens is rotated toward the patient's left, the left ureteral orifice is seen as a bolus of urine exits, leaving the orifice open. The ridge is less prominent laterally than it was on the right lateral wall (see Fig. 1-11).*

REFERENCES

1. Flocks, R. H. The arterial distribution within the prostate gland: Its role in transurethral prostatic resection. *J. Urol.* 37:524, 1937.
2. Hutch, J. A. A new theory of the anatomy of the internal urinary sphincter in the physiology of micturition. IV. The urinary sphincteric mechanism. *J. Urol.* 97:705, 1967.
3. Woodburne, R. T. Structure and function of the urinary bladder. *J. Urol.* 84:79, 1960.

SUGGESTED READINGS

Lich, R., Jr., Howerton, L. W., and Amin, M. Anatomy and Surgical Approach to the Urogenital Tract in the Male. In J. H. Harrison, et al. (Eds.), *Campbell's Urology* (4th ed.). Philadelphia: Saunders, 1978. Chap. 1, pp. 3–33.
Williams, P. L., and Warwick, R. (Eds.). *Gray's Anatomy* (36th ed.). Philadelphia: Saunders, 1980. Pp. 1404–1410.

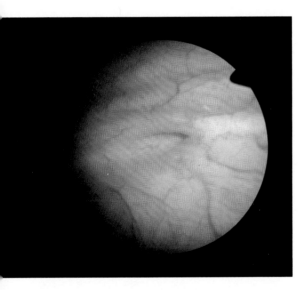

Figure 1-14. *The same orifice in Fig. 1-13 is viewed through the 70-degree telescope. In this patient, the orifice appears flatter but the same configuration of the os and vascular pattern is evident.*

The base, or fundus, of the bladder is located posterior to the trigone. The lateral walls of the bladder extend superiorly to the dome or vertex, as do the anterior and posterior walls. The normal vascular pattern and topographic appearance of the mucosa can be seen over the bladder musculature in these areas. When the bladder is distended, this pattern becomes relatively smooth unless there is prominent trabeculation.

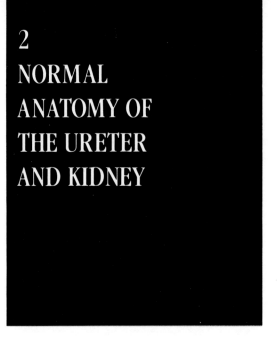

2
NORMAL ANATOMY OF THE URETER AND KIDNEY

Jeffry L. Huffman

Demetrius H. Bagley

Edward S. Lyon

The ureter and intrarenal collecting system constitute the upper portion of the urinary tract and function to transport urine from the nephron to the bladder. The anatomic relation of these structures, including the kidney itself, has been extensively studied and is vital to know when one performs surgery within the retroperitoneum or pelvis. Only recently has the in situ intraluminal surface anatomy of these structures been elucidated to the extent of the bladder and urethra. The addition of this endoscopic anatomy allows for a more complete description of the anatomy of the upper urinary system.

ANATOMIC RELATIONS OF THE URETER. The ureter is an entirely retroperitoneal structure extending from the renal pelvis to the bladder. The average length is 25 to 30 cm. It can be divided into pelvic and abdominal portions for descriptive purposes [4].

The *pelvic ureter* begins at the ureterovesical junction, which consists of the ureteral os and the submucosal and intramural portions of the ureter. From the ureteral orifice, the ureter courses submucosally, proximally, and posterolaterally within the bladder. It then passes through the musculature of the bladder wall at the detrusor hiatus in an oblique fashion. The ureterovesical junction is the narrowest portion of the ureter, with an average size of 3 to 4 mm [3].

The pelvic portion continues outside the bladder laterally and slightly posteriorly along the musculature of the lateral pelvic wall to the region of the ischial spine. The course then continues medially and anteriorly to the pelvic brim where it lies immediately anterior to the internal iliac artery and the obturator vessels (Figs. 2-1, 2-2). The pelvic portion of the ureter thus extends from the bladder to the pelvic brim.

The relation of the pelvic ureter to other pelvic organs varies in the male and female. In the male, as the ureter emerges from the bladder wall, it lies just anterior to the free end of the seminal vesicle and just lateral to the vas deferens. As it comes superiorly, it then is related dorsally to the obturator vessels and nerve. In the female, the ureter emerges from the bladder and courses slightly posteriorly and laterally to cross just caudally to the uterine artery. It then turns superiorly to run 8 to 12 mm anteriorly and parallel to the vaginal wall and cervix. It thus continues anterolaterally and superiorly to course posteriorly to the middle and superior vesical arteries and then posteriorly to the ovary.

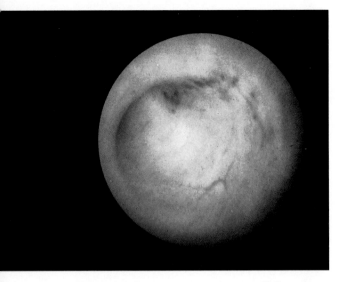

Figure 2-1. *The distal ureter courses medially and anteriorly after initially emerging from the bladder in a posterior and lateral direction. This and subsequent views in Chap. 2 are of the left ureter and kidney.*

The *abdominal ureter* extends superiorly beyond the true pelvis. It crosses the bifurcation of the common iliac artery anteriorly and the ventral surface of the transverse processes of the third to fifth lumbar vertebral bodies (Fig. 2-3). Superiorly, the ureter lies anterior to the psoas muscle and the genitofemoral nerve (Fig. 2-4). It then courses slightly laterally and posteriorly to the renal pelvis, which it joins at the ureteropelvic junction (Fig. 2-5). The average size of the abdominal portion of the ureter is 5 to 6 mm [4].

On the right, the abdominal ureter lies in close relation to the inferior vena cava medially and is crossed anteriorly by the gonadal vessels and the peritoneal attachment of the small bowel mesentery. Superiorly, it also lies dorsal to the descending portion of the duodenum. The left abdominal ureter lies just lateral to the aorta. It is crossed anteriorly by the gonadal vessels and the peritoneal attachment of the sigmoid mesocolon.

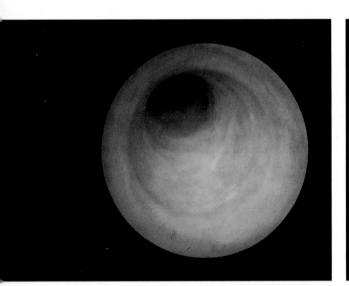

Figure 2-2. *The ureter courses anteriorly toward the pelvic brim. This relatively narrow portion of the ureter appears slightly stenotic and is relatively nondistensible.*

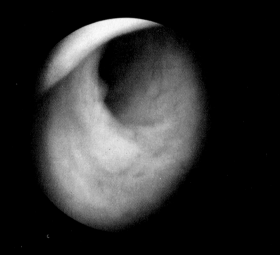

Figure 2-3. *After crossing the pelvic brim, the ureter lies in close relation anterior to the common iliac artery, the pulsations of which are seen moving the posteromedial portion of the ureteral wall.*

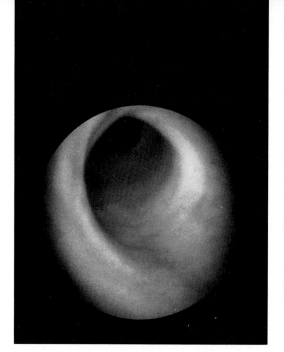

Figure 2-4. *Superiorly, the midureter is relatively straight and courses slightly anteriorly to cross the psoas muscle and genitofemoral nerve. This is the most anterior portion of the ureter and usually the most distensible.*

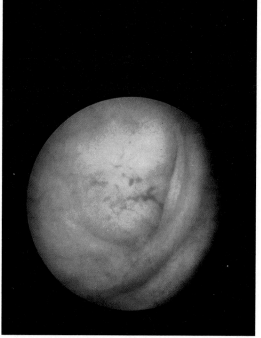

Figure 2-5. *The proximal ureter courses posteriorly toward the ureteropelvic junction. A lip of mucosa is visible posterolaterally, corresponding to the bending of the ureteropelvic junction with each respiration and downward movement of the kidney.*

ENDOSCOPIC ANATOMY OF THE URETER. Although the normal ureter is relatively uniform in size and easily distensible, there are three naturally narrow sites within the lumen: the ureteropelvic junction (Fig. 2-6), the pelvic brim (see Fig. 2-2), and the ureterovesical junction (see Figs. 15-6, 15-7). Although the narrowest portion, the ureterovesical junction, requires dilation prior to introducing the rigid ureteropyeloscope, the more proximal constrictions usually can be dilated with the pressure of the irrigation fluid and thus passed as the instrument is inserted.

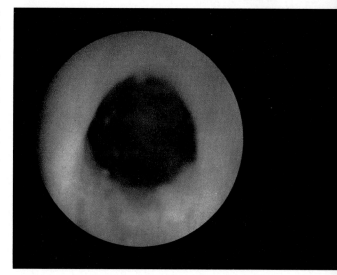

Figure 2-6. *The ureteropelvic junction is another relatively narrow portion of the ureter. The capacious renal pelvis is visible in the background.*

Besides these anatomic regions, which are readily identified endoscopically by a slightly stenotic appearance and relative nondistensibility, there are several other landmarks to observe since, in its course between the bladder and the kidney, the ureter conforms to the surrounding retroperitoneal structures. The portion of the ureter crossing the iliac vessels can be seen pulsating as the instrument ascends through the ureter out of the pelvis to this level (see Fig. 2-3). The midureter is relatively straight since it lies along the psoas muscle. As the proximal ureter is approached, it can be seen that the entire kidney and ureteropelvic junction lie posteriorly and the course of the ureter passes posteriorly and laterally over the psoas muscle (see Fig. 2-4). The excursion of the kidney with respiration is also readily apparent endoscopically as the instrument approaches the proximal ureter and the ureteropelvic junction. The ureter is a relatively fixed structure whereas the ureteropelvic junction and the renal pelvis are mobile and move in an axial plane cephalad or caudally with each movement of the diaphragm and kidney with respiration. Endoscopically, the peristaltic contractions of the ureter, along with the opening and closing of the ureteropelvic junction, can be observed (Figs. 2-5, 2-6).

The proximal ureter joins the renal pelvis at the ureteropelvic junction, which, as noted earlier, is one of the naturally narrow portions of the ureter. Endoscopically, it can be identified as a narrowing in the ureter when compared with the more distal ureter or the larger proximal renal pelvis (Fig. 2-6). Also, its movement with each excursion of the kidney with respiration is readily apparent. Occasionally, a lip is visible in the lumen posterolaterally near the region of the ureteropelvic junction (see Fig. 2-5). This bend of mucosa corresponds to the junction of the proximal ureter with the dependent portion of the pelvis and can be seen to accentuate with each downward movement of the kidney with respiration.

The inner surface of the ureter is lined by transitional epithelium, which is four to five cells thick and surrounded by the lamina propria[1]. This connective tissue structure forms thin longitudinal folds in the mucosal surface and causes the characteristic folded appearance of the nondistended ureteral lumen. The middle layer of the ureter is muscular and consists of inner longitudinal fibers and outer circular fibers, which account for the periodic contractions that propel urine to the bladder.

In the lower ureter, there is an additional outer longitudinal muscular layer extending into the bladder. The outer surface of the ureter is an adventitial layer of connective tissue and vessels, which entirely surrounds the smooth muscle coat and is covered by retroperitoneal fat.

ANATOMIC RELATIONS OF THE KIDNEY. The anatomic relations of the right and left kidney are different and become particularly important in performing percutaneous intrarenal procedures and endourologic techniques. The right renal hilus lies directly posterior to the descending portion of the duodenum and farther, anteriorly, toward the anterior abdominal wall are the right lobe of the liver and hepatic flexure of the colon. Immediately anterior to the renal pelvis are the renal artery and vein, which drain into the inferior vena cava medially. Posteriorly, the right kidney is in contact with the psoas, quadratus lumborum, and transversus adominus muscles from the medial to the lateral aspect. The adrenal gland overlies the superior and medial aspect of the upper pole, and the diaphragm and twelfth rib overlie the upper pole of the kidney posteriorly. The posterior segmental branch of the main renal artery also crosses directly behind the upper portion of the renal pelvis.

The left kidney has different relationships. Posteriorly, the same muscles are encountered and the diaphragm, along with the eleventh and twelfth ribs, overlies the upper pole. Anteriorly, however, the tail of the pancreas extends across the upper pole of the kidney, as does the inferior tip of the spleen. In a pattern similar to the relationship of the duodenum to the right kidney, the proximal portion of the jejunum and greater curvature of the stomach overlie the left renal hilus. Also, the splenic flexure of the colon extends across the lower pole of the left kidney anteriorly.

The anatomic relation of the intrarenal collecting system, which includes the renal pelvis and calyces, has been well described[2]. There are normally four to twelve minor calyces, which, except for the upper and lower pole calyces, are aligned in two distinct rows within the kidney anteriorly and posteriorly (see Fig. 15-9). The frontal plane of the kidney lies at a 30-degree angle posterior to the coronal axis of the body with the renal pelvis being most anterior and the convex lateral margin of the kidney being most posterior. The anterior row of calyces thus lies at an angle that is 40 degrees anterior to the coronal body plane, and the posterior row of calyces lies at an angle 50 degrees posterior to the coronal axis.

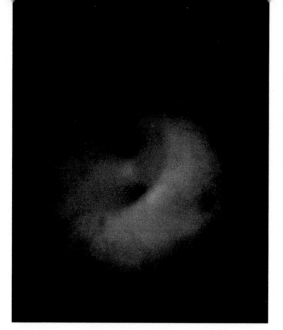

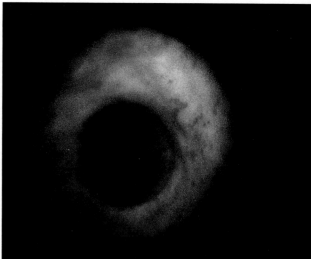

Figure 2-7. *On entering the renal pelvis, the first structures visualized are the ostia of the major calyces. These are circular openings with carinae separating individual calyces.*

Figure 2-8. *The infundibulum is a tubular structure extending from the ostium and connecting the renal pelvis with the minor calyces visible in the background.*

ENDOSCOPIC ANATOMY OF THE INTRARENAL COLLECTING SYSTEM. The endoscopic anatomy of the renal pelvis is extremely variable. There are many variations in size, shape, and location of the pelvis. Essentially, the normal pelvis can be thought of as conical in shape with the apex of the cone representing the ureteropelvic junction. Intrarenal pelvises are often small with short major calyces. They lie almost entirely within the renal sinus. Extrarenal pelvises are usually large and have long major calyceal infundibula and lie outside the renal sinus.

Endoscopically, as an instrument enters the renal pelvis, the ostia of the major calyces leading to the upper, middle, and lower poles of the kidney are the first structures visible (Fig. 2-7). They appear as circular openings branching from the pelvis, and often minor calyces with renal papillae are visible in the background. The long tubular portion, or *infundibulum,* connects the base, or *ostium,* to the apex of the major calyx (Fig. 2-8). Separating the major calyces into branches from the renal pelvis are *carinae.* Anatomically, calyceal branching is similar to the branching of the trachea into the right and left mainstem bronchi; it differs, however, in that there can be two or three major calyces with one or two carinae (see Fig. 2-7).

As the instrument then enters the infundibulum, the next structures visible are the minor calyces. There are usually four to twelve minor calyces, which coalesce to drain into two or three major calyces. Endoscopically, it is readily apparent that the calyces are dynamic structures. They contract intermittently to obliterate the lumen totally. Their muscular component, especially the outer circular muscle fibers, cause these intermittent sphincteric contractions. These circular fibers extend around the base of each papilla to form a muscular ring that controls and helps to propel urine from the papillary ducts into the minor calyces. Inner longitudinal muscle fibers end at the area where the minor calyx attaches to the renal papilla. As in the ureter, the muscular layer of the pelvis and calyces is surrounded by an adventitial layer of connective tissue.

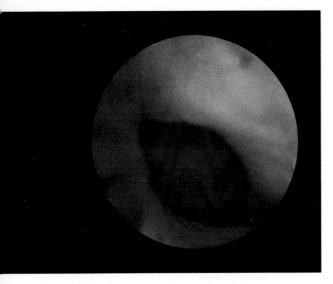

Figure 2-9. *The renal papilla is a pink convex disc surrounded by the pale epithelium of the calyceal fornix.*

REFERENCES

1. Bloom, W., and Fawcett, D. W. The Urinary System. In W. Bloom and D. W. Fawcett (Eds.), *A Textbook of Histology* (10th ed.). Philadelphia: Saunders, 1975. Pp. 766–804.
2. Kaye, K. W., and Goldberg, M. E. Applied anatomy of the kidney and ureter. *Urol. Clin. North Am.* 9:3, 1982.
3. Lich, R., Jr., Howerton, L. W., and Amin, M. Anatomy and Surgical Approach to the Urogenital Tract in the Male. In J. H. Harrison, et al. (Eds.), *Campbell's Urology* (4th ed.). Philadelphia: Saunders, 1978. Chap. 1, pp. 3–33.
4. Markee, J. E. The Urogenital System. In B. J. Anson (Ed.), *Morris' Human Anatomy* (12th ed.). New York: McGraw-Hill, 1966. Pp. 1457–1537.

The conical minor calyx surrounding the renal papilla is called the *calyceal fornix.* Occasionally, more than one papilla may project into a minor calyx to form a *compound calyx.* This situation is most common in the upper pole[3]. The minor calyx differs in its endoscopic appearance from the papilla by having a pale mucosal surface of epithelium consisting of transitional cells usually arranged in a layer only two to three cells thick (Figs. 2-8, 2-9). This type of transitional epithelium lines the remainder of the intrarenal collecting system and the entire ureter.

The papillae are the final structures visible. They appear endoscopically as a circular convex disc surrounded by the calyceal fornix with a pink, friable epithelium (Fig. 2-9). Unlike the remainder of the intrarenal collecting system and ureter, the papillae are lined by cuboidal epithelium[1]. The papillae form the apex of the renal pyramids and vary in number from four to twelve, depending on the individual. As urine is drained through the papillary ducts of Bellini within the renal pyramids, it exits into the minor calyces via these renal papillae. Occasionally, the papillary ducts of Bellini can be identified on the renal papillae. They can be seen as pinpoint openings and are dilated and more apparent in a patient with urinary obstruction.

II
ABNORMAL
ENDOSCOPIC
ANATOMY

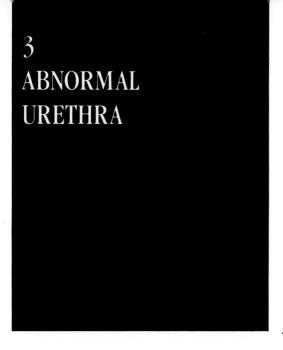

3
ABNORMAL URETHRA

Demetrius H. Bagley

Edward S. Lyon

Jeffry L. Huffman

Direct endoscopic visualization has a major role in the diagnosis and often the treatment of disorders of the urethra. Structural abnormalities that may have been reflected symptomatically can often be diagnosed endoscopically. Similarly, structural abnormalities that have remained asymptomatic, yet are of varying significance, may be discovered on endoscopic examination performed for other reasons. Evaluation for some diagnoses requires special endoscopic techniques while other suspected diagnoses represent contraindications to endoscopy.

URETHRITIS. Urethritis, an inflammation of the urethra, can result from several entities. These include infections either with bacteria such as gonococci or with other organisms such as mycoplasmas or chlamydiae. The inflammation may also be the result of foreign body irritation such as that seen with urethral catheterization or with noxious chemicals.

Clinical Presentation. The symptoms of urethritis are predominantly irritative. Burning, stinging, or itching within the urethra or at the urethral meatus may be described. The presence of a urethral discharge is variable: It may be absent, scant, or copious, as well as clear, white, or yellow. Patients with infective urethritis who complain of urgency or frequency often have involvement of the prostate as well.

Symptoms produced by the foreign body reaction of an indwelling catheter are often less severe since the urine is diverted by the catheter. The patient may complain of discomfort within the penis but the symptoms often become much more prominent after removal of the catheter. The patient usually complains of severe burning and discomfort during urination immediately after removal of the catheter. These symptoms usually subside after 3 to 5 voidings and usually disappear within 24 to 48 hours.

Diagnosis. The diagnosis of urethritis can be confirmed by microscopic examination of a Gram stain of the urethral discharge to examine for both leukocytes and bacteria, particularly intracellular bacteria. The presence of intracellular gram-negative diplococci is diagnostic for gonococcal urethritis. The diagnosis can also be made by microscopic examination of a three-glass urine specimen. This technique can localize the site of pyuria to the urethra in cases of urethritis.

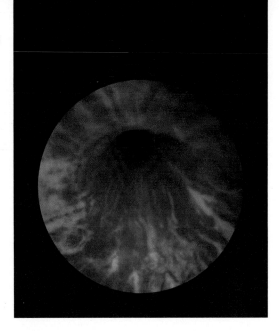

Figure 3-1. *The mucosa of the bulbous urethra is found markedly erythematous on urethroscopy after removal of a urethral catheter in this 60-year-old man.*

Endoscopic Appearance. Endoscopy should be avoided in patients in whom infective urethritis is suspected. An effort should be made to avoid dissemination of causative microorganisms by instrumentation. Nevertheless, endoscopy is often essential to clarify the differential diagnosis. The changes seen endoscopically in urethritis appear as a spectrum. The mildest inflammatory change may be manifest as erythema of the mucosa that can be seen at any site within the urethra (Fig. 3-1). There may be only fullness of the normally located vessels or increased vascularity. More severe inflammation appears as mucosal edema with formation of pseudopapillae. Diffuse mucosal fibrosis or stricture formation may be seen as a late result of urethritis of any variety.

Management. Treatment of urethritis is directed toward the cause. In infectious urethritis, antibiotic therapy is directed toward the gonococcus, chlamydia, or ureaplasma considered responsible for nonspecific urethritis. Foreign body urethritis can be treated by removal of the foreign body. If a catheter is present and the patient's symptoms from urethritis become intolerable, then an alternative form of diversion such as suprapubic cystostomy should be considered.

URETHRAL STRICTURE

Clinical Presentation. Since a urethral stricture results from contraction of a circumferential scar of the urethra, the presenting symptoms are those of lower urinary obstruction. The major complaints are slow, prolonged voiding and a thin, weak stream; reduced or intermittent urinary stream; or more irritative symptoms, such as nocturia, frequency, or urgency. In severe strictures, urinary retention may develop. Recurrent urinary infections are common with urethral strictures and often are responsible for the dominant symptoms.

Diagnosis. The diagnosis can be strengthened by additional functional, radiographic, and endoscopic studies. Determination of the urinary flow rate often detects more subtle changes in the stream than the patient can appreciate[1]. Although a low flow rate is not diagnostic of a urethral stricture, a higher flow rate (>15 ml/sec) is very strong evidence that no significant stricture is present. In a patient with obstructive symptoms, the diagnosis of urethral stricture can also be suggested by the inability to pass a catheter (16 or 18 Fr.) or an 18 or 20 Fr. sound. When being removed, the catheter may seem to "hang" or "grab" and be somewhat difficult to withdraw from the urethra. Conversely, the diagnosis can be excluded if an instrument of this caliber can pass easily. A sound smaller than 18 Fr. should not be used because of the possibility of perforating the urethra.

A retrograde urethrogram can be used to delineate the full extent of the urethral stricture. The retrograde urethrogram is performed by injection of radioopaque contrast material into the urethra via the urethral meatus. A dynamic urethrogram with films taken during the intraurethral instillation of contrast will routinely demonstrate the entire extent of a stricture (see Fig. 8-1)[2]. An aqueous contrast agent suitable for intravenous injection should be used for the retrograde urethrogram since contrast frequently enters the periurethral veins during the study.

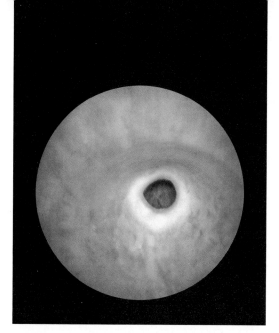

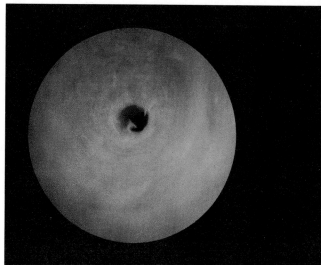

Figure 3-2. *A urethral stricture with a narrow lumen exhibits pallor of the surrounding scar tissue.*

Figure 3-3. *A stricture found in a 19-year-old male without any previous history of instrumentation was considered congenital. It appears less fibrous and less dense.*

If the retrograde urethrogram does not define the full extent of the urethral stricture, then contrast should be passed into the urethra in an antegrade fashion by voiding urethrogram. A fine catheter, such as a no. 8 pediatric feeding tube or a 5 Fr. ureteral catheter is passed transurethrally to allow instillation of contrast into the bladder. After removal of the catheter, the patient is asked to void, and x-ray films are taken for the voiding urethrogram. This should be done with fluoroscopy but can be performed adequately with individual radiographs taken during voiding. Combination of the retrograde and antegrade urethrograms will then define the proximal and distal extents of the urethral stricture.

Endoscopic Appearance. Direct visualization of a urethral stricture with the urethroscope or panendoscope with a forward viewing (0- to 30-degree) lens provides the most definitive diagnostic information. A severe traumatic or inflammatory stricture appears as a sudden narrowing of the urethral lumen with surrounding dense, white, fibrous scarring (Figs. 3-2, 3-3). Congenital strictures appear very similar, although less dense, fibrous scarring may be apparent. It is generally not possible to distinguish congenital from secondary strictures endoscopically, and the distinction must be made on an historic basis. No attempt should be made to pass the instrument through such a small, densely scarred area since the beak of the instrument may perforate the softer, normal urethral mucosa, creating a false passage.

Asymptomatic strictures may be found on urethroscopy. Surprisingly, small caliber strictures may be encountered in this way although, more commonly, less severe, larger caliber strictures are found in the asymptomatic patient (Fig. 3-4). Partially dilated strictures can also be seen endoscopically after catheter or filiform and follower dilation (Fig. 3-5). Once partially dilated, the lumen is often adequate to accept the endoscope.

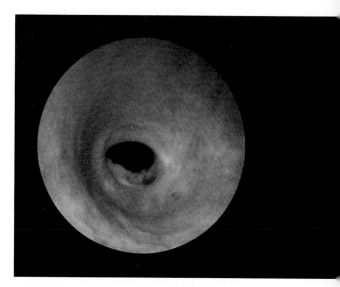

Figure 3-4. *A mild urethral stricture developed in a patient on self-intermittent catheterization. A 16 Fr. catheter readily passed through the lumen.*

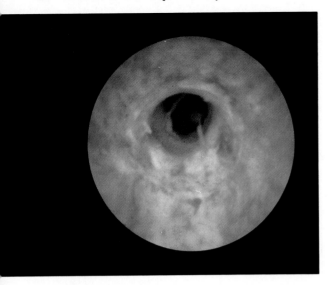

Figure 3-5. *A proximal urethral stricture has been dilated with urethral catheters. Narrowing of the lumen with residual fibrous bands is evident with the membranous urethra seen more proximally in the background.*

Management. Several different forms of therapy for urethral strictures have evolved. No single form of treatment will provide routinely successful results in all strictures. Therapy, therefore, should be individualized to each patient and the characteristics of the stricture in order to provide the best chance of cure. The treatment of urethral strictures is discussed further in Chapter 8.

URETHRAL CALCULI

Clinical Presentation. Symptomatic urethral calculi are uncommon. They may occur as a primary crystallization within the urethra or after migration from the bladder or kidney into the urethra. Primary urethral calculi usually form as a result of some abnormality within the urethra, either a diverticulum or an obstruction in association with chronic infection. They usually produce more chronic symptoms such as dysuria or decreased urinary stream in men. In women, symptoms are more often dysuria or perineal pain. Secondary stones, which migrate from a more proximal site of formation in the urinary tract, often cause more acute symptoms because of their sudden appearance within the urethra. Among published series, Amin's report from Kuwait [3] found that 88.9 percent of patients presented with acute urinary retention while only 1 of 47 patients described in the report from the Mayo Clinic [4] presented with retention.

Diagnosis. Radiographic demonstration of the calculus was made in only 42.5 percent of patients in the Mayo Clinic series. This low rate was seen because some calculi were relatively radiolucent and in some x-ray films the external genitalia were excluded from the field. Retrograde urethrography is of value in demonstrating calculi and any underlying disorders within the urethra, particularly in males.

Endoscopic Appearance. Urethroscopy often provides the diagnosis. Because of the confined lumen of the urethra, any calculus within the lumen can be visualized endoscopically. The calculus appears as a crystalline mass often surrounded by edematous, inflammatory tissue. The macroscopic structure of the calculus itself is typical of the chemical composition and is similar to that of an upper tract stone (described fully in Chap. 6).

Management. The management of calculi depends on their size and location as well as the associated underlying disease. Calculi can often be extracted endoscopically with a stone basket, although larger stones may require urethrotomy. In addition, any causative obstructive lesion within the urethra should be treated with internal urethrotomy if necessary. Posterior urethral calculi may be expressed in a retrograde fashion into the bladder with either an instrument or irrigation fluid passed through the urethroscope. They can then be fragmented within the larger volume of the bladder just as primary vesical stones. Calculi may also be disintegrated ultrasonically within the urethra as described for ureteral calculi (see Chap. 15).

URETHRAL TUMORS

Clinical Presentation. Tumors within the urethra present with local or voiding symptoms. The symptoms of carcinoma of the urethra vary with the sex of the patient and the site of the tumor in males. A urethral mass or obstructive symptoms are the most frequent presentations in men with primary carcinoma of the urethra (48%)[7,8]. Tumors located in the proximal bulbous, membranous, or prostatic urethra are more chronic and often associated with previous symptoms of existing urethral strictures, which, among the patients studied by Kaplan[7] and Ray[8], were present in 36 percent of men with bulbous urethral tumors. Urethral tumors should be given primary consideration in a patient who has a previous history of stricture and suddenly develops more severe or more frequent recurrence of the symptoms. In the series of Ray and colleagues[8], less than 25 percent of men with urethral tumors presented with pain or with hematuria. Urethral tumors in women more frequently cause urethral bleeding or spotting, dysuria, or a palpable urethral mass[5,6]. The most frequent symptom of transitional cell carcinoma developing in a residual urethra after previous cystectomy in men is bloody discharge[9]. Other presentations include penile or perineal mass or inguinal adenopathy.

Many urethral tumors are asymptomatic. They should be sought in patients who have other similar lesions that are at high risk for developing or implanting within the urethra. As an example, patients with numerous condylomas on the glans penis may develop condylomas within the urethra (Fig. 3-6). Also, patients with transitional cell carcinoma of the bladder are prone to develop urethral tumors (Fig. 3-7). In the series of Schellhammer and Whitmore[9], among those patients with a previous cystectomy, carcinoma developed in the urethra in 7 percent. Among patients who underwent urethrectomy at the same time as cystectomy, there was a 12.5-percent incidence of unsuspected carcinoma in the urethra in the resected specimen.

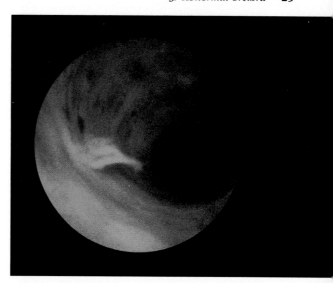

Figure 3-6. *A condyloma is located on the ventrolateral surface of the pendulous urethra in a patient with a history of a bloody urethral discharge.*

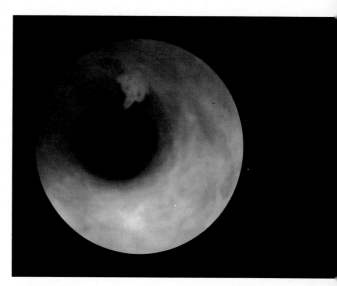

Figure 3-7. *A low-grade papillary transitional cell carcinoma was found on urethroscopy in a patient with an invasive bladder tumor.*

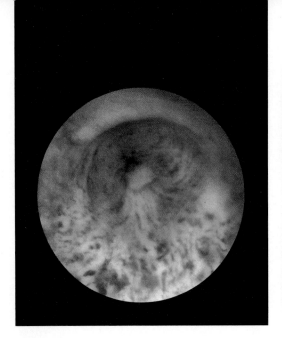

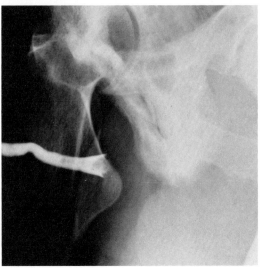

Figure 3-8. *A small benign tumor located at the external sphincter was histologically identical to a second papilloma located at the verumontanum. It was removed with the rigid biopsy forceps.*

Figure 3-9. *A retrograde urethrogram outlines the urethral tumor shown in Fig. 3-10. Two air bubbles can be seen in the urethra, distal to the nearly obstructing neoplasm.*

Pathology. The most common urethral tumor is a *condyloma acuminatum,* a benign verrucous lesion thought to be caused by a virus. The symptoms of intraurethral lesions are similar to those of other urethral tumors, and this lesion should be considered in any patient with condyloma of the genitalia who develops urinary or urethral symptoms. There are numerous other benign lesions such as fibrous or fibroepithelial polyps or, rarely, nephrogenic adenomas (Fig. 3-8).

A tumor of the transitional epithelium within the proximal portion of the urethra can either develop primarily or theoretically represent implantation of a lesion located more proximally within the bladder. Transitional cell tumors range from the very well differentiated low-stage papillomas, which can be considered benign, to the much more bizarre, cytologically high-grade and usually higher stage, malignant transitional cell carcinomas. Squamous cell carcinoma may be found mixed with these other lesions or may be found alone. Rare tumors of the urethra include malignant melanomas and carcinoids.

Diagnosis. Several studies can be employed to indicate the presence of a urethral tumor; endoscopic biopsy, however, is essential for confirmation of a final diagnosis. Retrograde urethrography may outline a large urethral tumor. It is often the first test employed to distinguish urethral stricture from urethral tumor, particularly in those patients with a previous history of stricture. The tumor appears as a filling defect on the urethrogram (Fig. 3-9). Examination of voided urine for cytologic abnormalities may reveal cells shed from the urethral tumor, but this study is more valuable with the higher grade tumors.

Radiologic study by urethrogram or endoscopic examination by direct urethroscopy does not always detect the neoplasm in the urethra retained after cystectomy. In the series by Schellhammer and Whitmore[9], only half of the urethral lesions could be detected on gross inspection of the urethral specimen. Cytologic examination was more accurate in determining the presence of these lesions. A technique to obtain material for cytologic examination by scraping the urethra with a resecting loop has been described.

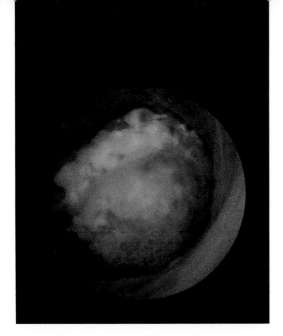

Figure 3-10. *A high-grade mixed transitional and squamous cell carcinoma is visualized in the bulbous urethra. The patient had a previous history of a urethral stricture.*

Endoscopic Appearance. Endoscopic examination of the urethra provides the most direct information regarding the presence of urethral tumors and should be employed in any patient either suspected of having a urethral tumor or at high risk of developing such a lesion. Benign intraurethral condyloma acuminata have an appearance similar to verrucous lesions elsewhere. The tumors are usually localized and have a broad base and irregular, often firm, epithelized surface. They may be difficult to distinguish from squamous carcinoma without biopsy.

Transitional cell carcinomas vary in appearance from low-grade, papillary tumors to high-grade, often invasive carcinomas. The low-grade papillary tumors may appear as individual or multiple fronds adherent to the urethral surface with a fine stalk (see Fig. 3-7). Sessile, solid lesions are more likely to be high-grade tumors with a higher propensity for invasion. These tumors can be mixed with squamous cell carcinoma (Fig. 3-10). Squamous cell carcinoma also develops in a pure form and appears either as solid lesions or flat, slightly raised tumors extending along the urethra. The keratinized surface can be seen as a white, firm epithelial surface.

Urethral tumors usually can be distinguished from pseudopapillary mucosal edema on gross inspection. A lesion characteristic of edema is more transparent with a single stalklike base. Any more complex or solid-appearing urethral lesions should be biopsied for diagnosis. The addition of microscopic cystoscopy may be a major aid in the differentiation of mucosal lesions (see Chap. 11).

In the female, endoscopic inspection of the urethra may be more difficult because the very short urethra will not distend well with irrigating fluid, and the redundant mucosa of the urethra may obscure small lesions. Despite these difficulties, tumors with the appearance described above can be detected within the urethra of the female. There is also the added advantage of the ability to palpate the urethra transvaginally with or without the urethroscope in position.

Management. The primary treatment of carcinoma of the urethra in the male includes surgical resection. Superficial lesions can be resected endoscopically while invasive tumors require open surgical resection with urethrectomy. The advisability of concomitant node dissection remains controversial. In the female, urethral tumors have been satisfactorily treated with combined intraurethral and external beam radiation [6].

URETHRAL DIVERTICULA IN THE MALE. Diverticula within the urethra may be either primary or secondary [11,12]. The primary diverticula may be congenital or, in the male, arise from cystic dilatation of Cowper's glands. The secondary or acquired urethral diverticula are much more common. They result from obstruction, infection, and instrumentation.

Congenital diverticula in the male can be divided into two types: (1) the wide-mouth, or saccular, and (2) the narrow-neck, or globular types (Fig. 3-11). The saccular variety appears along the ventral surface of the urethra from the pendulous to the bulbous urethra. The distal lip of the diverticulum may form an obstructive valve while the proximal margin is indistinct. The narrow-neck or globular diverticulum is usually located proximally within the bulbous urethra, again on the ventral surface, and has a well-defined mouth. These diverticula often obstruct the outflow of urine because of their tendency to collect volumes of urine during voiding but to drain poorly. They can often be palpated as a mass in the perineum and emptied manually by compressing the perineum. Because of the poor drainage, they tend to be a site of infection and calculus formation.

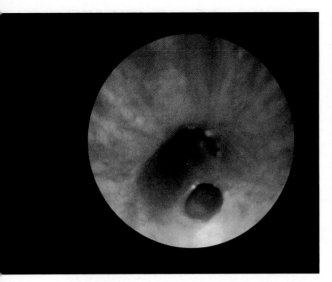

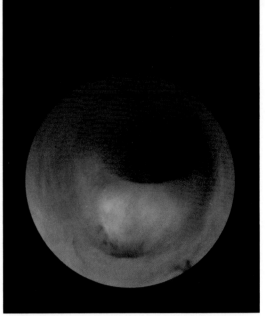

Figure 3-11. *A well-defined ostium of a midline ventral urethral diverticulum is shown in the proximal bulbous urethra. The 42-year-old male denied any previous pelvic trauma or urethral instrumentation. The diverticulum is of the primary or congenital type.*

Figure 3-13. *A large mouth of urethrocutaneous fistula is located ventrally within the distal bulbous urethra. The patient had a neurogenic bladder and had an indwelling urethral catheter for 5 years before developing a periurethral abscess and subsequently the urethrocutaneous fistula shown.*

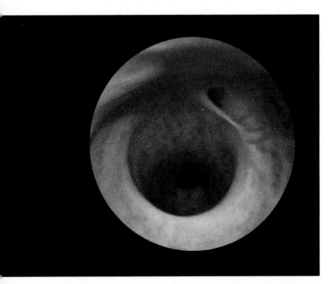

Figure 3-12. *The opening of a urethral diverticulum or healed false passage is located on the anterolateral aspect of the bulbous urethra. There is associated scarring and pallor of the bulbous urethra in this patient who had a previous pelvic fracture and long-term catheterization as well as a history of a urethral stricture dilated several years previously.*

Secondary or acquired urethral diverticula are much more common in both males and females. In males the diverticulum may be caused by an infection, including a periurethral or prostatic abscess or hematoma; obstruction from stricture, stone, or external compression, such as may occur with a condom catheter; and trauma, resulting from either external injury or instrumentation (Fig. 3-12). Patients with indwelling urethral catheters or those subjected to frequent instrumentation are at risk of developing urethral diverticula. The basis for this danger may be disruption of the urethra by misguided passage of the instrument or by pressure of the catheter associated with chronic infection within the urethra. A periurethral abscess may also rupture percutaneously and result in a urethrocutaneous fistula rather than a diverticulum (Fig. 3-13). Urethroplasty, particularly by the two-stage techniques, can result in a urethral diverticulum that has the added disadvantage of bearing hair, which can serve as a nidus for calculus formation (see Figs. 8-2, 8-3). Schistosomiasis is the most common cause of acquired diverticula in areas where it is endemic, such as Egypt.

Cysts of Cowper's ducts may also be found in the male urethra and may give rise to similar obstructive or irritative symptoms or hematuria. They can be differentiated from diverticula on urethroscopy because the ducts can be seen opening into the apex of the cyst (see Chap. 17).

An accessory urethral channel may also form a periurethral cavity. This may be difficult to distinguish from a saccular congenital diverticulum unless it is complicated by communication with the skin, the bladder, or the urethra at multiple sites.

Endoscopic Appearance. Congenital diverticula can be viewed on urethroscopy and are located on the ventral surface of the urethra. In the saccular type, the distal rim is usually well defined whereas the proximal margin may be rather indistinct. The small-mouth or globular type is also located on the ventral aspect of the urethra but usually in the proximal portion. Often there is a definite orifice with a narrow neck visible.

Acquired diverticula may be located at any site and have varying configurations. The mouth of the diverticulum is usually visible and well defined on urethroscopy. There is a large variation in size of the opening, which may range from a pinhole communication to a major channel difficult to distinguish from the urethra itself. A diverticulum formed from a scrotal urethroplasty is often characterized by the presence of hair emanating from its mouth (see Fig. 8-3). Some authors have emphasized the importance of intubation urethroscopy in identifying lesions, particularly Cowper's duct cysts.

Management. Treatment can be similar for several varieties of congenital or acquired diverticula, Cowper's duct cysts, or accessory urethral channels. If there is no evidence of a penile or scrotal bulge on micturition, it can be assumed that the corpus spongiosum is intact and there is sufficient support of the urethra to permit transurethral treatment. The diverticulum can be unroofed transurethrally with either the Bugbee electrode or the cutting stylet with a resectoscope.

Diverticula in the form of large cavities, which may not drain well; those that are insufficiently supported by the corpus spongiosum; and those with thick, inflexible anterior walls may require open excision and closure. Urethrocutaneous fistulas should be treated by open surgical incision. Small asymptomatic diverticula, regardless of pathogenesis, may not require any treatment.

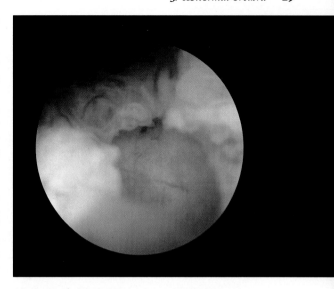

Figure 3-14. *The opening of a diverticulum on the posterolateral surface of a female urethra is shown at the center of the field extending toward 4 and 5 o'clock. The bladder neck is located at the 11 o'clock position. This 38-year-old female had recurrent irritative symptoms.*

URETHRAL DIVERTICULA IN THE FEMALE. Congenital diverticula are extremely rare in the female. Diverticula seen in the adult female urethra are almost exclusively of the acquired type. Presentation is usually with recurrent infections or recurrent irritative symptoms. Diagnosis can be made by voiding cystourethrography, urethrography, and urethroscopy. Treatment in a symptomatic patient consists of excision or, if the diverticulum is located quite distally within the urethra, drainage into the vagina.

In the female urethra accurate localization is useful in planning surgical therapy[10]. The ostium of a diverticulum may be seen directly on urethroscopy in some patients (Fig. 3-14). If the site of communication between the urethra and diverticulum is not readily identified, then the area of the diverticulum identified radiologically or as a palpable mass can be compressed manually through the anterior vaginal wall and, as purulent material is expressed from the diverticulum, the ostium can be identified endoscopically.

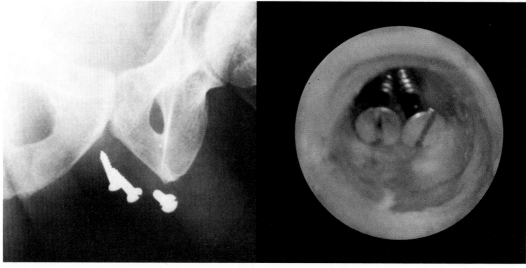

A

B

Figure 3-15. *Three metallic screws placed by a patient into his urethra are evident by (A) x-ray and (B) urethroscopy in the bulbous urethra. These foreign bodies were removed with a three-prong grasper endoscopically.*

FOREIGN BODIES IN THE URETHRA. Foreign bodies within the urethra may become symptomatic as a result of obstruction of the urinary flow or from the consequent inflammation or infection within the urethra. Foreign bodies may be self-induced and the patient may be reluctant to admit the presence of the agent until symptoms develop and require medical attention.

Diagnosis. Radioopaque foreign bodies can be detected within the urethra by plain radiographs (Fig. 3-15). Urinalysis will usually reveal hematuria and pyuria.

Endoscopic Appearance. The foreign body within the urethra can be demonstrated on urethroscopy (Fig. 3-15). It can then be grasped with flexible or rigid grasping, or foreign body, forceps and removed. A long object, such as wire or tubing, introduced within the urethra may coil and become knotted within the bladder and require cystotomy for removal.

Endoscopic vision may be obscured by bleeding or inflammation. Although irrigation will usually provide a sufficiently clear visual field, temporary urinary diversion may be required before endoscopic removal is possible.

REFERENCES

Urethral Stricture

1. Cole, A. T., Peterson, D. D., Biddle, W. S., and Fried, F. A. Uroflowmetry: A useful technique in the management of urethral strictures. *J. Urol.* 112 : 483, 1974.
2. McCallum, R. W., and Colapinto, V. The role of urethrography in urethral disease: Part IA. Accurate radiological localization of the membranous urethra and distal sphincters in normal male subjects. *J. Urol.* 122 : 607, 1979.

Urethral Calculi

3. Amin, H. A. Urethral calculi. *Br. J. Urol.* 45 : 192, 1973.
4. Paulk, S. C., Khan, A. U., Malek, R. S., and Greene, L. F. Urethral calculi. *J. Urol.* 116 : 436, 1976.

Urethral Tumors

5. Bracken, R. B., et al. Primary carcinoma of the female urethra. *J. Urol.* 116 : 188, 1976.
6. Johnson, D. E., and O'Connell, J. R. Primary carcinoma of the female urethra. *Urology* 21 : 42, 1983.
7. Kaplan, G. W., Bulkley, G. J., and Grayhack, J. T. Carcinoma of the male urethra. *J. Urol.* 98 : 365, 1967.
8. Ray, B., Canto, A. R., and Whitmore, W. F. Experience with primary carcinoma of the male urethra. *J. Urol.* 117 : 591, 1977.
9. Schellhammer, P. F., and Whitmore, W. F. Transitional cell carcinoma of the urethra in men having cystectomy for bladder cancer. *J. Urol.* 115 : 56, 1976.

Diverticula

10. Appell, R. A., and Suarez, B. D. Experience with a laterally based vaginal flap approach for urethral diverticulum. *J. Urol.* 127 : 677, 1982.
11. Firlit, C. Urethral abnormalities. *Urol. Clin. North Am.* 5 : 31, 1978.
12. Ortlip, S. A., Gonzalez, R., and Williams, R. D. Diverticula of the male urethra. *J. Urol.* 124 : 350, 1980.

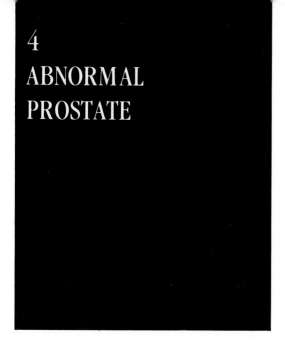

4
ABNORMAL PROSTATE

Jeffry L. Huffman

Edward S. Lyon

Demetrius H. Bagley

INFLAMMATORY CONDITIONS OF THE PROSTATE. Inflammatory conditions of the prostate are very common. Although the diagnosis of acute prostatitis is usually apparent from the clinical presentation, urinalysis, and specific cultures, the differential diagnosis of the various chronic prostatitis syndromes is often very difficult. The common syndromes include bacterial prostatitis (acute and chronic), nonbacterial prostatitis, and prostatodynia. Less commonly, fungal prostatitis or tuberculous prostatitis may occur.

Acute and Chronic Bacterial Prostatitis

CLINICAL PRESENTATION. The patient with acute bacterial prostatitis presents with irritative voiding symptoms of urgency, frequency, and dysuria, accompanied by either suprapubic or low back pain. Usually the patient also has fever and chills and occasionally varying degrees of obstructive symptoms.

On rectal examination, the prostate is extremely tender, boggy, and edematous. Vigorous examination of the prostate should be avoided because of pain and the possibility of bacteremia. For these same reasons, manipulation of the urethra is contraindicated and cystoscopy or urethral catheterization should not be performed.

The presentation of patients with chronic bacterial prostatitis varies significantly. Most commonly, they have relapsing urinary tract infections; a history of acute prostatitis may or may not be found. Although they usually do not have chills and fever, most patients have irritative voiding symptoms with dysuria, urgency, and frequency. Pain with ejaculation is another common complaint.

The diagnosis of bacterial prostatitis is established by performing quantitative localization cultures. This procedure has been outlined by Meares and Stamey[14] and entails obtaining three split volumes of voided urine (VB1, VB2, and VB3) and the expressed prostatic secretions (EPS). For the diagnosis of bacterial prostatitis, the EPS and VB3 sample should have colony counts of pathogenic bacteria that exceed 10-fold the count of the VB1 sample.

The most common organism cultured in cases of bacterial prostatitis is *Escherichia coli*. Other gram-negative organisms such as species of *Klebsiella, Enterobacter, Proteus, Pseudomonas,* or *Serratia* may be implicated. The only common gram-positive organism causing bacterial prostatitis is *Streptococcus faecalis* (enterococcus)[13].

Nonbacterial Prostatitis. Nonbacterial prostatitis is the most common prostatitis syndrome encountered. Patients present with symptoms very similar to those of chronic bacterial prostatitis. Despite having 10 WBC per high-power field (HPF) in the expressed prostatic secretions, however, they very rarely have positive localization cultures for pathogens. *Ureaplasma urealyticum* and *Chlamydia trachomatis* have been implicated as pathogens in this syndrome, although they cannot be isolated in every case[13].

Prostatodynia. *Prostatodynia* is a term proposed by some investigators to differentiate a syndrome of prostatitis caused by noninfectious agents from other infectious prostatitis syndromes. Patients generally have irritative voiding symptoms with dysuria, frequency, and urgency; however, they do not have inflammatory cell reactions in their EPS samples and have negative localization cultures.

Fungal Prostatitis. Fungal prostatitis is a very rare clinical entity. Orr[18] reported on 150 patients who had documented systemic fungal infection and found that only 4 of these patients had prostatic involvement. Fungal prostatitis is thought to spread by hematogenous means, usually from a pulmonary focus where the primary infection exists. The patient may present with symptoms comparable to chronic bacterial prostatitis or may be referred for evaluation of an abnormally indurated prostate by rectal examination.

The diagnosis should be suspected when the prostatic biopsy is suggestive of granulomatous prostatitis. A final diagnosis is based on positive fungal cultures or smears. The most common pathogens are *Blastomyces, Cryptococcus,* and *Histoplasma.* It has been shown that colony counts for fungal infections are of no importance since there is no correlation between colony count and presence or severity of infection[19].

Tuberculous Prostatitis. Tuberculous (TB) prostatitis affects 3 to 15 percent of all patients, 15 to 20 years after they have undergone successful treatment of pulmonary tuberculosis[10]. The prostate is involved in one-third of cases of genitourinary tract tuberculosis, and usually (25–50% of cases) the patients present with prostatic nodules. The diagnosis of TB prostatitis is based on finding acid-fast organisms in the urine and sterile pyuria with positive cultures for TB.

Endoscopic Appearance. Acute bacterial prostatitis is characterized by prostatic tissue that is markedly inflamed and friable. The overlying prostatic mucosa is erythematous and edematous, and there is associated cystitis and bulbar urethritis. Endoscopy should be avoided when prostatitis is thought to be present unless there are other strong indications for the procedure.

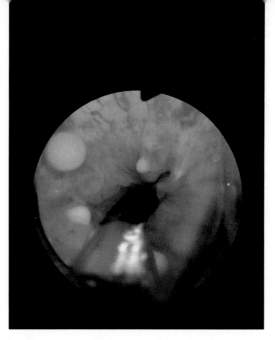

Figure 4-1. *An inflammatory vesicular reaction of the prostatic mucosa is demonstrated in this patient with a urethral stricture and previous urinary infection. The blade of the urethrotome is evident in the right and lower fields.*

There is no characteristic appearance of chronic bacterial prostatitis, nonbacterial prostatitis, prostatodynia, or fungal prostatitis. Nonspecific inflammation and edema may be present but the prostate will frequently appear normal (Fig. 4-1). Mucosal inflammation resulting from catheterization often cannot be distinguished from other inflammatory lesions (Fig. 4-2).

The appearance of TB prostatitis has been well described by Lattimer[9]. He characterized the prostatic urethra as beefy red initially with superficial ulcerations. With chronic involvement, the floor of the urethra is drawn into longitudinal folds with a dark red velvety surface, and the prostatic ducts become markedly dilated.

Management. The treatment of acute bacterial prostatitis depends on the results of culture and sensitivity testing. While awaiting these findings, however, therapy with trimethoprim-sulfamethoxazole orally or gentamicin plus ampicillin parenterally in the septic patient should be started.

Many drugs penetrate the intensely inflamed prostatic tissue in acute prostatitis; in chronic prostatitis, only lipid-soluble antibiotics achieve desirable levels. Treatment with trimethoprim-sulfamethoxazole, tetracycline, or carbenicillin indanyl sodium is usually recommended pending results of culture and sensitivity tests. Long-term (12 wk) therapy achieves better cure rates.

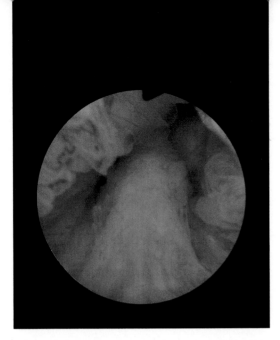

Figure 4-2. *Marked mucosal edema and inflammation are present in the prostatic urethra after catheterization. The mucosal edema is evident as translucent bullae of protruding mucosa.*

Occasionally, transurethral prostatectomy is used to treat chronic bacterial prostatitis, especially in patients who have infected prostatic calculi. When this form of therapy is selected, all areas of infected prostatic tissue and calculi must be removed.

For patients with nonbacterial prostatitis it is recommended that a trial of tetracycline therapy be given for 2 weeks. If there is no response, the patients should be reassured and maintained on a regimen to give symptomatic relief of their irritative voiding symptoms.

The therapy of prostatodynia is not antimicrobial. The patients are treated symptomatically and occasionally alpha-blocking agents such as phenoxybenzamine provide relief of symptoms.

The recommended treatment for systemic fungal disease is amphotericin B. Surgical removal of infected prostatic tissue is not recommended because of the possibility of dissemination[18]. Another antifungal drug, 5-fluorocytosine, has been reported to produce good results in treating cryptococcal infection of the prostate[2]. Triple drug chemotherapy for 2 years is recommended for treatment of genitourinary TB[10]. The drugs commonly used are isoniazid, rifampin, and ethambutol, with pyridoxine added to help prevent the peripheral neuropathy often caused by isoniazid.

Prostatic Calculi. Prostatic calculi are common and only occasionally clinically important. They can be either endogenous, arising from within the prostate, or exogenous, arising from the urine.

Endogenous calculi result from partial prostatic ductal obstruction causing accumulation of inspissated prostatic secretions and desquamated epithelial cells. The corpora amylacea then undergo cyclic growth causing further ductal obstruction and further deposition of inspissated secretions. The calculi are usually multiple and can vary greatly in size from 1 mm to 5 cm. They characteristically are located in the plane between the surgical capsule and the true prostate, and on removal generally indicate the margin of resection followed when performing transurethral resection of prostatic adenoma.

Exogenous calculi are less common. They form in the urine and are usually the result of urinary stasis within the prostatic fossa or bladder.

CLINICAL PRESENTATION. Patients with prostatic calculi generally develop symptoms comparable to those of chronic bacterial prostatitis. Occasionally the calculi may be palpated during digital examination of the prostate or sounded during passage of a urethral catheter or sound. Often the calculi are unsuspected and identifiable only through transurethral prostatectomy or plain roentgenography of the pelvis.

ENDOSCOPIC APPEARANCE. The endogenous prostatic calculi are generally grouped together with faceted surfaces. They may be round, ovoid, or triangular and vary in color from grayish white to dark brown. Usually they are identified during a transurethral resection of the prostate in the plane between the true prostate and the surgical capsule.

Exogenous calculi are similar in appearance to bladder calculi. They are usually yellow orange in color, depending on their chemical composition.

MANAGEMENT. Prostatic calculi are usually removed endoscopically during transurethral resection of prostatic adenomas. They are uncovered and removed with a cold loop or irrigated from the bladder after being dislodged from the prostatic fossa. Occasionally the removal of large prostatic calculi requires some form of lithopaxy.

IATROGENIC ABNORMALITIES OF THE PROSTATE. Abnormalities of the prostate that result from traumatic injuries occurring at the time of an endoscopic procedure or urethral manipulation include vesical neck contracture following transurethral prostatectomy and false passages within the prostatic urethra.

Vesical Neck Contracture. Greene[8] has suggested that vesical neck contractures result from resection of the smooth muscle at the bladder neck when removing prostatic adenomas. Proper resection of adenomas results in an incidence of bladder neck contracture of approximately 2 percent; the risk of contracture can be lowered by maintaining proper boundaries of proximal resection and avoiding excessive fulguration of the bladder neck (see Chap. 9).

CLINICAL PRESENTATION. The patient with a vesical neck contracture usually notices symptoms several months following a transurethral prostatectomy. The progressive narrowing of the bladder neck leads to symptoms of bladder outlet obstruction, such as diminution of urinary stream, hesitancy, and postmicturition dribbling. Irritative voiding symptoms are occasionally present as well.

ENDOSCOPIC APPEARANCE. A vesical neck contracture is a concentric fibrous scar at the level of the bladder neck or occasionally in the proximal prostatic urethra. The lumen may be partially occluded or have only a pinpoint opening for passage of urine (see Figs. 9-15, 8-10). The overlying mucosa is pale, and the scar is extremely dense and relatively immobile.

MANAGEMENT. The treatment of a vesical neck contracture includes (1) dilation with filiforms and followers or urethral sounds, (2) transurethral resection, (3) cold-punch resection, or (4) visual internal incision. Greene[8] has also advocated steroid injection circumferentially following transurethral resection. These procedures are discussed in other chapters.

False Passages of the Prostatic Urethra. False passages within the prostatic urethra result from errant attempts to catheterize the bladder or other forms of instrumental perforation. Forceful passage of a urethral catheter, sounds, or filiforms and followers can perforate the prostatic urethra in the region of the posterior bladder neck. This injury usually occurs when there is marked elevation of the posterior bladder neck resulting from vesical contracture or benign prostatic hypertrophy.

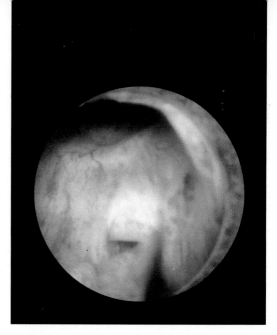

Figure 4-3. *A false passage within the prostatic urethra is present at the 6 o'clock position. The bladder neck is evident in the upper field of view. The patient had a long history of urethral stricture, which had been dilated previously, and the false passage probably resulted from misguided sound. The blade of the urethrotome is shown at the 6 o'clock position.*

CLINICAL PRESENTATION. The patient with a false passage may have no referable symptoms. The injury is usually found incidentally during a subsequent endoscopic procedure or during retrograde urethrography. If the false passage is large enough, however, stasis of urine may occur with resulting infection and possible calculus formation.

ENDOSCOPIC APPEARANCE. A false passage can appear as a tiny slit or a large opening, usually on the floor of the prostatic urethra. A recently formed false passage may show active bleeding at the site of the mucosal defect with otherwise normal-appearing prostatic tissue. An older, well-healed false passage is firm and pale and surrounded by scar tissue (Figs. 4-3, 4-4).

MANAGEMENT. False passages that heal as well-defined diverticula usually need no further therapy. It is incumbent on the urologist, however, to ensure urinary drainage by proper catheter placement, either transurethrally or suprapubically, when a false passage has been created acutely.

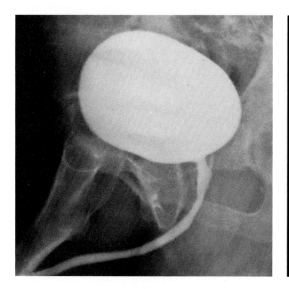

Figure 4-4. *The prostatic urethral false passage fills with contrast during retrograde urethrography.*

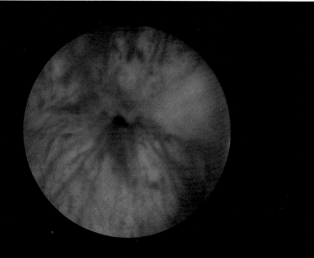

Figure 4-5. *An obstructive bladder neck is almost entirely occlusive even in the presence of active fluid irrigation.*

BENIGN PROSTATIC HYPERTROPHY. Benign prostatic hypertrophy (BPH) is a progressive pathologic condition associated with aging. Lytton's series[11] showed that a 50-year-old male had a 10-percent chance of having a prostatectomy during his lifetime due to BPH and that seldom did this disease affect males less than 40 years of life. Franks' report[5] on 211 autopsies in Great Britain provided similar conclusions. After separating BPH into four categories — none, possible, small or microscopic, and, lastly, large or macroscopic — Franks found that by age 80, 53 percent of the autopsy subjects had large or macroscopic BPH and 32 percent had microscopic BPH.

Clinical Presentation. Patients with BPH commonly present with symptoms of bladder outlet obstruction. Often the symptom complex known as *prostatism* will incorporate both irritative and obstructive symptoms. Irritative symptoms include dysuria, nocturia, urgency, and urgency incontinence. Obstructive symptoms include diminution of urinary stream, hesitancy, postmicturition dribbling, and a feeling of incomplete emptying.

Acute urinary retention is also not uncommon in the natural history of BPH. In Lytton's series[11], 10 to 15 percent of the patients undergoing surgery presented with acute retention. Craigen's series[3] showed that 44 percent of patients presented with retention while 54 percent presented with symptoms of prostatism.

For the clinician, the differential diagnosis of benign prostatic hypertrophy is difficult. Many disorders, such as vesical neck obstruction secondary to detrusor-sphincter dyssynergy[23], or contracture, prostatic carcinoma, squamous cell carcinoma, sarcoma of the prostate, and urethral obstruction secondary to urethral stricture, can cause bladder outlet obstruction and simulate this benign condition. To differentiate BPH from other disorders, the rectal examination, excretory urogram, cystoscopy, postvoid residual determination, and possibly prostatic biopsy should be included in the evaluation of the patient.

The urinary flow rate has also been shown to decline with progressive prostatic enlargement. Drach[4] has showed a decrease in the flow rate with aging of 2.1 cc/sec/10 yr in normal men. In a report of patients undergoing prostatectomy, there was a change in flow rate from 13.2 cc per second initially to 8.1 cc per second at the time of surgery[1].

The symptoms of BPH are nonspecific, and prostatic obstruction must be differentiated from other obstructive lesions such as urethral stricture and bladder neck stenosis (Fig. 4-5) or contracture.

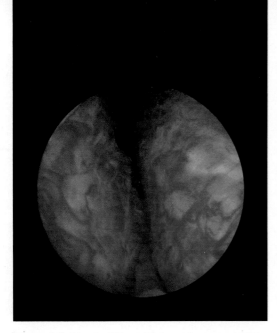

Figure 4-6. *Massive bilateral lobar enlargement of the prostate obscures vision within the prostatic urethra from the level of the verumontanum. There was prominent vascularity of the mucosa bilaterally.*

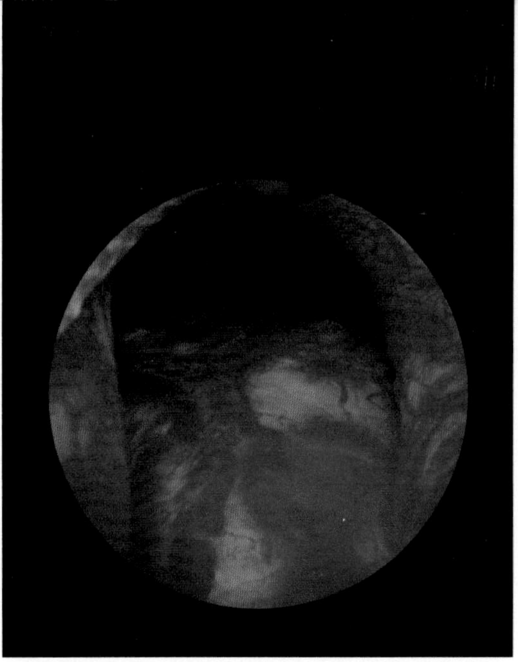

Figure 4-7. *As the urethroscope is advanced proximally within the prostatic urethra, a large median lobe is evident. Numerous large vessels course over the surface of the adenoma.*

Pathology. BPH originates from the periurethral portion of the lateral and middle prostatic lobes and compresses the true prostate peripherally. The compressed subcapsular zone is separated from the region of BPH by a fine muscular capsule termed the *surgical capsule*. Essentially, the surgical capsule is a benign growth composed of varying proportions of the fibromuscular and glandular components of the prostate. The gland may be soft and boggy due to a greater component of glandular hyperplasia, or it may be firm due to a higher degree of fibromuscular growth.

The microscopic appearance of the nodular hyperplasia of the prostate associated with BPH has been described as varying degrees of glandular and stromal hyperplasia. Franks[6] has classified BPH into five types: (1) stromal, (2) fibromuscular, (3) muscular, (4) fibroadenomatous, and (5) fibromyoadenomatous hyperplasia. The most common component of BPH found in man is fibromyoadenomatous hyperplasia.

Endoscopic Appearance. The appearance of BPH varies greatly according to the type, amount, and particularly the lobar distribution of hypertrophy. The classic adenomatous hypertrophy generally appears salmon gray with a soft, fluffy texture. Varying numbers of dilated blood vessels appear on the urethral surface, which may be pale to beefy red depending on the extent of associated inflammation in the prostatic urethra (Figs. 4-6 to 4-10).

Many combinations and patterns of prostatic lobar hyperplasia occur. The nature of these hypertrophied glands relative to their transurethral removal is discussed in greater detail in Chapter 9.

The most frequently observed pattern of hypertrophy shows a trilobar distribution with enlargement of the median and both lateral lobes. With moderate enlargement, the urethral lumen will be only partially occluded. There is little intravesical extension of the growth and only minor variations in the normal anatomy of the bladder neck and trigone. With more severe hyperplasia, the lobes extend intravesically, displacing the bladder neck and distorting the trigonal anatomy. The urethral lumen may become either totally occluded to visual inspection with the tip of the instrument located at the verumontanum, or the prostatic lumen may assume the appearance of an inverted V due to the anterior connection of the lateral lobes.

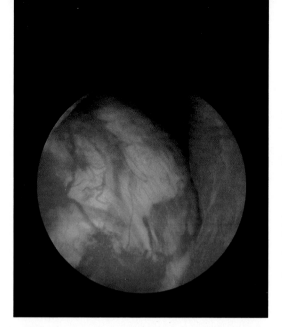

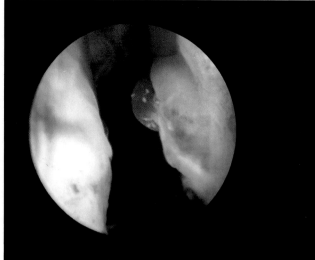

Figure 4-8. *There is a sharp distinction between the median lobe and the bladder neck at their junction in this patient. This view alone, without benefit of inspection from the point shown in Fig. 4-7, could appear to indicate only lateral lobe enlargement. Full endoscopic inspection of the prostatic urethra, however, reveals the presence of median lobe enlargement. Resection should be started with the median lobe initially.*

Figure 4-10. *The prostatic adenoma has regrown after a previous transurethral resection. Edematous mucosal bullae are present.*

Lobar enlargement may also appear to be limited to a single lobe or to affect the lobes asymmetrically. A very large intravesical median lobe with relatively smaller lateral lobes may be present, or the lateral lobes, either singly or bilaterally, may have significant intravesical components. Permanent elevation of the bladder neck and trigone may develop with hypertrophy of the subcervical lobe.

As discussed in Chapter 9, recognition of the type and extent of hyperplastic prostatic enlargement allows transurethral resection of the obstructive tissue in a safe and successful fashion.

Management. Indications for the treatment of benign prostatic hypertrophy are varied. The patient who presents with hydronephrosis and azotemia secondary to acute urinary retention from BPH has an obvious indication for relief of bladder outlet obstruction. Many other patients with varying degrees of prostatism, however, have less obvious indications for surgical treatment. These patients are discussed in greater detail in Chapter 9. The procedures that can be performed to remove the prostate include transurethral resection with removal of the periurethral adenoma to the surgical capsule, and suprapubic, retropubic, and perineal prostatectomy. The choice of procedure for relief of outlet obstruction depends on the individual patient and his associated complicating factors, the size of the hypertrophied gland, and the preference of the urologist.

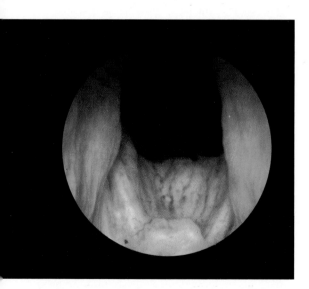

Figure 4-9. *Nearly the entire prostatic urethra can be seen in a single field in this patient with previous bladder neck resection. The verumontanum is evident at the 6 o'clock position, and minimal lateral lobe enlargement is seen on each side.*

MALIGNANT TUMORS OF THE PROSTATE. Prostatic cancer is the second most common malignancy in man and the third most common cause of cancer death in men over 55 years of age. The incidence increases with advancing age with autopsy series reporting the presence of prostatic carcinoma in 12 to 46 percent of males over 50 years. The cancer appears to be most common in American blacks and definitely less common in Japanese males[24].

The role of BPH in prostatic cancer is controversial. It is very difficult to evaluate BPH as a risk factor since both cancer and BPH occur in older age groups, making it hard to find a comparison group of patients in the same age group without BPH. As a result, no definite relationship can be proved at this time.

Clinical Presentation. Prostatic cancer is generally asymptomatic in its early stages and only later will patients develop symptoms of urinary outflow obstruction or metastatic disease. Disease outside the prostatic capsule (stage C or D), will affect 70 to 80 percent of patients, whereas only 20 to 30 percent will present with stage A or B disease, limited to the prostate. Of patients operated on for benign prostatic hypertrophy, 6.3 percent (ages 40–49 yr) and 28.7 percent (ages 70–79 yr) will be found to have prostatic carcinoma[20].

The physical examination of the patient with prostatic cancer is the most important factor in the diagnosis. The most sensitive finding for prostatic cancer on the physical examination appears to be the digital examination of the prostate. Often, indistinct findings such as induration will be found on biopsy to represent prostatic cancer[17].

Although there are many ancillary methods used for diagnosis of prostatic cancer, such as serum acid phosphatase, transrectal ultrasonography, and digital examination, the final diagnosis rests on prostatic biopsy[24]. The different methods used to obtain tissue include transperineal, transrectal, or transurethral biopsy.

Pathology. Carcinoma of the prostate arises from the periphery of the prostate gland. This subcapsular region is the portion displaced peripherally by benign prostatic hyperplasia in the periurethral tissue, a finding reached by the examination of radical prostatectomy specimens in which all cancers were located peripherally and all BPH located periurethrally[12].

The types of tumors encountered are adenocarcinoma (95% of cases), transitional cell or squamous cell carcinoma, and sarcoma or tumor of the verumontanum. Leukemia is a common secondary tumor of the prostate.

The histologic diagnosis of adenocarcinoma of the prostate is based on cellular anaplasia, histochemical changes, invasion, and architectural disturbances[17]. Because of the varied patterns of growth in its different regions, the tumor is often difficult to grade. The Gleason grading system assigns a grade from 1 to 5 (depending on dedifferentiation) to the most extensive and the less extensive regions of the tumor. The sum of these two grades, 2 to 10, can then be used to help predict the biologic behavior of the cancer[7].

Transitional cell and squamous cell carcinomas are rare. Transitional cell carcinomas arise from the distal regions of the prostatic ducts, which are normally lined with transitional epithelium. Squamous cell carcinomas may arise within the prostatic epithelium or occasionally within müllerian duct remnants[21].

Carcinoma of the verumontanum (a müllerian duct remnant) or endometrioid carcinoma is composed of columnar cells with cilia, which tend to form glands. These carcinomas are often papillary or polypoid and can invade the prostate directly[16].

Sarcomas of the prostate are also very rare, and only 25 percent of the patients affected are older than 40 years. Histologically, these sarcomas can be pure, such as leiomyosarcomas or rhabdomyosarcomas, or mixed, such as carcinosarcomas[22].

Very uncommonly, the prostate may be involved secondarily by leukemia. One series reported the presence in 4 of 17 leukemia patients of prostatic involvement diagnosed after prostatectomy[15]. In this series, as in others, the most common type of leukemia was chronic lymphocytic.

Endoscopic Appearance. It is often impossible to differentiate prostatic carcinoma in its early stages from benign hyperplasia by endoscopic means (Fig. 4-11). This is exemplified by the frequent diagnosis of carcinoma pathologically after transurethral resection of an apparently benign gland. Also, as discussed previously, the carcinoma arises posteriorly and usually does not involve the luminal surface, which therefore initially appears normal. In the carcinoma's more advanced stages, the urethral surface may be involved and appear as an assymetric nodular growth (Fig. 4-12). The cut surface of the tissue appears more yellow than the pale, benign adenomatous tissue and will be rather solid as compared with the fluffy, benign tissue.

Endometrioid carcinomas have a characteristic location near the verumontanum within the prostatic urethra. They appear as whitish gray, finger-like projections extending into the urethral lumen (Fig. 4-13).

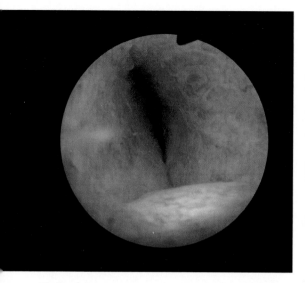

Figure 4-11. *Bilateral lobar enlargement is evident in this patient with a less prominent verumontanum. The lobes are visually obstructive and there is mild edema of the mucosa as a result of previous catheterization. Adenocarcinoma was present in the prostate of this patient but could not be distinguished endoscopically.*

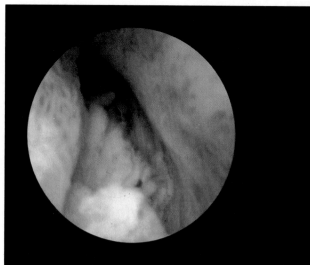

Figure 4-13. *An adenomatoid tumor of the verumontanum appears as a white, fluffy mass of tissue in the floor of the prostatic urethra, adherent to the verumontanum. It was treated successfully by transurethral resection.*

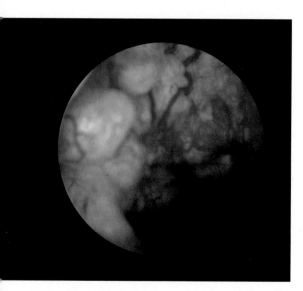

Figure 4-12. *Recurrent adenocarcinoma of the prostate is evident at the proximal portion of the prostatic fossa and the bladder neck. There is nodular regrowth of the tumor.*

Management. The treatment of adenocarcinoma of the prostate is based primarily on the stage of the tumor. Other factors of importance include the tumor grade and the patient's age and overall medical condition. The treatment modalities include external beam radiation, interstitial radiation, radical prostatectomy, hormonal manipulation, and observation alone. It is beyond the scope of this manual to discuss the current rationale for each type of therapy.

REFERENCES

1. Ball, A. J., Fenely, R. C. L., and Abrams, P. H. The natural history of untreated prostatism. *Br. J. Urol.* 53:613, 1981.
2. Brock, D. J., and Grieco, M. H. Cryptococcal prostatitis in a patient with sarcoidosis: Response to 5-fluorocytosine. *J. Urol.* 107:1017, 1972.
3. Craigen, A. A., Hickling, J. B., Sanders, C. R. G., and Carpenter, R. G. Natural history of prostatic obstruction. *J. R. Coll. Gen. Pract.* 18:226, 1969.
4. Drach, G. W., Layton, T. N., and Binard, W. J. Male peak urinary flow rate: Relationships to volume voided and age. *J. Urol.* 122:210, 1979.
5. Franks, L. M. Latent carcinoma of the prostate. *J. Pathol. Bacteriol.* 68:603, 1954.
6. Franks, L. M. The Prostate. In W. A. Anderson and J. M. Kissane (Eds.), *Pathology* (7th ed.). St. Louis: Mosby, 1977. Pp. 999–1012.

7. Gleason, D. F. Veterans Administration Cooperative Urological Research Group: Histologic Grading and Clinical Staging of Prostatic Carcinoma. In M. Tannenbaum (Ed.), *Urologic Pathology: The Prostate.* Philadelphia: Lea & Febiger, 1977.

8. Greene, L. F., and Segura, J. W. Transurethral Prostatic Resection: Delayed Post-operative Complications. In L. F. Greene and J. W. Segura (Eds.), *Transurethral Surgery.* Philadelphia: Saunders, 1979. Pp. 208–209.

9. Lattimer, J. K. Tuberculous prostatic urethritis: A suggestive diagnostic sign. *J. Urol.* 59:326, 1948.

10. Lattimer, J. K., and Wechsler, M. Genitourinary Tuberculosis. In J. H. Harrison, et al. (Eds.), *Campbell's Urology* (4th ed.). Philadelphia: Saunders, 1978. Pp. 557–575.

11. Lytton, B., Emery, J. M., and Harvard, B. M. The incidence of benign prostatic obstruction. *J. Urol.* 99:639, 1968.

12. McNeal, J. E. The prostate and prostatic urethra: A morphologic synthesis. *J. Urol.* 107:1008, 1972.

13. Meares, E. M., Jr., and Barbalias, G. A. Prostatitis: Bacterial, non-bacterial, and prostatodynia. *Semin. Urol.* 1(2):146, 1983.

14. Meares, E. M., Jr., and Stamey, T. A. Bacteriologic localization patterns in bacterial prostatitis and urethritis. *Invest. Urol.* 5:492, 1968.

15. Melchior, J., Valk, W. L., Foret, J. D., and Mebust, W. K. The prostate in leukemia: Evaluation and review of the literature. *J. Urol.* 111:647, 1974.

16. Melicow, M. M., and Tannenbaum, M. Endometrial carcinoma of the uterus masculinus (prostatic utricle). Report of six cases. *J. Urol.* 106:892, 1971.

17. Mostofi, F. K. Grading of prostatic carcinoma. *Cancer Chemother. Rep.* 59:111, 1975.

18. Orr, W. A., Mulholland, S. G., and Walzak, M. P. Genitourinary tract involvement with systemic mycosis. *J. Urol.* 107:1047, 1972.

19. Schonebeck, J., and Anselm, S. The occurrence of yeast-like fungi in the urine under normal conditions and in various types of urinary tract pathology. *Scand. J. Urol. Nephrol.* 6:123, 1972.

20. Sheldon, C. A., Williams, R. D., and Fraley, E. E. Incidental carcinoma of the prostate: A review of the literature and critical reappraisal of classification. *J. Urol.* 124:626, 1980.

21. Szemes, G. C., and Rubin, D. J. Squamous cell carcinoma in a müllerian duct cyst. *J. Urol.* 100:40, 1968.

22. Tripathi, V. N. P., and Dick, V. S. Primary sarcoma of the urogenital system in adults. *J. Urol.* 101:898, 1969.

23. Turner-Warwick, R., Whiteside, C. G., Worth, P. H. L., Milroy, E. J. G., and Bates, C. P. A urodynamic view of the clinical problems associated with bladder neck dysfunction and its treatment by endoscopic incision and transtrigonal posterior prostatectomy. *Br. J. Urol.* 45:44, 1973.

24. von Eschenbach, A. C. Needle Biopsy of the Prostate. In D. E. Johnson and M. A. Boileau (Eds.), *Genitourinary Tumors.* New York: Grune & Stratton, 1982. Pp. 33–41.

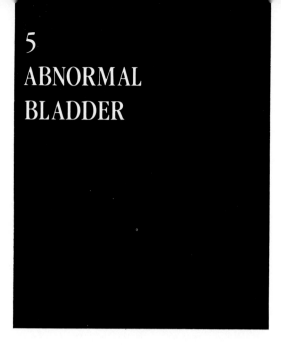

5
ABNORMAL BLADDER

Demetrius H. Bagley

Jeffry L. Huffman

Edward S. Lyon

CONGENITAL ANOMALIES. Congenital anomalies within the bladder are rarely detected endoscopically in the adult. The majority of these structural abnormalities become manifest through urinary symptoms and the appropriate urologic investigation in children. Other congenital lesions of the bladder are reviewed in Chapter 18.

PATENT URACHUS. The urachus is a vestigial remnant of the allantois. It is usually obliterated so that only fibrous bands remain. If the lumen persists at any portion, however, the urachus may form a urachal cyst, a vesical diverticulum, or even a vesicoumbilical fistula. A cyst is usually asymptomatic but may present as a suprapubic mass, while a persistent fistula may present with umbilical drainage of urine. Although a persistent diverticulum may serve as a site for residual urine and a focus for infection, persistence of the urachus at the level of the bladder is more often noted incidentally on endoscopy as a diverticulum or fistula at the dome of the bladder. The diagnosis can be made with a cystogram demonstrating the vesical lesion or by cytoscopy. Treatment is not necessary for the asymptomatic lesion.

URACHAL CARCINOMA. Urachal carcinomas are rare, accounting for less than 1 in 1,400 bladder tumors[1]. These tumors are mucus-secreting adenocarcinomas located at the bladder dome. Any adenocarcinoma at that site should be suspicious for having arisen in a urachal remnant, and consideration for treatment should extend to the total urachus. Local treatment by transurethral resection, therefore, may not be adequate and excision of the tract of the urachus to the umbilicus should be considered.

CYSTITIS. Cystitis, broadly defined, includes all inflammatory abnormalities of the bladder. These range from the very common episodes of infectious cystitis, which do not require endoscopic evaluation, to the more unusual lesions requiring biopsy for diagnosis. Endoscopically, the classic findings of inflammation, including erythema and edema, are readily apparent. It may be impossible to distinguish these lesions solely on the basis of clinical symptoms or endoscopic findings, and often the final diagnosis is based on the entire clinical pattern, cultures, and occasionally biopsy of the bladder[4].

Bacterial Cystitis

CLINICAL PRESENTATION. Patients with bacterial cystitis typically present with urinary frequency, urgency, and dysuria. Hematuria may develop, thus allowing the subclassification of hemorrhagic cystitis.

On physical examination, there may be suprapubic tenderness and, in the female, anterior vaginal tenderness may be elicited with palpation of the bladder on pelvic examination. Urinalysis will usually show pyuria and often hematuria. Bacteria often are also seen on microscopic examination. Radiologic studies usually are unrevealing, although some irregularity of the bladder may be seen and considered consistent with mucosal edema on the cystogram obtained with the excretory urogram.

ENDOSCOPIC APPEARANCE. Endoscopically, the appearance of the bladder may vary with the severity of the infection. A mild cystitis evidenced by voiding symptoms and a positive urine culture may exhibit a relatively normal-appearing bladder. There may be some dulling of the mucosa with loss of the sharp vascular pattern because of the presence of mucosal edema. With hemorrhagic cystitis there may be large confluent mucosal hemorrhages or patchy hemorrhagic areas. Because of the possibility of disseminating causative organisms during endoscopy, instrumentation should be avoided if infection is suspected.

Pathologic examination of biopsies from the involved bladder show interstitial edema, acute and chronic inflammatory cellular infiltrates, and interstitial hemorrhage in the hemorrhagic areas.

MANAGEMENT. Treatment consists of administration of appropriate antimicrobial agents based on the culture and sensitivity of the organism. An agent such as phenazopyridine (Pyridium) often relieves the irritative symptoms.

Pseudomembranous Trigonitis.
Pseudomembranous trigonitis is a common, normal finding in women, although it is almost never seen in men. On the trigonal mucosa is a white, patchy elevation, which does not scrape off or slough spontaneously. Histologically, this is a squamous epithelium that, like the vaginal epithelium, changes appearance with the menstrual period. It has been considered either squamous metaplasia or more probably ectopic vaginal epithelium. It is not associated with urinary infections or irritative symptoms and requires neither biopsy nor treatment.

Cystitis Cystica and Cystitis Glandularis.
Recurrent and chronic infections may be associated with other inflammatory lesions within the bladder. Subepithelial islands of transitional cells, also referred to as *Brunn's nests,* can degenerate to form cystic lesions lined by layers of one or, at most, two cells in the bladder mucosa. Such lesions also occur elsewhere in the urinary tract—for example, pyelitis cystica and ureteritis cystica, which are also usually associated with recurrent and chronic infections. If these nests contain several layers of cells, including mucus-secreting cells within the epithelium, then a lesion that appears similar grossly, known as *cystitis glandularis,* results.

Endoscopically, cystitis cystica and cystitis glandularis can sometimes be recognized as small, clear, mucosal cysts. They can be masked by associated inflammatory changes and thus be indistinguishable from cystitis or carcinoma in situ. Although tumors may arise in these cells, the lesions are not considered precancerous and do not require aggressive extirpative therapy (Fig. 5-1).

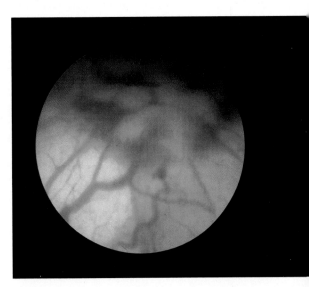

Figure 5-1. *Cystitis glandularis can appear as a localized erythematous patch. In this patient the "glandular" portion is quite prominent and can be seen endoscopically.*

Cystitis Follicularis. Another pattern that can be seen, particularly in patients with chronic bacterial cystitis, is called *cystitis follicularis.* Numerous small, white elevations can be seen in the mucosa, often scattered throughout the hyperemic and hemorrhagic areas. These lesions have been shown to be lymphoid follicles[4]. No specific therapy is necessary other than to treat the primary infection.

Urinary Tuberculosis

CLINICAL PRESENTATION. Tuberculosis of the urinary tract may present with a wide variety of symptoms. In one series, epididymitis was the most frequent early indication of renal tuberculosis in males[8]. Another major group of patients had symptoms of cystitis, including urinary frequency and dysuria. Irritative lower tract symptoms were more common among females, but hematuria was seen more often in males. The degree of involvement of the kidneys or lower urinary tract is not always related directly to the extent of symptoms.

DIAGNOSIS. The diagnosis of urinary tuberculosis can be made by finding tubercle bacilli in the urine. A valuable technique for recovering the bacteria is to obtain three morning urine specimens on successive days. Urine should be obtained for specific culture for tuberculosis in any patient in whom tuberculosis is suspected. In turn, tuberculosis should be considered in all patients with sterile pyuria, in those with urinary symptoms who fail to develop typical bacterial infections, or in patients with ureteral strictures that are otherwise unexplained. On physical examination there may be few findings in the female patient. In males, concurrent tuberculous involvement of the prostate may produce a shrunken, firm, irregular gland or small firm nodules. The epididymis may contain numerous firm, beadlike areas.

ENDOSCOPIC APPEARANCE. Endoscopy can provide valuable clues in the diagnosis of tuberculosis. As the endoscope passes through the prostate, marked velvety erythema of the prostatic urethra with indurated ridges proximal to the verumontanum may be seen with dilated prostatic ducts. Prostatic involvement may advance to caseation. As the instrument enters the bladder, ulcerations in the mucosa may be seen with surface exudate. Ureteral orifices may be quite erythematous with an erythematous patch below each orifice. As the disease advances, contracture of the bladder may be noted, particularly at the dome. Ureteral involvement with tight stricture formation is a serious potential complication.

MANAGEMENT. Treatment involves multiple-drug, antituberculous chemotherapy. The regimens may include isoniazid, ethambutol, and rifampin. Other drugs that have been used include streptomycin, *para*-aminosalicylic acid (PAS), cycloserine, and kanamycin. Severely contracted bladders can be augmented by interposition of patches or segments of large bowel or by bypass with an appropriate diversion. Ureteral strictures should be treated initially when possible by dilation with ureteral catheters, bulbs, or angioplastic balloon catheters.

Radiation Cystitis

CLINICAL PRESENTATION. Radiation to a field that includes the bladder may result in the injury known as *radiation cystitis.* Radiation injuries can be divided into two phases: (1) The early phase, which occurs during or immediately after treatment, may present as acute cystitis with urinary frequency, urgency, dysuria, and possibly hematuria. (2) The later phase, occurring months to years later, may develop with similar irritative symptoms or may progress to severe urinary frequency because of severe contraction and fibrosis of the bladder (Figs. 5-2, 5-3). A prominent symptom of radiation cystitis, and not an infrequent problem confronting the urologist, is hematuria. This may be of variable severity, ranging from microscopic hematuria to massive bleeding, which is life threatening and requires emergency therapy.

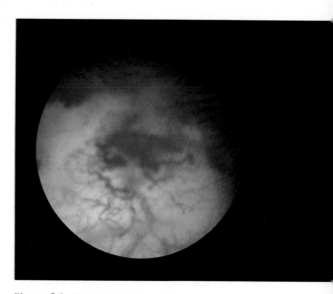

Figure 5-2. *Acute radiation cystitis appears as submucosal hemorrhage often with ulceration and confluence of the hemorrhagic patches.*

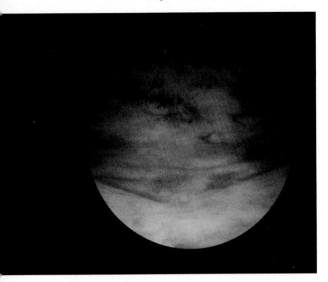

Figure 5-3. *Radiation injury to the bladder results in diffuse fibrosis as demonstrated in this patient 10 years after radiation for carcinoma of the cervix. Hemorrhagic patches remain on the posterior bladder wall while the trigone exhibits the pallor of fibrosis.*

DIAGNOSIS. The diagnosis can be made on the basis of the patient's history and endoscopic findings, including biopsy. Localized or confluent areas within the bladder may be hemorrhagic and interspersed with other mucosal areas showing fibrosis and scarring. Years after radiation, severe fibrosis can develop; vascular telangiectactic lesions can be seen. If the field of radiation has not involved the entire bladder, a sharp demarcation between the involved and the normal bladder is often demonstrated.

MANAGEMENT. Rarely, individual sites of arterial bleeding are seen and can be controlled by fulguration. More often there is bleeding from a larger area, which cannot be controlled endoscopically. Small patches of hemorrhagic mucosa can be fulgurated with control of bleeding. Massive diffuse hemorrhage has been treated with intravesical instillation of silver nitrate, formalin, or other caustic agents. In rare patients, massive bleeding cannot be controlled intravesically and requires drastic therapy, such as embolization or ligation of the internal iliac arteries, or even cystectomy.

Interstitial Cystitis

CLINICAL PRESENTATION. The typical symptoms of presentation in patients with interstitial cystitis are those of an irritable, painful bladder. Characteristically, urinary frequency and urgency are unrelenting. Pain is usually suprapubic, particularly after emptying of the bladder. Patients have usually had a long history of similar complaints and have been treated for infection on numerous occasions without documentation of active bacterial infection. Laboratory studies are unrevealing in these patients. The urine is normal on microscopic examination and cultures are sterile. Similarly, radiologic examinations are negative.

DIAGNOSIS AND ENDOSCOPIC APPEARANCE. The diagnosis of interstitial cystitis can be made on the basis of the clinical history and cystoscopic findings. It is valuable to use anesthesia, either general or spinal, for cystoscopy since the procedure is quite painful, particularly with distention of the bladder. The bladder should be observed during filling, then emptied and refilled. Often the bladder appears normal on initial inspection, but there may be some blood tinging of the irrigant when drained. On repeat filling, small submucosal hemorrhages may be detected. The most typical lesion, however, is a linear crack noted when the bladder is filled nearly to capacity (Fig. 5-4). Blood may exude from this crack. In the later stages of the disease, the mucosal surface may be quite pale with linear scars of earlier lesions and stellate scars radiating from a central ulceration (Fig. 5-5). These ulcers are actually quite rare, although the term *Hunner's ulcer* has become synonymous with interstitial cystitis. In advanced cases, there may be fibrosis of the full thickness of the bladder with diminished capacity.

It is essential to biopsy the bladder at several sites, mainly to distinguish interstitial cystitis from carcinoma in situ. Pathologically, the bladder wall is thickened with vascular injection of the serosa. There may be loss of the mucosa. In the submucosal layer, inflammatory changes are seen with edema, vascular congestion, perivascular hemorrhage, and cellular infiltration.

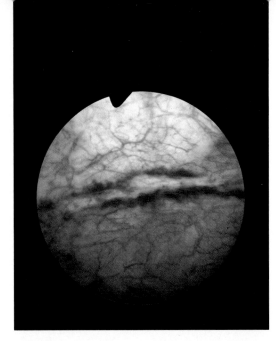

Figure 5-4. *The typical mucosal lesion of interstitial cystitis is a linear fissure in the mucosa that appears after distention or on repeated distention of the bladder. There is usually only mild bleeding from the fissure.*

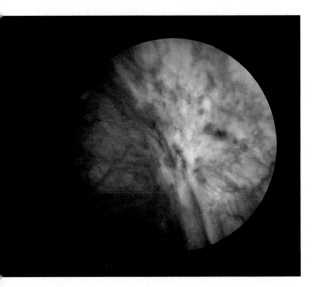

Figure 5-5. *Advanced interstitial cystitis is characterized by stellate scarring of the bladder.*

MANAGEMENT. Treatment includes numerous techniques, which may provide temporary palliative relief of symptoms. Local treatment with bladder distention is often successful in reducing pain and frequency on either a temporary or a long-term basis. Infiltration of the bladder wall with steroids has been reported to provide relief. Transurethral resection and fulguration of localized mucosal lesions have also been successful in some hands [3].

Instillation of silver nitrate, oxychlorosene (Clorpactin), dimethyl sulfoxide, or pentosan polysulfate [6] has provided relief in some patients. More extensive surgical treatment with denervation or bladder substitution has been employed in patients with severe symptoms.

Chronic Eosinophilic Cystitis. Chronic eosinophilic cystitis is extremely rare. The presentation is one of irritative bladder symptoms but the course may be more protracted than that of acute bacterial cystitis. Endoscopic appearance is nondiagnostic; the diagnosis, however, depends on histologic examination of biopsy of the bladder wall, which shows marked eosinophilic filtration.

Cystitis from Drug Ingestion. Acute or chronic cystitis may develop after ingestion of toxic agents, the best known example being cyclophosphamide. Diffuse hemorrhagic cystitis may be produced by the administration and subsequent excretion of this drug in the urine. Patients receiving cyclophosphamide are often receiving a combination of other chemotherapeutic agents. The hematuria is often exacerbated by thrombocytopenia. Radiologic and endoscopic studies are nonspecific. Treatment, in addition to cessation of the causative drug, is directed at controlling the symptoms, usually hemorrhage. Focal bleeding, although uncommon, may be controlled by local fulguration cystoscopically. More diffuse bleeding can be controlled by instillation of a caustic agent such as formalin, by Helmstein balloon pressure therapy, and possibly, when thrombocytopenia is not an associated complicating factor, by administration of epsilon-aminocaproic acid.

Malacoplakia of the Bladder

CLINICAL PRESENTATION. Malacoplakia is a disease that affects many body tissues but most often involves the urinary tract. Of the 153 cases reviewed by Stanton and Maxted [7], the urinary tract was involved in 58 percent. Of these, the bladder was involved in 40 percent, the ureter in 11 percent, the renal pelvis in 10 percent, and the ureteropelvic junction in 3 patients. There is a female predominance with approximately a 4 : 1 female-male ratio.

Generally, the presentation of patients with bladder malacoplakia is that of bladder irritability and hematuria. In as many as 76 percent of the patients, there is a coliform infection of the urine. There are also many patients who are malnourished, cachetic, or have a concurrent systemic disease. There is some tendency for involvement of the lower ureter and renal pelvis as well.

CLINICAL FINDINGS. There are few findings on physical examination of patients with malacoplakia. An associated *E. coli* urinary tract infection can be present in up to 89 percent of the patients who have urinary cultures performed. Other organisms such as *Klebsiella, Enterobacter, Proteus,* and *Pseudomonas* may be present. The serum urea nitrogen and creatinine are usually normal. An excretory urogram, although usually not helpful, may demonstrate some irregularity consistent with edema of the bladder mucosa.

ENDOSCOPIC APPEARANCE. Endoscopically, these lesions appear as pink brown, flat nodules or yellow nodular lesions similar to amyloid deposits (Fig. 5-6). They may also appear as yellow brown, soft plaques with central umbilication, ulceration, and peripheral hyperemia. They may be 1 mm to 3 cm in diameter. Initially, the overlying epithelium remains intact and only slight erythema of the mucosa may be seen.

PATHOLOGY. Malacoplakia probably results from defective intracellular digestion of bacteria. There is impaired intracellular killing of bacteria and an overloading of the digestive capacity of the phagocytes. The accumulation and subsequent mineralization of bacterial cell wall fragments lead to the formation of the Michaelis-Gutmann bodies [5, 7].

Histologically, there are dense aggregates of large mononuclear phagocytes, which are also von Hanseman cells. These are associated with Michaelis-Gutmann bodies and scanty connective tissue stroma infiltrated by lymphocytes and plasma cells (Fig. 5-7).

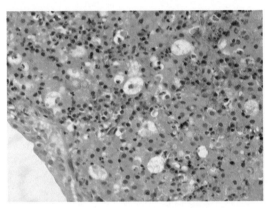

Figure 5-7. *Biopsy of the area demonstrates the histologic changes characteristic of malacoplakia. Note the large cells containing Michaelis-Gutmann bodies.*

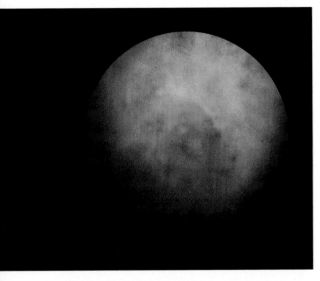

Figure 5-6. *Malacoplakia may be localized as a yellowish or reddish mucosal lesion as found on the posterior wall of this 45-year-old female with a history of irritative voiding symptoms.*

MANAGEMENT. There has been little experience in treating patients with malacoplakia; many researchers, however, have suggested different forms of treatment. Since the disease involves defective, intracellular digestion of bacteria, in order to treat the disease, antibiotics must penetrate the cell membrane. Rifampin and trimethoprim enter the phagocyte and can assist in intracellular killing of bacteria. Long-term treatment of patients with trimethoprim and sulfamethoxazole may therefore lead to cure. Cholinergic agents such as bethanechol can relieve symptoms but histologically the lesions persist. Ascorbic acid may also be used to treat these lesions. It acts by increasing the ratio of intracellular cyclic guanine monophosphate to cyclic adenosine monophosphate and favors the assembly and increased function of microtubules. The currently recommended therapy consists of combining an intracellularly active antibiotic such as trimethoprim, sulfamethoxazole, or rifampin with bethanechol and ascorbic acid.

Surgical Treatment. It may be necessary to eradicate the local lesion or divert the urine if the disease progresses despite the medical regimen.

Vesicoenteric Fistulae

CLINICAL PRESENTATION. Patients with vesicoenteric fistulae characteristically complain of symptoms of pneumaturia and recurrent urinary infection. They may also notice the passage of feces with urine from the bladder. Infections with multiple organisms that persist despite antimicrobial therapy are one of the key findings in the history of patients with vesicoenteric fistulae.

Vesicoenteric fistulae are usually associated with a specific gastrointestinal lesion. These include diverticulitis, colonic tumors, or Crohn's disease. Less frequently, fistulae may develop with spontaneous penetration of pelvic abscesses into both the bowel and the bladder and, very rarely, by perforation of a foreign body from the lumen of the bowel transmurally into the bladder.

DIAGNOSIS. Radiographic studies may define the fistula and its location and are essential both to rule out other possible abnormalities and to define the underlying bowel disease. A cystogram may demonstrate contrast medium passing from the bladder into the bowel. Barium within the lumen of the bowel may also demonstrate the site of communication but is more important to define the status of the bowel and to rule out a colonic neoplasm or Crohn's disease. An excretory urogram should be obtained to define the status of the upper collecting system.

ENDOSCOPIC APPEARANCE. Cystoscopy is the most valuable technique for diagnosing vesicoenteric fistulae. Although in the presence of infection a generalized cystitis may be seen, there is usually a marked local inflammatory reaction with bullous edema at the site of the fistula. Rarely, bowel content may be seen exuding from the fistulous tract into the bladder, particularly on manual compression of the abdomen (Fig. 5-8).

MANAGEMENT. In treating a patient with a vesicoenteric fistula resulting from gastrointestinal disease, the major problems for management are those associated with therapy of the intestinal disease. Closure of the tract into the bladder is usually a relatively simple procedure with a high rate of success after treatment of the primary bowel disease. Treatment of vesicoenteric fistulae resulting from radiation injury is a more complex problem. Dissection of the involved fistulous tract on both the bladder and the bowel sides must be accomplished and normal tissue interspaced for optimal healing. Endoscopy plays a role only in the diagnosis of these lesions.

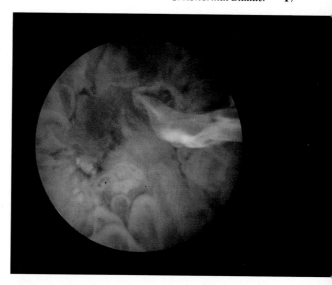

Figure 5-8. *The ostium of a vesicocolonic fistula is surrounded by edematous mucosa, and yellow brown intestinal content with particulate matter streams into the bladder.*

Vesicovaginal Fistulae

CLINICAL PRESENTATION. Vesicovaginal fistulae can result from local trauma to the anterior vaginal and posterior vesical wall. In medically modern societies, the most common cause of vesicovaginal fistulae is gynecologic surgery. In less developed countries, the most common cause is protracted labor during childbirth.

The patient with a vesicovaginal fistula presents with urinary incontinence. Urinary leakage is usually constant although in the presence of a small fistula it can be intermittent and may relate to pooling within the vagina. The fistula may develop immediately or after several days.

DIAGNOSIS. Diagnosis is assisted with excretory urography, which is essential to evaluate the upper tracts in order to rule out a ureteral fistula. Cystography may demonstrate the site of leakage. The two-dye test may be helpful in differentiating vesicovaginal from ureterovaginal fistulae. Physical examination alone will often reveal the presence of the fistula.

ENDOSCOPIC APPEARANCE. Endoscopic examination of the bladder is essential for the diagnosis of vesicovaginal fistulae. If the fistula is quite large, it may be difficult to distend the bladder adequately because of loss of the irrigating fluid through the fistula. In that case, the fistula can be occluded vaginally by manual compression or with a large Foley catheter placed into the vagina with the balloon inflated. The fistula can be identified as the opening in the mucosa, and can range in size from a pinhole opening to a large defect of several centimeters diameter. It may be obscured by folds of mucosa and seen only with distention of the bladder. The extent of inflammation around the fistulous tract should be evaluated, and the fistula's exact location accurately determined. Careful inspection should be made to exclude any additional fistulae.

MANAGEMENT. In the very early, small fistula, coagulation into the fistula coupled with urinary drainage may rarely promote closure. More often, surgical closure is necessary. If the fistula is located near the ureteral orifice, ureteral catheters should be placed endoscopically to identify the ureters during repair.

Intravesical Foreign Bodies. A foreign body within the bladder can serve as an irritant resulting in a general or localized inflammatory reaction. The patients' symptoms often vary but frequently are those of bladder irritation with urgency, frequency, and dysuria. The major examples of foreign bodies are bladder calculi, sutures, and indwelling catheters (see Figs. 5-15, 5-16).

Catheter Cystitis. Catheter, or polypoid, cystitis develops in the presence of an indwelling urethral catheter. A patient may develop an inflammatory reaction within the bladder even in the presence of sterile urine. This may appear as diffuse, bullous edema of the mucosa, but local irritation is a much more common appearance (Figs. 5-9 to 5-12). Because the dome and posterior wall of the bladder collapse onto the catheter, the tip of the catheter lies in direct contact with the bladder at a single or several discrete areas. As a result, a very localized edematous reaction develops. This area is usually translucent and limited to the mucosa. Occasionally, however, it is difficult to distinguish these lesions from bladder tumors. The inflammatory lesions are usually translucent, lack the multiple papillary configurations of low-grade tumors, and are located at a typical position at the posterior wall of the bladder [2]. Biopsy is occasionally necessary. Magnification chromocystoscopy may prove to be of value for the in vivo differential diagnosis of these lesions. The inflammatory exudate may coalesce and form a nidus for calculus formation (Fig. 5-13).

The only treatment required is removal of the foreign body as well as therapy for any concurrent infection.

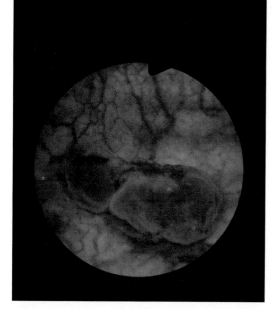

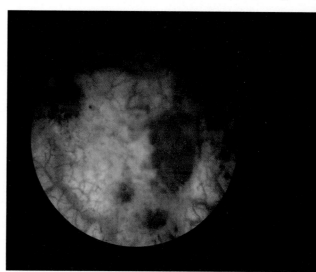

Figure 5-9. *Catheter cystitis and resultant edema of the bladder mucosa can take the several forms shown in Figs. 5-9 to 5-12. Here, edema is localized to the area directly traumatized by the catheter tip. Large edematous mucosal bullae are formed.*

Figure 5-10. *Several hemorrhagic submucosal areas have developed after urethral catheterization of several days' duration.*

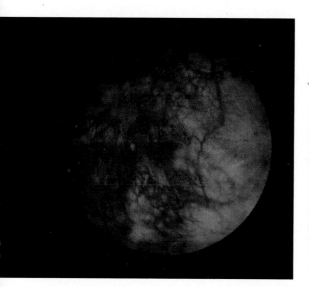

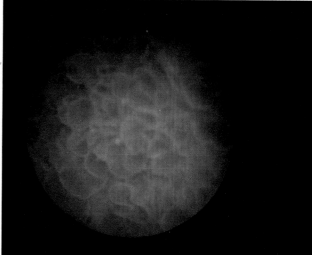

Figure 5-11. *There is diffuse scarring and inflammation of the bladder in this elderly male catheterized for several months.*

Figure 5-12. *Nearly the entire surface of the bladder is involved with diffuse pseudopapillary mucosal edema. This patient had a suprapubic latex Foley catheter for several months.*

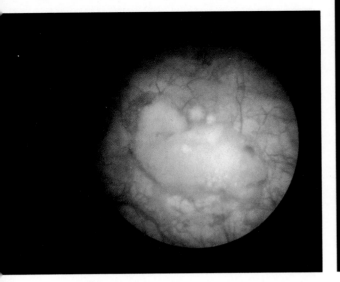

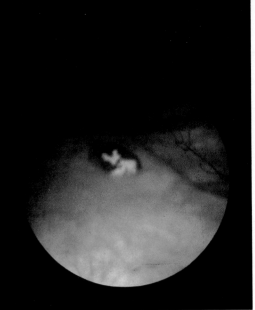

Figure 5-13. *Encrustations may develop on a catheter within the bladder, where they may remain after removal of the catheter. These encrustations are characteristically yellow, soft, amorphous masses. If left within the bladder, they may serve as a nidus for crystallization and stone formation and, therefore, should be removed when seen.*

Figure 5-14. *A renal calculus has been passed spontaneously to the right ureteral orifice where it can be seen. Such a calculus can often be removed with grasping forceps but may require prior ureteral meatotomy.*

Calculi

CLINICAL PRESENTATION. Bladder calculi develop as a result of urinary stasis secondary to outlet obstruction or neurogenic bladder dysfunction, or form on an abnormal surface such as a foreign body. Stones passing from the upper collecting system usually exit from a normal bladder without difficulty (Fig. 5-14). Individual or multiple calculi can occur. The symptoms are usually irritative but often can be related to the initiating factor leading to formation of the calculi. For example, in a patient with prostatic hypertrophy and lower urinary obstruction, calculi can form with urinary stasis, and the symptoms are those of lower urinary obstruction. Often bladder calculi are asymptomatic. Almost any foreign body within the bladder will serve as a nidus for calculus formation (Fig. 5-15). As an example, a suture from a previous operation passing through the wall of the bladder or a fragment of catheter or other instrument placed into the bladder will serve as a basis for a calculus (Fig. 5-16).

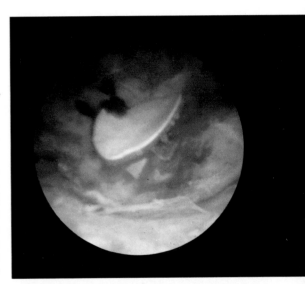

Figure 5-15. *Foreign bodies within the bladder become encrusted with crystals. A fragment of latex from a Foley catheter balloon had been in the bladder of this patient for 18 months and was entirely encrusted until the stone was disintegrated with the electrohydraulic lithotriptor. The fragment of latex could then be removed with the grasping forceps.*

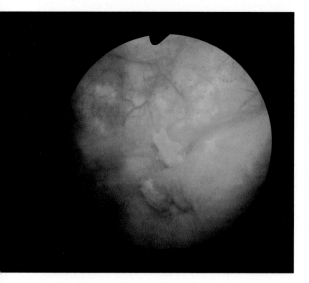

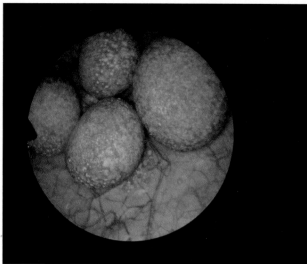

Figure 5-16. *A suture from a previous gynecologic procedure passed entirely through the bladder wall. It was the site for calculus formation. The calculus before its removal is shown in Fig. 12-6.*

Figure 5-18. *Four calculi and several smaller bits of gravel were found in the bladder of a patient with prostatic obstruction.*

DIAGNOSIS. Bladder calculi often are first detected radiographically. Radioopaque calculi can be seen on a plain x-ray as a centrally placed opacity overlying the bladder area (Fig. 5-17). Radiolucent calculi appearing on an intravenous pyelogram (IVP) as a filling defect within the bladder can be diagnosed with ultrasound since calculi exhibit a typical pattern of high-level surface echoes with acoustic shadowing.

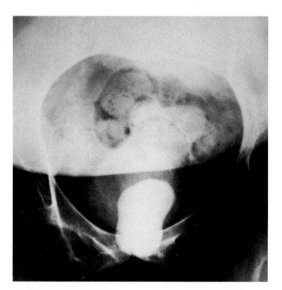

Figure 5-17. *A large radioopaque bladder calculus formed in a patient with a neurogenic bladder. It was removed entirely in a single procedure by electrohydraulic lithotripsy.*

ENDOSCOPIC APPEARANCE. The most direct method for diagnosing bladder calculi is endoscopy. With the cystoscope within the bladder, the calculi can be visualized directly (Fig. 5-18). They may be single or multiple, and smooth and round or, as in the example of the "jackstone" calculus (Fig. 5-19), irregular. The composition of the calculi is often evident from their appearance. For example, uric acid stones are usually orange yellow or gold, while infection or struvite stones may be white to brown and break easily. Calcium oxalate monohydrate calculi have a dark brown, relatively smooth surface with small mammilations and are very hard. Calcium oxalate dihydrate calculi exhibit a highly crystalline surface, almost jewel-like in appearance. The appearance is the same as that of ureteral calculi, which are reviewed extensively in Chapter 6.

The endoscopic treatment of bladder calculi is reviewed in Chapter 12.

Diverticula of the Bladder. Bladder diverticula can be grouped into congenital and acquired forms. The congenital diverticula include paraureteral diverticula, also known as *Hutch diverticula* and *urachal diverticula.* The acquired diverticula are the more common type and usually result from outlet obstruction or neurogenic dysfunction, although they have also been seen after surgical procedures.

The symptoms of bladder diverticula arise from the retention of urine. Urinary infection with its attendant irritative symptoms may develop. Urinary frequency and the need for double voiding may develop with large retentive diverticula.

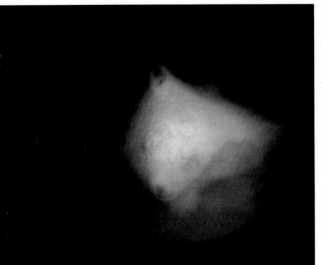

Figure 5-19. *Several papillations have formed on this bladder calculus in a pattern referred to as a "jackstone."*

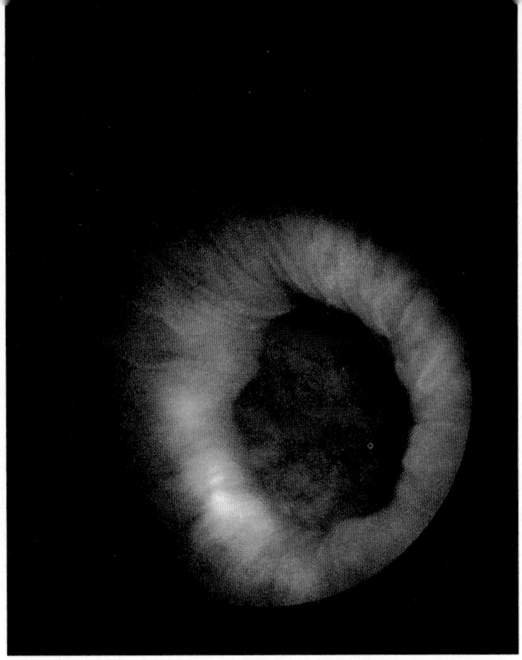

Figure 5-20. *Outpouching of vesical mucosa between the muscular bands results in a diverticulum with a well-defined ostium. Such diverticula may be the sites of calculi or tumors.*

DIAGNOSIS. Diverticula can be diagnosed radiographically with a cystogram or more accurately with a voiding cystogram. Multiple views may be necessary to demonstrate the diverticulum and avoid overlapping contrast shadows. In the case of bladder outlet obstruction, a cystogram may demonstrate both the irregularity of bladder trabeculation and multiple diverticula.

ENDOSCOPIC APPEARANCE. Cystoscopic examination of the surface of the bladder reveals the orifice of the diverticulum (Fig. 5-20). In the presence of severe trabeculation (Fig. 5-21), it is helpful to know the approximate position of the ostium of the diverticulum in question since multiple cellules and smaller diverticula may be present. It may be difficult to distinguish the diverticulum by direct examination alone. The ostium of the diverticulum can be either inconspicuous or a prominent, large opening surrounded circumferentially by well-defined musculature.

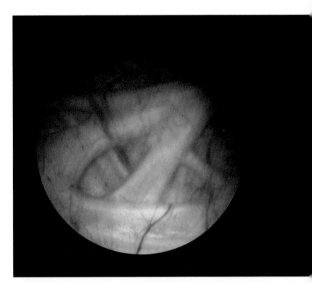

Figure 5-21. *As the bladder works to overcome outlet obstruction, the muscle hypertrophies and forms a pattern recognized as trabeculation.*

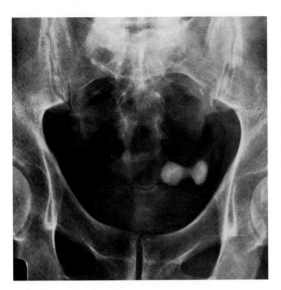

Figure 5-22. *A calculus has formed within a diverticulum and extends into the bladder with a dumbbell shape.*

MANAGEMENT. The need for treating bladder diverticula is based on the patient's symptomatology and any associated complicating factors. Asymptomatic nonobstructive diverticula may not require treatment. Diverticulum of the bladder can be treated adequately by open resection with direct closure of the ostium. The presence of a calculus or tumor in the diverticulum must be determined and treated appropriately (Fig. 5-22).

Interest has recently been revived in transurethral resection of the mouth of the diverticulum to provide adequate drainage[9]. While there is some risk of perforation with this technique, adequate drainage is often achieved. To prevent recurrence or the development of other diverticula, any associated outlet obstruction must also be relieved. The endoscopic technique should not be employed when other factors such as calculi, which cannot be removed, are present.

Bladder Tumors

CLINICAL PRESENTATION. The most frequent single symptom of bladder tumors is hematuria. Usually the patient complains of an episode of total gross hematuria, which is painless; sometimes, however, the patient presents with asymptomatic microscopic hematuria. A small fraction of patients with bladder tumors present with irritative symptoms such as urinary frequency, urgency, even dysuria or postvoiding discomfort. It is quite clear that all patients presenting with gross, painless hematuria must have a thorough urologic evaluation to exclude the presence of urothelial malignancy. The evaluation of microscopic hematuria is more controversial.

CLINICAL EVALUATION. On evaluation of the patient with a bladder tumor, physical examination is often unrevealing unless a large tumor mass within the bladder or a large metastatic lesion is present. Low-grade intravesical tumors usually cannot be palpated on physical examination, even with anesthesia. Bimanual examination with anesthesia, however, is valuable for staging bladder tumors in an effort to determine the presence of a solid mass lesion, bladder wall invasion, or nodal enlargement.

The single most important laboratory study is the urinalysis. This will often show hematuria, which may be intermittent. Cytologic examination of the urine may reveal tumor cells, particularly those of high-grade tumors. Several radiologic studies have proved valuable in the patient with a bladder malignancy. Among them, the excretory urogram remains the most important. In addition to giving some indication of bladder involvement on the cystographic portion of the study, and implying invasion by the tumor when ureteral obstruction exists, it provides information on the remainder of the urothelium in the upper tracts (Fig. 5-23). According to some early reports, staging of bladder tumors has been assisted by both ultrasound and computerized tomography (CT) scans of the bladder and pelvis. These modalities may indicate the depth of invasion within the bladder wall as well as the presence of pelvic nodal metastases.

Endoscopic inspection remains the major technique for the diagnosis of bladder tumors. Any patient suspected of having a bladder tumor, whether because of an episode of gross hematuria or a previous bladder tumor, must be examined cystoscopically. Cystoscopy permits not only the diagnosis of the presence or absence of a bladder tumor but also the number and position of the tumors. Inspection of the lesions will also offer some evidence of the stage and frequently the grade of the tumor.

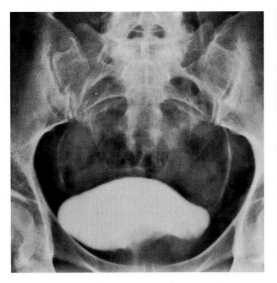

Figure 5-23. *A cystogram obtained with the excretory urogram of a patient with an invasive high-grade transitional carcinoma of the bladder demonstrates the irregular filling defect on the floor and lateral wall of the bladder corresponding to the tumor in Fig. 5-29.*

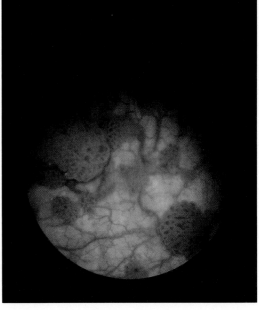

Figure 5-24. *Multiple low-grade, low-stage transitional cell carcinomas have circumscribed papillary configurations and appear as mulberries on the bladder surface.*

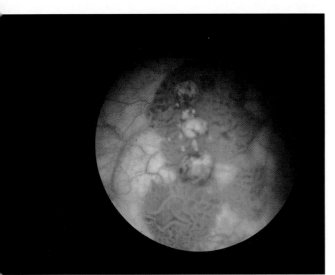

Figure 5-25. *Crystals may coalesce to form calculi on the abnormal surfaces of bladder tumors.*

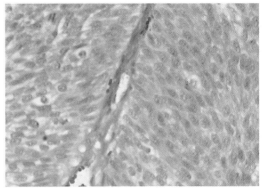

Figure 5-26. *Histologically, low-grade tumors are cytologically uniform and have a central stalk in the papillary configuration.*

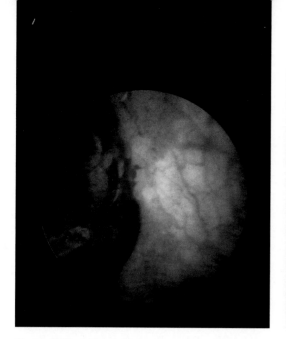

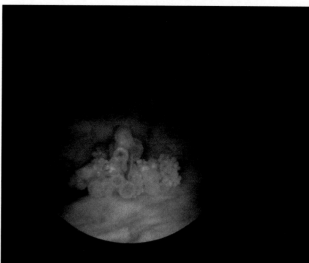

Figure 5-27. *A blood clot is seen within the bladder in the left lateral field. It is adherent to a low-grade tumor evident at the 12 and 6 o'clock positions.*

Figure 5-28. *A bizarre configuration of a transitional cell carcinoma in a young male.*

ENDOSCOPIC APPEARANCE. Bladder tumors vary widely in their endoscopic appearance (Figs. 5-24 to 5-34). The form of the lesion correlates well with the grade and often the stage of the tumor. Papillary lesions with well-defined fronds, which can be individually identified, are usually low grade and low stage as well (Fig. 5-24). These papillary tumors can be solitary or multiple. They are often located just lateral to the ureteral orifice but can be found anywhere within the bladder. Individual lesions may appear as individual fronds but more often as nearly spherical masses of tumor fronds. They also may appear as flat patches of low-lying fronds on the mucosa. A more solid-appearing mass of tumor, possibly with a wide base, is much more likely to be high grade and high stage (Figs. 5-29, 5-32). This variety in appearance from a papillary to a sessile tumor represents a spectrum of morphology, and various patterns and combinations may be seen within the same tumor.

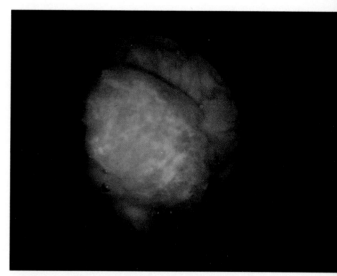

Figure 5-29. *The solid-appearing or sessile bladder tumor is a high-grade (III-IV) transitional cell carcinoma.*

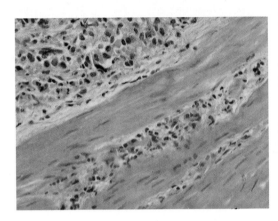

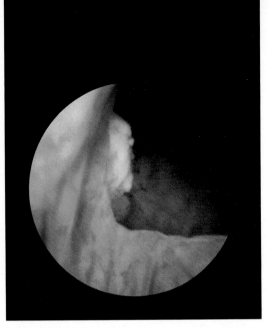

Figure 5-30. *The high-grade tumor shown in Fig. 5-29 is seen here invading muscle of the bladder wall. The cells have a wide variation in configuration and size, and mitoses can be seen.*

Figure 5-31. *A bladder tumor with adherent calculus is partially obscured on the right bladder wall adjacent to the bladder neck. It can be seen better with the 70- or 90-degree lens.*

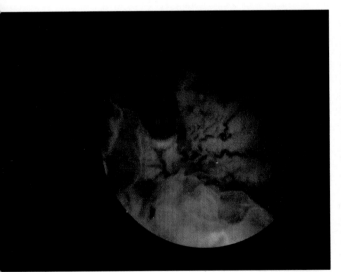

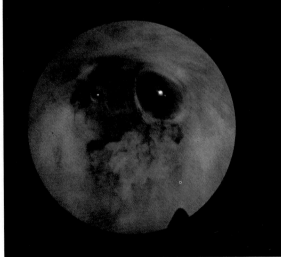

Figure 5-32. *A high-grade bladder tumor presents an irregular appearance on the surface of the bladder. This tumor appears solid, firm, and irregular, and there is edema of the mucosa. There is no papillary appearance of the tumor.*

Figure 5-33. *A bladder tumor (transitional cell carcinoma grade III-IV) has developed at the site where a suprapubic cystostomy tube entered the bladder.*

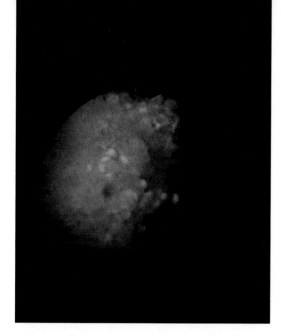

Figure 5-34. *Adenocarcinoma may have a papillary or sessile appearance and often cannot be distinguished endoscopically from other histologic types.*

PATHOLOGY. Histologically, the vast majority of bladder tumors are transitional cell carcinomas. Squamous carcinoma represents less than 5 percent of the total number of bladder tumors while adenocarcinoma accounts for less than 2 percent of the total and sarcoma of the bladder is even less frequent (Fig. 5-34).

Pathologic evaluation of bladder tumors includes their staging and grading, which are of paramount importance in assessing prognosis and determining therapy. Grading is based on cytologic and architectural abnormalities within the tumor. The papilloma that is considered benign is an uncommon lesion. The term is reserved for the papillary lesion with a well-defined fibrovascular stalk and cytologically normal epithelium.

In transitional cell carcinoma, there is increasing abnormality of individual cells and cellular pattern with increases in grade [12]. In addition to this increase in cytologic abnormality from grades I to IV, there is increasing loss of the normal pattern of maturation and intercellular relationships. There is some correlation of grade to the propensity for invasion and to the stage of the tumor. In bladder tumors, the depth of invasion into the bladder wall is expressed in the staging and can be determined by transurethral biopsy and resection of the lesion [10].

The treatment of urothelial tumors is discussed in Chapter 10.

Carcinoma In Situ. Carcinoma in situ of the urothelium deserves separate attention. In the past several years, the significance of high-grade carcinoma in situ has been recognized for its poor prognosis and need for individualized treatment. This lesion is often found in association with frank invasive carcinoma. There has been a propensity for these lesions to metastasize but the probability of their progression to invasive lesions is unknown.

Patients with carcinoma in situ may be asymptomatic or present with hematuria or, more frequently, have various degrees of irritative symptoms including urgency, urinary frequency, and dysuria. These symptoms often mimic those of cystitis, and carcinoma in situ may be impossible to differentiate from interstitial cystitis without biopsy and histologic confirmation. The diagnosis can be made with urinary cytology and bladder biopsy.

DIAGNOSIS. Cytologic examination of the urine has been most valuable in indicating the presence of carcinoma in situ. The diagnosis is confirmed by biopsy. Radiologic tests have not been of value. Early carcinoma in situ may appear essentially normal or have only nonspecific erythematous areas possibly with increased vascular prominence. The more classic appearance of carcinoma in situ, however, is usually a patchy, granular, slightly raised or velvety lesion, which is characteristically defined. The borders may be seen on biopsy to extend into areas of hyperplasia or atypia [11].

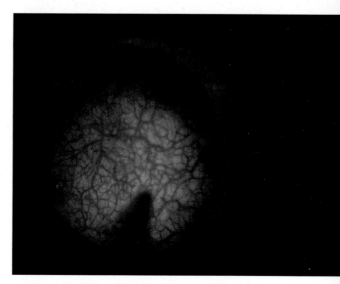

Figure 5-35. *Generalized hyperemia of the mucosa may appear after overdistention of the bladder. This patient had a urethral stricture, which was incised with the urethrotome blade evident in the 6 o'clock position.*

These lesions may be indistinguishable from other erythematous lesions such as hemorrhagic cystitis, cystitis glandularis, or interstitial cystitis. Any suspicious lesions should be biopsied. In the presence of urinary cytology indicating malignant cells but without evidence of gross tumor within the bladder, multiple, random biopsies should be taken since they may reveal carcinoma in situ despite inconclusive endoscopic appearance of the mucosa.

Optimal visualization has been reported when the mucosa is examined in profile with the cystoscopic lens close to the mucosa and the bladder filled to only one-third capacity. Overdistention of the bladder must be avoided since the resultant hyperemia may mask areas of carcinoma (Fig. 5-35). Microscopic cystoscopy has added a new dimension and may be of considerable value in the endoscopic diagnosis of carcinoma in situ (see Chap. 11).

MANAGEMENT. The optimal treatment of carcinoma in situ remains unclear at present. Some authors recommend early cystectomy while others have advocated intravesical chemotherapy or immunotherapy.

REFERENCES

Congenital Anomalies

1. Beck, A. D., Gaudin, H. J., and Bonham, D. G. Carcinoma of the urachus. *Br. J. Urol.* 42:555, 1970.

Inflammation of the Bladder

2. Ekelund, P., Anderstrom, C., Johansson, S. L., and Larsson, P. The reversibility of catheter-associated polypoid cystitis. *J. Urol.* 130:456, 1983.
3. Greenberg, E., Barnes, R., Stewart, S., and Furnish, T. Transurethral resection of Hunner's ulcer. *J. Urol.* 111:764, 1974.
4. Marsh, F. P., Banerjee, R., and Panchamia, P. The relationship between urinary infection, cystoscopic appearances and pathology of the bladder in man. *J. Clin. Pathol.* 27:297, 1974.
5. McClure, J. Malacoplakia of the urinary tract. *Br. J. Urol.* 54:181, 1982.
6. Parsons, C. L., Schmidt, J. H., and Pollen, J. J. Successful treatment of interstitial cystitis with sodium pentosanpolysulfate. *J. Urol.* 130:51, 1983.
7. Stanton, M. J., and Maxted, W. Malacoplakia: A study of the literature and current concepts of pathogenesis, diagnosis and treatment. *J. Urol.* 125:139, 1981.
8. Wechsler, H., Westfall, M., and Lattimer, J. K. The earliest signs and symptoms in 127 male patients with genitourinary tuberculosis. *J. Urol.* 83:801, 1960.

Diverticula

9. Vitale, P. J., and Woodside, J. R. Management of bladder diverticulum by transurethral resection: Re-evaluation of an old technique. *J. Urol.* 122:744, 1979.

Neoplasms

10. American Joint Committee on Cancer. Bladder. In American Joint Committee on Cancer, *Manual for Staging of Cancer.* Philadelphia: Lippincott, 1983. Pp. 171–176.
11. Herr, H. Carcinoma in situ of the bladder. *Semin. Urol.* 1:15, 1983.
12. Pugh, R. C. B. Lower Urinary Tract. In W. A. Anderson and J. M. Kissane (Eds.), *Pathology* (7th ed.). St. Louis: Mosby, 1977. Pp. 977–998.

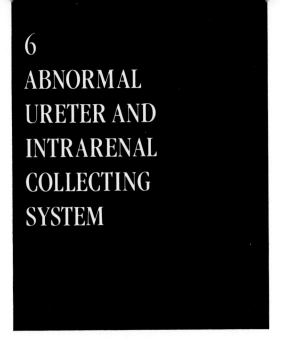

6
ABNORMAL URETER AND INTRARENAL COLLECTING SYSTEM

Jeffry L. Huffman
Demetrius H. Bagley
Edward S. Lyon

CONGENITAL ANOMALIES OF THE URETER AND PELVIS

Clinical Presentation. Congenital abnormalities of the ureter are common, with the reported incidence varying from 2 to 10 percent [1]. Congenital duplication of the ureter and pelvis is the most common of the anomalies, accounting for as many as 20 percent [2].

Often the diagnosis is made incidentally; in childhood, however, complications resulting from malformations, especially duplication, are common.

COMPLETE URETERAL DUPLICATION. Complete duplication of the ureter—two separate ureteral orifices with two pelvises—is a result of two separate ureteral buds arising from the Wolffian duct. Usually, the pelvises drain renal masses that are fused to become one kidney.

When located in the bladder, the orifice situated lower and more medial is associated with the upper renal pelvis. The higher, more laterally located orifice drains the lower pelvis (Weigert-Meyer law).

INCOMPLETE URETERAL DUPLICATION. The splitting of the ureteral bud embryologically results in the formation of two ureters with a common ureteral orifice. The branching of the ureter (bifid ureter) can occur anywhere along its course and can be identified endoscopically. If it occurs just below the ureteropelvic junction, a bifid pelvis results.

BLIND-ENDING URETER. Rarely, a segment of ureter will be blind-ending and not associated with any renal parenchyma. This abnormality usually occurs with one of a pair of duplicated or bifid ureters.

URETERAL AGENESIS. A totally absent ureter probably results from embryologic failure of the ureteral bud. This condition results in hemiatrophy of the bladder trigone, which can be diagnosed cystoscopically.

RETROCAVAL URETER. A retrocaval ureter results from an embryologic error in the formation of the inferior vena cava. In this unusual condition, the ureter wraps around the vena cava. It has a normal position proximally, then crosses posteriorly behind the vena cava before turning anteriorly to come between the aorta and vena cava. It then crosses laterally over the vena cava to take its normal position distally.

Endoscopic Appearance. Complete ureteral duplication results in two separate orifices. The orthotopic orifice draining the lower pole of the kidney generally appears near its normal location in the bladder whereas the ectopic orifice draining the upper pole is more medial and inferior on the trigone (see Fig. 18-14). Occasionally, the ectopic orifice is formed in locations outside the bladder, including the posterior urethra (see Fig. 18-13); the seminal vesicles, vas deferens, and ejaculatory ducts in the male; or the vestibule, urethra, vagina, and uterus in the female. The ectopic orifice is often also associated with a *ureterocele,* a thin-walled cystic structure that protrudes into the bladder or urethra when distended (see Fig. 18-17).

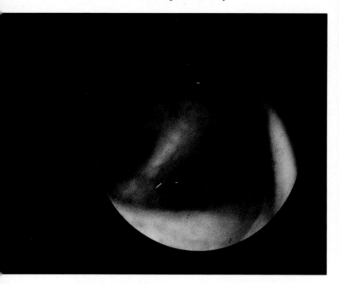

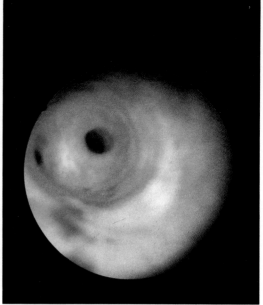

Figure 6-1. *A calcium oxalate monohydrate stone lodged in the medial segment of this V-shaped bifid ureter is characterized by its smooth, dark brown, noncrystalline external surface.*

Figure 6-2. *A U-shaped bifurcation located in the proximal ureter. The individual ostia are much smaller in caliber than those of the common ureter distally. (Second orifice partially obscured at 9 o'clock position.)*

A bifid ureter appears endoscopically as a branching of a common ureteral lumen into two separate ureteral lumen. This branching may be V-shaped with a thin separation of the lumen (Fig. 6-1) or U-shaped with a wider separation and two distinct smaller caliber ostia (Fig. 6-2). A blind-ending ureter is often found in conjunction with one of the branches of a bifid ureter. In these structures, the normal-appearing ureteral lumen will become obliterated with no visible proximal lumen.

Complete ureteral agenesis has a characteristic appearance cystoscopically. In these cases only a hemitrigone will be identified on the side of the existing kidney and ureter. The other portion of the trigone corresponding to the absent kidney and ureter is atrophic with no visible interureteric ridge or orifice.

A retrocaval ureter is difficult to examine endoscopically. There may be narrow regions in the ureter corresponding to the passage of the ureter behind the vena cava.

Management. The treatment of these congenital anomalies is surgery as necessary. For example, the upper pole of a completely duplicated collecting system is often obstructed by an ectopic ureterocele and surgical intervention is usually required. Similarly, surgical intervention may be needed to treat the lower pole segment of a complete duplication, which often is associated with high-grade vesicoureteral reflux.

URETERAL AND RENAL PELVIC CALCULI

Clinical Presentation. Calculi of the ureter and renal pelvis represent a common urologic problem. Often, an underlying metabolic disorder can be identified in these patients. Hypercalcemia from hyperparathyroidism or sarcoidosis with resultant hypercalciuria may be found. Also, patients with gout or those undergoing chemotherapy for a variety of malignant diseases may develop uric acid calculi. Hereditary factors are present in patients with cystine stones or stones resultant from renal tubular acidosis[3].

The patient with a ureteral or renal pelvic calculus most commonly presents with renal colic. The stone becomes lodged in a narrow portion of the ureter, usually either the ureteropelvic junction (UPJ), the pelvic brim, or the ureterovesical junction, resulting in obstruction and pain. The pain, typically, is acute in onset and located in the flank region with radiation anteriorly to the inguinal canal and testicle in the male or the round ligament and labia majora in the female; it is often associated with nausea.

If the stone has been impacted in the ureter for a prolonged time, there may be a local inflammatory reaction and a localized area of tenderness. Often, if the stone is near the bladder, the patient will have irritative voiding symptoms.

Gross hematuria may or may not be present but microscopic hematuria is the rule. In severe cases, the pain is usually associated with vomiting.

Clinical Findings

PHYSICAL EXAMINATION. On physical examination, it is typical for the patient to have flank tenderness over the region of the kidney on the side of the calculus. Fever may be present if there is an associated urinary tract infection with the obstruction. Bimanual examination may reveal an inflammatory mass or localized tenderness if the stone is impacted in the lower ureter, in either male or female patients.

LABORATORY STUDIES. Examination of the urine is essential in the diagnosis of a patient with a ureteral or renal pelvic stone. The dipstick analysis of urine for urinary pH and occult blood, along with the microscopic examination for cells and crystals, may be helpful. Identification of the stone type by observation of the crystals present in the sediment is crucial to successful stone management. Uric acid and cystine calculi are associated with an acid urine whereas magnesium ammonia phosphate and calcium phosphate calculi are usually present in an alkaline urine.

Microscopically, hematuria is usually present; it is not essential, however, and, in the case of a completely obstructing calculus, may not be present at all. Pyuria is an important finding and indicates the need for close observation of a urine culture for signs of infection and sepsis.

Often, on examination of the urine, crystals are found. Calcium oxalate, cystine, or uric acid crystals may be identified on a freshly voided urine. Although the presence of a normal contralateral kidney will normalize the blood urea nitrogen (BUN) and creatinine, bilateral stones or a stone in a solitary kidney with obstruction may lead to azotemia.

RADIOLOGIC STUDIES. Essential in evaluation of the patient with a suspected calculus is the plain film of the abdomen (KUB). Although the KUB cannot definitely verify the presence of a stone in the urinary system, it will show any suspicious calcifications overlying the renal shadow or in the region of the ureter. Stones that do not opacify well, such as uric acid or cystine stones, will be difficult or impossible to identify on a plain film.

Following the plain film, an excretory urogram (IVP) is essential. The IVP will verify whether the opacity is lodged within the urinary system, will document the degree of the urinary tract obstruction, and may outline a radiolucent stone. Often a retrograde study should be done to verify the presence of a nonopaque stone and to identify the ureter distal to the calculus since this portion of the ureter may not visualize on the excretory urogram with an obstructing stone proximally.

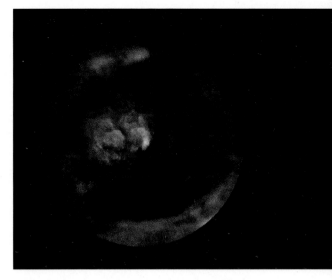

Figure 6-3. *This calcium oxalate stone partially obscured by blood clot is located in the distal ureter. There is a relatively narrow area in the ureter that appears as a rim of mucosa immediately distal to the stone along with inflamed edematous mucosa consistent with acute ureteritis. The stone is a mixture of monohydrate and dihydrate crystals.*

Renal ultrasound is especially useful in the patient with suspected calculus. The ultrasound will identify hydronephrosis and often, if there is a renal pelvic calculus, the stone can be diagnosed by ultrasound alone if the examination demonstrates the characteristic high-intensity echoes from the stone with a definite acoustic shadow beyond.

Endoscopic Appearance

CALCIUM OXALATE STONES. Calcium oxalate stones are commonly composed of a mixture of monohydrate and dihydrate crystals with the smaller stones tending to take mostly one or the other form (Fig. 6-3). Monohydrate calculi are characteristically smooth, dark, almost noncrystalline. Endoscopically, they appear honey brown to reddish brown, or occasionally dark brown. Most commonly, they have a smooth external surface with a varnished appearance that does not exhibit recognizable crystals (Fig. 6-1). Less often, they appear as "mulberry" stones with irregular mammillary processes. The so-called jackstone is a mixed stone combining the two hydrates with a central mass and radiating spicules.

Calcium oxalate dihydrate calculi are lighter in color than the monohydrate form. They have a pale, yellowish white to honey brown color with well-formed crystals on their surface. Individual granular crystals may be visible or larger interlocking aggregates may be present to form a more coarsely crystallized surface (Fig. 6-4).

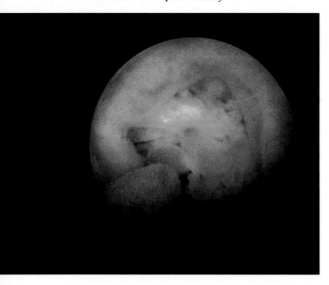

Figure 6-4. *Just proximal to a relatively narrow region in the ureter is this well-crystallized, yellow calcium oxalate dihydrate stone. A ureteral catheter is visible in the foreground along with several bullous inflammatory polyps consistent with chronic ureteritis.*

URIC ACID STONES. Uric acid stones usually appear as a shade of brown or orange yellow, or a combination of the two. These stones may have a smooth, fine-grained structure with an oblong or flattened pebble shape (Fig. 6-5) or appear quite crystalline as one approaches the surface.

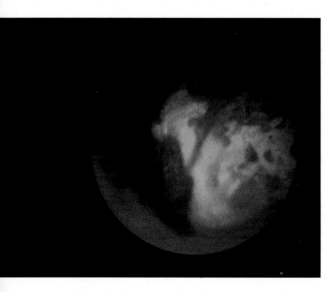

Figure 6-5. *A uric acid stone lodged in an upper pole renal calyx. The stone is yellow orange and brown with a smooth, fine grain surface.*

CYSTINE STONES. Cystine stones appear honey yellow to yellowish white. They have a waxy appearance with a soft, pearly luster and usually a very prominent crystalline appearance (Fig. 6-6).

STRUVITE STONES. Endoscopically, struvite or magnesium ammonia phosphate stones appear dirty white to creamy white. Although their surface may appear relatively smooth, it is actually densely granular and irregular (Fig. 6-7) as a result of contact with the adjacent urothelium.

Pathology. Pathologically, the different types of stones exhibit representative crystalline structures under the stereoscopic dissecting microscope. Optical crystallography, using a polarizing stereoscope, allows the individual crystalline substances of a calculus to be identified [4]. The immersion method of matching a crystal's index of refraction to that of known liquids enables identification of minute amounts of material that would be too small for chemical analysis. These methods combined make the identification of a urinary calculus accurate and simple. Another accurate method of determining the composition of calculi is quantitative chemical analysis, but this approach requires a larger sample. X-ray diffraction studies also yield accurate results and require only small amounts of material. Although these techniques may require sophisticated and expensive equipment, they do lead to accurate determinations [5].

Management. The management of ureteral and renal pelvic stones is often expectant. Up to 90 percent of all ureteral stones, especially those that are 4 to 5 mm or less in size, will pass spontaneously and not require urologic intervention. In the presence of intractable pain, urinary tract infection, impending sepsis, or a stone in a solitary kidney, however, urologic intervention is necessary.

With an obstructing calculus and pyonephrosis proximal to the stone, the crucial method of treatment is to provide drainage of the obstructed kidney. This is performed by passing a ureteral catheter in a retrograde fashion past the stone by standard cystoscopic techniques. Also, using ureteroscopic techniques, the stone can be visualized and a catheter passed under direct vision (see Fig. 15-15). A second method to provide upper tract drainage is to perform a percutaneous nephrostomy. These procedures can often be used to temporize a very ill patient and allow definitive treatment of the stone once the patient has stabilized.

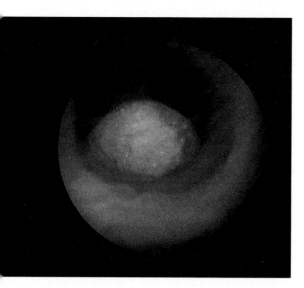

Figure 6-6. *A cystine stone in the proximal ureter. It is characteristically honey yellow with a soft pearly luster and a prominent crystalline surface. The appearance is often described as resembling maple sugar candy.*

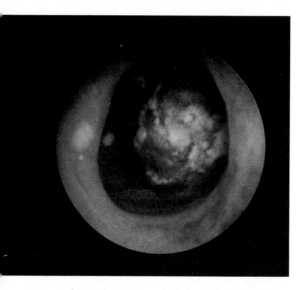

Figure 6-7. *This struvite stone located in the distal left ureter is dirty white with a densely granular irregular surface. Again, there is a relatively narrow region in the ureter immediately distal to the stone.*

Standard pyelolithotomy or ureterolithotomy is often the definitive treatment for removal of calculi. Both the ureter and kidney can be approached in a retroperitoneal fashion and the stone's position verified with radiographs or fluoroscopy. In the case of ureteral stones, it is critical that both proximal and distal control of the ureter be attained prior to manipulation of the stone. This ensures that the stone will not migrate proximally or pass farther distally once the calculus has been identified.

ENDOSCOPIC REMOVAL OF URETERAL STONES. The standard approach to small stones in the distal ureter has been blind endoscopic manipulation. This procedure has been done by urologists for years and can be performed with a variety of catheters. Most commonly, a stone basket is passed through standard cystoscopic approaches into the ureter and past the stone. The basket is then withdrawn in an open position in order to engage the stone, and then gently removed by traction. This technique can be facilitated by using intraoperative fluoroscopy to identify the stone and ensure that it is being engaged in the basket. Many complications with this technique have been reported; however, urologists routinely perform this procedure, often with excellent results.

Another type of catheter that is often used is the Davis loop extractor. This catheter has a fine nylon string passing from its tip to the proximal end of the catheter. The catheter is passed proximal to the stone into the renal pelvis where a loop is formed at the tip of the catheter by pulling on the nylon thread. The catheter with the loop at the end is then drawn to the level of the stone, at which point the stone is trapped in the center of the loop. Then, using gentle traction on the catheter, the stone is slowly extracted. Traction can be performed at the time of the initial procedure or gentle traction can be maintained following the procedure for stone removal.

Recently the ureteroscopic approach to ureteral and renal calculus has made significant advances. Using the ultrasonic techniques for stone disintegration, larger stones can be treated in the proximal ureter and renal pelvis. This technique is described in detail in Chapters 15 and 16.

INFLAMMATORY CONDITIONS
OF THE URETER AND RENAL PELVIS

Clinical Presentation. Inflammation of the ureter (ureteritis) or renal pelvis (pyelitis) usually occurs as a secondary complication of bacterial infection within the kidney or bladder, that is, pyelonephritis or cystitis. It may also be associated with mechanical irritation following either passage of a calculus or instrumentation of the ureter with a ureteral catheter or stone basket.

Patients with an acute inflammatory process present with fever and either flank pain or suprapubic pain, depending on the origin of the infection. Hematuria is also a common presenting symptom.

A chronic inflammation may lead to stricture formation and ureteral obstruction. These patients present with symptoms of chronic ureteral obstruction, which include intermittent flank pain with radiation along the course of the ureter. Because of a common autonomic and sensory nerve supply from the upper urinary tract and gastrointestinal system, the patient may also have significant gastrointestinal symptoms with nausea, vomiting, and distention. If bilateral obstruction exists, symptoms of uremia, such as lethargy, weight loss, poor appetite, and vomiting, occur.

Clinical Findings

PHYSICAL EXAMINATION. Examination of the patient yields findings similar to those of acute pyelonephritis or cystitis. The patient may have temperature elevation, tenderness in the flank or suprapubic region, or, if hydronephrosis is present, possibly a mass in the flank.

LABORATORY STUDIES. The two most important laboratory studies are the urine microscopic examination and the urine culture. Infection spreads from the bladder and kidney by urine. Coliforms, staphylococci, enterococci, and gram-negative bacilli are the most common organisms cultured.

RADIOLOGIC STUDIES. Depending on the size of the lesion involved, the excretory urogram may show filling defects or obstruction on the side of the lesion. The kidney on the affected side may be edematous and enlarged in cases of acute pyelonephritis or may show calyceal clubbing with renal cortical defects if chronic pyelonephritis coexists. Retrograde pyelography will show similar findings of a filling defect and possible obstruction from the lesion.

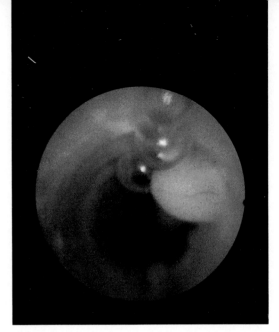

Figure 6-8. *An inflammatory lesion consistent with ureteritis cystica was identified in the proximal ureter. A guidewire has been placed through the ureteral lumen (6 o'clock position), and several air bubbles have accumulated at the 12 o'clock position.*

Endoscopic Appearance. Ureteritis and pyelitis may be difficult to distinguish endoscopically from benign and malignant tumors, and often biopsy is necessary to make the diagnosis. Initially, the mucosa will appear edematous, thickened, and inflamed (see Fig. 6-3). More severe forms, such as ulcerative gangrenous ureteritis, will have superficial ulceration and possibly areas of necrosis. In chronic cases, hyperplastic mucosa will be apparent and there may be narrowing of the ureteral lumen and stricture formation (see Fig. 6-4).

Ureteritis cystica appears as fine submucosal cysts, which can be from 0.1 to 0.5 cm in diameter. These lesions are usually located in the upper third of the ureter and are often associated with similar findings in the bladder (Figs. 6-8, 15-13).

Follicular ureteritis is less common. This condition is characterized by the formation of fine pink or red, slightly raised nodular areas on the mucosal surface.

Pathology. The microscopic appearance of these lesions is that of acute or chronic inflammation. Edema, congestion, and infiltration of acute or chronic inflammatory cells will be present. With chronic infection, *Brunn's nests* — discrete masses of cells beneath the epithelium that are formed by downward growth of hyperplastic transitional epithelium — may be identified.

The cysts of ureteritis cystica are formed by the degeneration of Brunn's nests and are lined by cuboidal epithelial cells. Follicular ureteritis consists of nodules that contain aggregates of lymphocytes in the subepithelial region.

Management. Once these lesions have been identified radiographically or endoscopically, they can be biopsied for diagnosis. It is essential to differentiate these lesions from a malignancy of the upper urinary tract. After an inflammatory lesion has been confirmed, treatment consists of eradicating the underlying infection or removing the source of chronic irritation, such as a stone or catheter. Specific antimicrobial therapy can be started after the pathogen has been identified by urine culture.

URETERAL STRICTURES. A *ureteral stricture* has been defined as a constriction in the ureteral lumen that prohibits normal flow of urine and causes a rise in hydrostatic pressure of the proximal collecting system. This increase in pressure is clinically manifested by hydronephrosis with resulting renal colic. With endoscopic access to the upper urinary tract now readily available and routinely used, however, many relatively narrow nondistensible areas are identified within the ureter that previously were inapparent. These narrowings are "subclinical" strictures in that they often do not obstruct the flow of urine significantly enough to increase proximal hydrostatic pressure and produce renal colic and hydronephrosis. They may become clinically significant in certain instances, however, such as stone passage if they obstruct the progress of the stone (see Figs. 6-3, 6-4, 6-7) or ureteroscopy if their caliber is smaller than that of the instruments. This section discusses those entities causing strictures that present clinically as either partial or complete ureteral obstruction. Chapter 15 discusses the subclinical strictures that are encountered endoscopically during passage of the ureteroscope or extraction of ureteral stones.

Clinical Presentation. The presentation of ureteral strictures is that of ureteral obstruction. The patient may have flank pain, hematuria, nausea, vomiting, or abdominal distention. As noted earlier, the gastrointestinal symptoms result from a common autonomic and sensory nerve supply with that of the ureter and kidney.

Occasionally, slowly progressive unilateral strictures may be silent and are diagnosed only when radiographic studies are performed for other reasons. Conversely, the presentation may be that of oliguria and uremia if a stricture occurs either in a solitary collecting system or bilaterally.

Ureteral strictures may result from either congenital or acquired conditions. The ureteropelvic junction is the most common site of congenital strictures while the remainder occur at the ureterovesical junction. Acquired strictures result from chronic inflammatory conditions such as those associated with chronic ureteritis, tuberculosis, or an impacted calculus. Tumors, along with scarring from surgery or penetrating trauma, may also lead to ureteral strictures.

Ureteral involvement in patients with genitourinary tuberculosis is common, affecting 34 to 46 percent of such patients in reported series[6,7,8,9]. The resultant stricture frequently is silent and may even progress during treatment for TB. Often patients present with symptoms of tuberculous involvement in other areas of the genitourinary system, such as the prostate, epididymis, or bladder.

Clinical Findings

PHYSICAL EXAMINATION. On physical examination, the patient will have findings of ureteral obstruction. There may be flank tenderness and a palpable mass. If infection exists in the urine, fever may be present.

LABORATORY STUDIES. Examination of the urine may reveal the presence of microscopic hematuria or pyuria. Urinary cytologic studies may also be positive for malignant cells if the stricture results from a malignant process in the urothelium.

The urine of a patient with genitourinary tuberculosis shows pyuria, hematuria, and proteinuria. Although the diagnosis is confirmed bacteriologically by culture or histologic examination, often patients will have concomitant nontuberculous bacterial infections[8].

RADIOLOGIC STUDIES. On excretory urography, a stricture presents as ureteral obstruction. The affected kidney may have delayed function with hydronephrosis or no function at all if the obstruction has been chronic and complete. In the case of a poorly functioning kidney, a retrograde study performed cystoscopically will help to identify the site of a stricture and show the anatomy of the ureter distal to the lesion.

Occasionally, a stricture will become apparent only during passage of a ureteral calculus. In such cases, the narrowing of the ureter is not significant enough to cause proximal dilation of the pelvis and calyces, yet it still prohibits stone passage.

The radiographic findings of a patient with renal TB are very typical[9]. Often the plain abdominal film will show calcifications in the region of the kidney, ureter, or bladder. The pyelographic features of renal TB include stricture of the renal infundibula with cavitation of the papilla and cortical scarring. There may also be a stricture at the ureteropelvic junction or, more commonly, near the lower end of the ureter, with resultant hydronephrosis.

Endoscopic Appearance. Endoscopically, a stricture appears as a concentric narrowing in the ureteral lumen (Fig. 6-9). The mucosa may be smooth and pale if the stricture is congenital or caused by previous scarring, or irregular and papillary if the stricture has resulted from a transitional cell carcinoma. If the stricture is secondary to an inflammatory process, ureteritis cystica or follicular ureteritis will be observed.

The initial appearance of tuberculosis of the ureter is similar to that of tuberculosis of the bladder, with inflamed and ulcerated urothelium. In later stages of healing, however, stricture formation with dense scarring and narrowing of the ureteral lumen will be apparent.

Pathology. The pathology of ureteral strictures depends on the etiology. A stricture resulting from scarring will show proliferation of fibrous tissue or possibly a chronic inflammatory infiltrate. If it has been caused by a carcinoma, malignant cells will be observed. The pathology of malignant tumors is considered in the subsequent section, Malignant Tumors of the Ureter and Renal Pelvis.

The stricture that results from urinary tract involvement by tuberculosis must be considered as a local manifestation of a disseminated disease that usually begins in the lung. Tubercles initially are formed in the glomerulus. They coalesce and erode into the renal papilla. Eventually, the caseous material within the tubercles is sloughed into the calyces and urine. It is in this descending fashion that the ureters, bladder, prostate, and epididymis become involved.

Management. Two main issues need to be considered when treating ureteral strictures. The first is the etiology of the process. It is essential preoperatively to have made a diagnosis by either direct vision ureteroscopic biopsy, cytologic brush biopsy, or possibly radiographic appearance. Secondly, once the diagnosis has been achieved, a therapeutic approach is planned, directed toward not only adequately treating the lesion but also conserving renal tissue wherever possible.

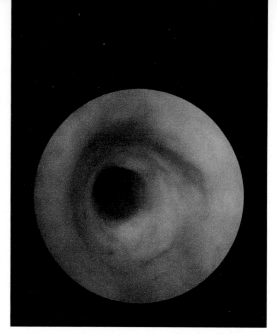

Figure 6-9. *A ureteral stricture identified during ureteroscopy in the midureter. There is a concentric narrowing of the ureteral lumen, which, compared to the normal ureter, is relatively nondistensible.*

The treatment of congenital strictures and many benign acquired strictures is surgical. Ureteropelvic junction obstruction can be treated by a variety of open procedures. Ureterovesical junction obstruction and low ureteral strictures are best treated by excision and ureteral reimplantation.

If the stricture is not a malignant process, often internal ureteral stents can be used to bypass the lesion and drain the obstructed kidney, thereby preserving renal function. Double pigtail or double J stents are used for this purpose (see Chap. 13).

Benign strictures can also be treated by balloon dilation under direct vision or under fluoroscopy. This can be done with angioplastic balloon catheters either through an antegrade approach with percutaneous nephrostomy techniques or in a retrograde fashion with ureteroscopic techniques (see Chap. 15).

The treatment of tuberculous ureteral strictures is directed toward conserving renal tissue. They most commonly occur in the distal ureter and, if not treated promptly, will progress to complete ureteral obstruction and possibly autonephrectomy[9,10]. Often the lower ureter can be dilated with successively larger ureteral catheters and possibly angioplastic balloon-dilating catheters. If surgery is required once all conservative methods have failed, the recommended procedure is ureteral reimplantation.

MALACOPLAKIA OF THE URETER AND RENAL PELVIS

Clinical Presentation. Malacoplakia can affect the ureter and renal pelvis as well as the bladder. In the series reported by Stanton and Maxted[12], the ureter was involved in 11 percent of patients, the renal pelvis in 10 percent, and the ureteropelvic junction in 5 percent. Patients usually present with symptoms associated with bladder inflammation, but hematuria may also be found. An associated coliform infection is detected in the urine of as many as 76 percent of patients.

Clinical Findings

PHYSICAL EXAMINATION. There are few findings on physical examination in the patient with malacoplakia of the upper urinary tract. If ureteral stenosis has developed, however, obstruction of the urinary tract may occur and the patient may have signs or symptoms of urinary tract obstruction[11], including flank tenderness and possibly a flank mass resulting from hydronephrosis.

LABORATORY STUDIES. A coliform infection of the urine can often be detected in patients when urine cultures are performed. The serum urea nitrogen and creatinine are usually normal although, if malacoplakia occurs in a solitary collecting system or bilaterally, obstruction may impair renal function.

RADIOLOGIC STUDIES. Excretory urography may reveal multiple filling defects in the renal pelvis or ureter and often may demonstrate obstruction resulting from stenosis or stricture of the ureter. Retrograde studies may also show filling defects. Differential diagnosis in these cases includes multiple small tumors or ureteropyelitis cystica.

Endoscopic Appearance and Pathology. Endoscopically, these lesions are similar to those seen in the bladder. They may appear as pink brown, flat nodules; yellow nodular lesions similar to amyloid deposits; or yellow brown, soft plaques with central umbilication, ulceration, and peripheral hyperemia. They may be 1 mm to 3 cm in diameter. Initially, the overlying epithelium remains intact and there may be only slight erythema of the mucosa.

The etiology and histologic appearance of malacoplakia of the upper urinary tract are similar to those reported for malacoplakia of the bladder (see Chap. 5).

Management. Treatment of patients with malacoplakia of the upper urinary system is similar to that reported for malacoplakia of the bladder. Ureteral lesions may necessitate early diversion, ureteral catheterization, or stenting for relief of obstruction.

ENDOMETRIOSIS OF THE URETER

Clinical Presentation. Involvement of the ureter by endometriosis is a rare clinical finding. When it does occur, it usually is found in premenopausal women but has also been reported in men[15]. Extrinsic endometriosis, which is more common, is present in premenopausal women and represents extension from endometriosis in adjacent pelvic organs. Presenting symptoms include ureteral obstruction, colic, and possibly hematuria.

Intrinsic involvement of the ureter is less common. These patients also present with hematuria and renal colic. Other possible symptoms include pelvic pain, dyspareunia, and dysmenorrhea.

Clinical Findings

PHYSICAL EXAMINATION. On physical examination, the patient may have tenderness in the flank on the affected side or tenderness on examination of the pelvic organs. A pelvic mass may also be present with extrinsic endometriosis.

LABORATORY STUDIES. Urinalysis usually shows hematuria, especially with the intrinsic lesions. If the process involves a solitary collecting system or is bilateral, azotemia may be present.

RADIOLOGIC STUDIES. The radiographic findings of endometriosis of the urinary tract sometimes differ for intrinsic and extrinsic lesions; findings, however, often are similar[14]. The IVP may show ureteral obstruction from an extrinsic process or may show an intraluminal filling defect in the ureter with associated hydroureter and hydronephrosis.

Endoscopic Appearance and Pathology. The appearance of endometriosis is similar to that seen at laparotomy or laparoscopy. The lesion will be seen as a hemorrhagic mass eroding through the mucosa and possibly producing luminal obstruction. Endoscopically, it may be difficult to distinguish from malignant processes of the ureter, and biopsy is needed to secure the diagnosis.

Typical endometrial glands and accompanying stroma are found on microscopic section. Varying amounts of focal stromal hemorrhage are also present.

Management. Endometriosis of the urinary tract can be treated medically or surgically. The medical treatment is with agents that suppress ovarian function as well as the formation of uterine and ectopic endometrium, such as danazol, which decreases the levels of follicle-stimulating hormone (FSH) and luteinizing hormone (LH)[13]. Estrogen-progestogen combinations can also be used to suppress ovarian function; these agents, however, often initially stimulate ectopic endometrial tissue and exacerbate symptoms.

Surgery is the major form of treatment and all of the involved mass can usually be removed. Often, ureterolysis can be performed or the involved portion of ureter can be removed by partial ureterectomy with a primary reanastomosis. Ureteroneocystostomy can be performed for disease involving only the lower ureter.

MALIGNANT TUMORS OF THE URETER AND RENAL PELVIS

Clinical Presentation. Upper tract urothelial tumors account for 1 percent of all upper urinary tract tumors. The peak age range is from 45 to 65 years. More frequently, the lower third of the ureter is involved (60–80%), and often these tumors are multiple and multicentric[21].

The most common presentation is gross hematuria, which occurs in approximately 80 percent of all patients. A complaint of flank pain on the involved side with or without fever or previous infection is also common. Irritative voiding symptoms occur more often in patients with ureteral tumors than those with pelvic tumors.

Clinical Findings

PHYSICAL EXAMINATION. On physical examination there are often no abnormalities. Rarely, with an extensive advanced malignant tumor of the upper urinary tract, a mass may be palpable.

LABORATORY STUDIES. The most common positive finding from a laboratory study is hematuria on the urinalysis. In the series of Murphy, Zincke, and Furlow[22] on 175 patients, hematuria was found in 73 percent of patients while microscopic hematuria was the only finding in 11 percent.

Positive urinary cytology is another possible finding. In a series of 101 patients with filling defects depicted in the ureter and renal pelvis by radiographic studies, it was possible to recognize 29 of 36 tumors (80.5%) by preoperative lavage cytology[20]. There were no false-positive diagnoses made in this study.

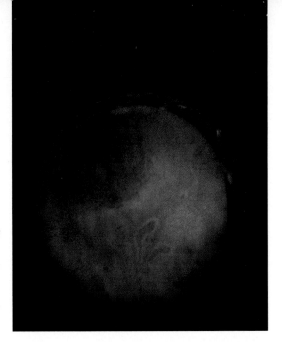

Figure 6-10. *A grade I papillary transitional cell tumor located in the midureter. Characteristics of a low-grade tumor are pink fingerlike projections with a central vascular core. (Lumen of proximal ureter at 11 o'clock position.)*

RADIOLOGIC STUDIES. Excretory urography usually shows an abnormality. Nonvisualization, obstruction, and a filling defect are the most common findings. Of the 175 patients with high-grade (II–IV) upper tract tumors reviewed by Murphy's group[22], only 1 patient had a normal IVP. Of the remainder, 45 percent had a filling defect in the ureter or pelvis, 31 percent had nonvisualization on one side, 10 percent had ureteropyelocaliectasis, and 8 percent had a renal mass. The same authors also reported on 48 patients with grade I tumors[23]. Of these patients, 3 had normal IVPs, while 26 had a filling defect, 9 had nonvisualization, 8 had hydronephrosis, and 2 had a renal mass.

Retrograde studies are also diagnostic, and in one series[26] 23 of 23 tumors had filling defects on retrograde ureteropyelography.

Endoscopic Appearance. The endoscopic appearance of these tumors depends on the epithelial origin. Transitional cell tumors typically have a papillary appearance similar to that seen in the bladder. The tumors are tan pink, bulky, and usually have numerous translucent filiform projections (Figs. 6-10, 6-11). They may be sessile or pedunculated, and occasionally have a more lobular external surface (Figs. 6-12, 6-13). They may be seen as small lesions rising from the mucosa or as larger lesions totally obliterating the ureteral or pelvic lumen (Fig. 6-14).

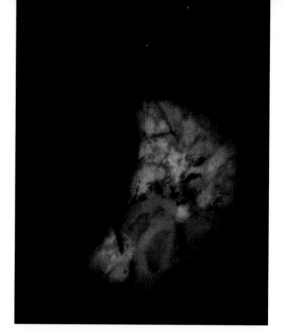

Figure 6-11. *Several papillary transitional cell tumors (grade I) identified in the infundibulum of an upper pole renal calyx. The translucent papillary projections are readily differentiated from the normal-appearing mucosa of the infundibulum.*

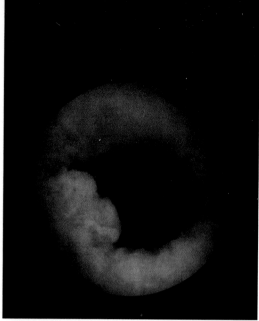

Figure 6-13. *A grade II transitional cell tumor located at the ureteropelvic junction. The sessile, lobular-appearing tumor is protruding from the ureteral wall with the dark capacious renal pelvis visible in the background. The tumors shown in Figs. 6-10, 6-11, and 6-13 were not detected by excretory or retrograde urography.*

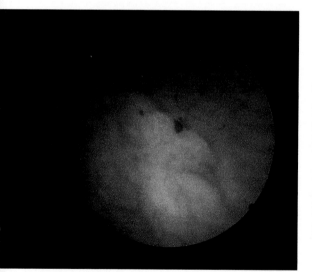

Figure 6-12. *A grade II transitional cell tumor located in the lower ureter. It has a sessile lobular arrangement of the papillary fronds.*

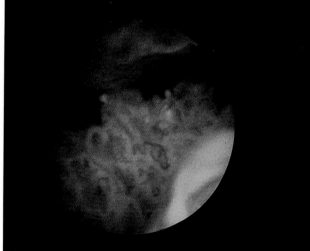

Figure 6-14. *A large grade III transitional cell tumor extending throughout the renal pelvis and proximal ureter. Papillary fronds are visible along with solid-appearing, high-grade tumors.*

Squamous cell carcinomas are solid and only slightly raised from the surrounding mucosa. There is often associated ulceration, fibrosis, and inflammation. Adenocarcinomas are very rare. They appear as glistening polypoid masses with delicate fronds and thin fibrovascular cores[18].

Carcinoma in situ of the upper urinary tract has a similar appearance to that found in the bladder. Often only irregularities of the mucosa are observed with hyperemic epithelium and focal hemorrhage.

Pathology. Transitional cell carcinoma is the most common tumor encountered, although squamous cell carcinoma and adenocarcinoma also occur. Histologically, these tumors can be graded into four separate groups, as outlined by Broders[19], or three, as suggested by the AFIP (Table 6-1)[31,32]. The staging of these tumors has not been unified. Two methods of classifying ureteral and pelvic tumors according to the extent of invasion are outlined in Table 6-2[17,31,32].

Table 6-1. Classification of Tumors by Grade

Grade	Description
BRODERS	
I	Well-differentiated; few mitoses
II	Less well-differentiated; irregular cells; crowding; atypical nuclei; mitoses
III	More sessile; composed of sheets, cords, and nests of malignant cells with marked nuclear and cellular irregularity
IV	Anaplastic; composed of infiltrating cords of cells; exhibit keratinization and intracellular bridge formation
AFIP	
I	Malignant cells; slightly anaplastic
II	Intermediate anaplastic malignant cells
III	Marked anaplastic cells

Histologically, papillary transitional cell carcinomas differ from benign papillomas in that they tend to be larger than papillomas with thicker villi and broader bases. There is irregular stratification of their epithelial layers with loss of polarity and sequential maturation. The more anaplastic forms show increased cellular atypia and occasionally sarcomatoid changes.

Table 6-2. Classification of Ureteral and Renal Pelvic Tumors by Stage

Stage	Description
BATATA AND GRABSTALD (1975)	
0	Mucosa involvement only
A	Submucosal infiltration (limited to lamina propia)
B	Muscularis invasion
C	Periureteral fat involvement
D	Extension outside the ureter to adjacent structures, lymph nodes, or distant metastases
AFIP (1975)	
I	Same as stage 0
II	Same as stage A
III	Same as stage B but may extend beyond muscularis in intrarenal portions of pelvis if confined to kidney
IV	Same as stages C and D

Squamous cell carcinomas are composed of rounded to polygonal cells infiltrating the stroma as branching projections. Cells in the basal layer usually are small with hyperchromatic nuclei while cells farther from the basal areas show features typical of normal maturation and normal squamous epithelial cells. Nearly 20 percent of squamous cell tumors of the renal pelvis are associated with long-standing renal pelvic stones.

Adenocarcinomas may show little anaplasia and are often difficult to distinguish from transitional cell carcinomas with mucinous metaplasia. Typically, they are composed of cuboid or columnar cells, many containing mucin.

Management. In discussing the management of tumors of the ureter and renal pelvis, several factors must be considered. It is difficult to diagnose these tumors at an early stage and also to determine accurately the histologic grade and depth of invasion prior to surgical exploration and excision. This is especially critical if any procedure less than total nephroureterectomy is planned. Pyeloscopy performed during an open exploration has been suggested as a method of obtaining tissue; however, an alarming number of local recurrences follow this procedure[25]. Brush biopsy, using cystoscopic techniques, has proved valuable in obtaining cytologic tissue by the closed endoscopic approach (see Chap. 14). In addition, our recent work with ureteropyeloscopic approach has been promising for diagnosing, treating, and following patients with upper tract tumors or those in whom previous partial ureterectomies have been performed.

Another factor of importance is the multicentricity of the tumors. Often more than one area of the urinary tract is involved, and it is difficult to determine the benign nature of any urothelium that is being conserved following surgical removal of a portion of the ureter or renal pelvis. Strong and Pearse[24] found a 30-percent rate of tumor recurrence in the ureter distal to the excision site of the original tumor.

A method of evaluating the entire ureter and renal pelvis preoperatively, such as ureteropyeloscopy, would help to identify those patients with a normal ureter distal to the main tumor, who could then be treated by removing only the involved urothelium. Endoscopic surveillance of the remaining stumps could also be achieved.

The method of treatment of patients with invasive upper tract tumors without evidence of metastatic spread remains total nephroureterectomy with resection of a cuff of the bladder. In the absence of a normal contralateral kidney, however, or in patients who are of advanced age or have significant underlying medical problems, certainly a less radical procedure should be attempted.

As suggested by Babaian and Johnson[16], patients with low-grade, noninvasive tumors involving only the distal ureter appear to be treated adequately by partial ureterectomy with reimplantation alone. This more conservative approach is also suggested by Murphy and colleagues[23], who found no differences in survival in patients with these low-grade tumors. These patients are the ones in whom ureteroscopy may permit endoscopic resection as a method of therapy with easy access for follow-up and without risk of tumor spillage at operation.

BENIGN TUMORS OF THE URETER AND RENAL PELVIS

Clinical Presentation. Because benign tumors usually present with symptoms similar to those of malignant tumors, including urinary frequency, suprapubic discomfort, and, most commonly, hematuria, often the differential diagnosis is difficult. Tumors such as papillomas, fibroepithelial polyps[27,29], inverted papillomas[28], or cholesteatomas[30] must be considered.

Clinical Findings

PHYSICAL EXAMINATION. The examination may show tenderness on the side of the lesion if obstruction exists. Rarely, a mass may be palpable. Although urinary cultures are usually negative, microscopic hematuria may be detected.

RADIOGRAPHIC STUDIES. The most common radiographic finding is a filling defect or obstruction at the site of the lesion. Retrograde ureteropyelography may also show filling defects or obstruction.

Endoscopic Appearance. The papillomas that occur in the ureter and renal pelvis appear identical to those identified in the bladder. They have long villous processes arising from a narrow base with a central fibrovascular core. Their color is indistinguishable from normal transitional epithelium. The fibroepithelial polyps are lobulated with a thin stalk and very smooth, pale gray mucosa. They are usually found in the proximal ureter.

Inverted papillomas are pendunculated or sessile polypoid lesions of the urothelium. They have a smooth, gray surface less than 3 cm in length with no papillary components.

Cholesteatomas appear as a cheesy, pasty material. These lesions are whitish gray in color and adhere firmly to the wall of the ureter or renal pelvis.

Often it is difficult to differentiate benign lesions from malignant tumors. Therefore, diagnostic procedures such as ureteropyeloscopy or brush biopsy prior to surgical removal are necessary to provide tissue for cytologic or histologic examination.

Pathology. Microscopically, papillomas are very similar to well-differentiated papillary transitional cell carcinomas. They are covered, however, by normal transitional epithelium with normal maturation patterns, normal cell size and shape, and a normal number of mitoses. Any pleomorphism or increased frequency of mitoses would be suspicious for papillary carcinoma.

Fibroepithelial polyps are characterized histologically by a normal-appearing transitional epithelium with a loose fibrovascular stroma.

Inverted papillomas are nonpapillary, noninvasive lesions formed by cords or nests of cells in the lamina propria of the ureter. The urothelium forms a continuous surface over these inverting cells. Urothelial carcinoma has been reported in association with inverted papillomas; however, transformation of an inverted papilloma into a carcinoma has not been documented[28].

Cholesteatomas appear microscopically as desquamated squamous epithelial cells with keratin lamellae and cholesterol crystals. Cholesteatomas have been confused pathologically with squamous metaplasia, leukoplakia, and squamous cell carcinoma. Since they have never been associated with squamous cell carcinoma, however, cholesteatomas are probably not premalignant lesions[30].

Management. Conservative management of these nonmalignant lesions is preferred. Local excision or partial ureterectomy can be performed for solitary lesions while nephroureterectomy can be reserved for multiple lesions or those causing severe hydronephrosis. Ureteroscopic resection may also prove useful in the treatment of small localized lesions.

REFERENCES

Congenital Anomalies of the Ureter and Pelvis

1. Dees, J. E. The clinical importance of congenital anomalies of the upper urinary tract. *J. Urol.* 46:659, 1941.
2. Smith, E. C., and Orkin, L. A. A clinical and statistical study of 471 congenital anomalies of the kidney and ureter. *J. Urol.* 53:11, 1945.

Ureteral and Renal Pelvic Calculi

3. Drach, G. W. Urinary Lithiasis. In J. E. Harrison, et al. (Eds.), *Campbell's Urology* (4th ed.). Philadelphia: Saunders, 1978. Pp. 779–878.
4. Prien, E. L., and Frondel, C. Studies in urolithiasis: I. The composition of urinary calculi. *J. Urol.* 57:949, 1947.
5. Schneider, H. J., Berenyi, M., and Hesse, A. Comparative urinary stone analysis. Quantitative chemical, x-ray diffraction, infrared spectroscopy, and thermoanalytical procedures. *Int. Urol. Nephrol.* 5:9, 1973.

Tuberculosis of the Ureter and Renal Pelvis

6. Cinman, A. C. Genitourinary tuberculosis. *Urology* 20:353, 1982.
7. Cos, L. S., and Cockett, A. T. K. Genitourinary tuberculosis revisited. *Urology* 20:111, 1982.
8. Feldstein, M. S., Sullivan, M. J., and Banowsky, L. H. Ureteral involvement in genitourinary tuberculosis. *Urology* 6:175, 1975.
9. Lattimer, J. K., and Wechsler, M. Genitourinary Tuberculosis. In J. H. Harrison, et al. (Eds.), *Campbell's Urology* (4th ed.). Philadelphia: Saunders, 1978. Pp. 557–575.
10. Wechsler, M., and Lattimer, J. K. An evaluation of the current therapeutic regimen for renal tuberculosis. *J. Urol.* 113:760, 1975.

Malacoplakia of the Ureter

11. Sexton, C. C., Lowman, R. M., Nyongo, A. O., and Baskin, A. N. Malacoplakia presenting as complete unilateral ureteral obstruction. *J. Urol.* 128:139, 1982.
12. Stanton, M. J., and Maxted, W. Malacoplakia: A study of the literature and current concepts of pathogenesis, diagnosis and treatment. *J. Urol.* 125:139, 1981.

Endometriosis of the Ureter

13. Gardner, B., and Whitaker, R. H. The use of Danazol for ureteral obstruction caused by endometriosis. *J. Urol.* 125:117, 1981.
14. Pollack, H. M., and Wills, J. S. Radiographic features of ureteral endometriosis. *Am. J. Roentgen.* 131:627, 1978.
15. Schrodt, G. R., Alcorn, M. O., and Ibanez, J. Endometriosis of the male urinary system: A case report. *J. Urol.* 124:722, 1980.

Malignant Tumors of the Ureter and Renal Pelvis

16. Babaian, R. J., and Johnson, D. E. Primary carcinoma of the ureter. *J. Urol.* 123:357, 1980.
17. Batata, M. A., Whitmore, W. F., Jr., Hilaris, B. S., Tokita, N., and Grabstald, H. Primary carcinoma of the ureter: A prognostic study. *Cancer* 35:1626, 1975.
18. Brawer, M. K., and Waisman, J. Mucinous adenocarcinoma probably arising in the renal pelvis and ureter: A case report. *J. Urol.* 123:424, 1980.
19. Broders, A. C. Epithelioma of the genitourinary organs. *Am. J. Surg.* 75:574, 1922.
20. Leistenschneider, W., and Nagel, R. Lavage cytology of the renal pelvis and ureter with special reference to tumors. *J. Urol.* 124:597, 1980.
21. Mills, C., and Vaughan, E. D., Jr. Carcinoma of the ureter: Natural history and management and five year survival. *J. Urol.* 129:275, 1983.
22. Murphy, D. M., Zincke, H., and Furlow, W. L. Management of high grade transitional cell cancer of the upper urinary tract. *J. Urol.* 125:25, 1981.
23. Murphy, D. M., Zincke, H., and Furlow, W. L. Primary grade I transitional cell carcinoma of the renal pelvis and ureter. *J. Urol.* 123:629, 1980.
24. Strong, D. W., and Pearse, H. D. Recurrent urothelial tumor following surgery for transitional cell carcinoma of the upper urinary tract. *Cancer* 38:2178, 1976.
25. Tomera, K. M., Leary, F. J., and Zincke, H. Pyeloscopy in urothelial tumors. *J. Urol.* 127:1088, 1982.
26. Werth, D. D., Weigel, J. W., and Mebust, W. K. Primary neoplasms of the ureter. *J. Urol.* 125:628, 1981.

Benign Tumors of the Ureter and Renal Pelvis

27. Fiorelli, C., Durval, A., DiCello, V., Rizzo, M., and Nicita, G. Ureteral intussusception by a fibroepithelial polyp. *J. Urol.* 126:110, 1981.
28. Fromowitz, F. B., et al. Inverted papilloma of the ureter. *J. Urol.* 126:113, 1981.
29. Stuppler, S. A., and Kandzari, S. J. Fibroepithelial polyps of ureter: A benign ureteral tumor. *Urology* 5:553, 1975.
30. Taguchi, Y., Kotha, V., Tomka, B., and Seemayer, T. Conserving nephrons in cholesteatoma. *J. Urol.* 123:258, 1980.

General

31. Bennington, J. L., and Beckwith, J. B. Tumors of the Kidney, Renal Pelvis and Ureter. In Armed Forces Institute of Pathology, *Atlas of Tumor Pathology.* Washington, D.C.: Armed Forces Institute of Pathology, 1975. Fascicle 12.
32. Jones, D. B. Kidneys. In W. A. D. Anderson and J. M. Kissane (Eds.), *Pathology* (7th ed.). St. Louis: Mosby, 1977. Pp. 928–976.
33. Pugh, R. C. B. Lower Urinary Tract. In W. A. D. Anderson and J. M. Kissane (Eds.), *Pathology* (7th ed.). St. Louis: Mosby, 1977. Pp. 977–998.

III
ENDOSCOPIC
TECHNIQUES

7
CYSTOURETHROSCOPY

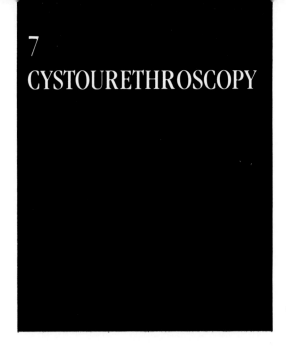

Demetrius H. Bagley

Jeffry L. Huffman

Edward S. Lyon

Cystourethroscopy, or endoscopic examination of the urethra and bladder, is the most common urologic procedure and that which most characterizes the field of urology. It is the major diagnostic and operative endoscopic procedure in the urinary tract. Advances in instrumentation and development of new endoscopic techniques have continued to expand and enhance the role of endoscopy in the urologist's armamentarium.

HISTORY. The forerunner of the modern cystoscope was constructed in 1877 by Max Nitze (1848–1906) of Dresden[1]. He developed a model for a lens system telescope and, with the help of an optical craftsman, an optician of Vienna named Beneche, was able to work out the details of the lens system that is still the foundation for modern cystoscopic telescopes. This lens system telescope provided a magnified image of the bladder, but one with a very limited field of vision. To illuminate the interior of the bladder, Nitze incorporated a platinum wire heated electrically to incandescence at the end of the cystoscope, the sheath of which was cooled by water. The platinum filament had been used 10 years previously by a dentist from Breslau, Julius Bruck. Bruck had used this light source attached to his "diaphanoscope," an instrument that he inserted into the rectum in an attempt to illuminate the bladder. This method, however, enabled him to see only a tiny portion of the bladder wall from the transmitted light.

Prior to Nitze's invention in 1877, there had been several attempts to visualize the interior of the urethra and bladder. As early as 1806, Bozzini demonstrated his "*lichtleiter*" to the Academy of Medicine in Vienna. This instrument had a round window to which could be attached a urethral speculum. The window was divided vertically by a mirror, with a candle for a light source on one half and the other half shielded for viewing through an observation eyepiece. Because of its poorly controllable and insufficient light source, along with its lack of magnification, the *lichtleiter* did not receive much endorsement.

In 1826, Pierre Segalos introduced his "urethral-cystic speculum" for the purpose of viewing the interior of the urethra and bladder. This instrument consisted of two silver tubes. The outer tube served to conduct light (which was provided by two candles and projected along the tube by conical mirrors), and the inner tube was used for observation. This same principle was followed by John Fisher from Boston, a year later. His instrument allowed light to reflect off two mirrors to make two 90-degree turns through cylindrical tubes. The field was viewed through a window and the more proximal mirror and a system of lenses was used to provide a sharp image.

An endoscope designed by Desormeaux in 1853 proved successful in Europe and America, where it was found superior to its predecessors because of its lighting system[2]. A bright flame was produced by a mixture of alcohol and turpentine, and light was focused on a mirror that reflected along the viewing axis of the endoscope. This instrument was used by Desormeaux mainly for observation and surgery of the urethra.

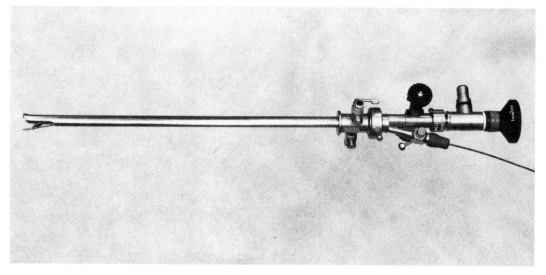

Figure 7-1. *The sheath of the cystourethroscope has both inflow and outflow irrigation channels. The telescope is attached through a bridge with, in this example, a working channel.*

The next major contribution to urologic endoscopy, following Nitze's cystoscope in 1877, was the development of the incandescent lamp by Thomas Edison in 1879. Edison used a carbon filament in a vacuum within a glass envelope, powered by electricity, which produced a reliable lamp that was not too hot to be used inside a patient's bladder. This lamp could be mounted at a 30-degree angle to the distal end of the cystoscope to provide ample illumination for visualization of the bladder wall. David Newman of Glasgow in 1883 was actually the first person to adapt the Edison electric lamp to a cystoscope, and it was not until 1887 that this light source was incorporated into the Nitze-Leader cystoscope. (Leader was a Viennese instrument maker with whom Nitze, soon after introducing his original cystoscope, collaborated.)

Later in 1887, Brenner improved the Nitze-Leader cystoscope by adding an irrigating channel through which water could pass into the bladder. This channel was also found very useful for introducing the catheter into the ureteral orifice, and Dr. James Brown of Baltimore is given credit for being the first American surgeon to catheterize the ureter using Brenner's apparatus.

Another advancement in the lighting system was developed by Charles Preston of Rochester, New York in 1898. He designed a "cold" lamp for illumination as contrasted to the hot incandescent lamp previously used. This lamp was adapted to almost every type of endoscope in use.

Tildon Brown in 1899 constructed a double catheterizing cystoscope patterned after Brenner's idea. In 1901 he introduced the two-telescope concept — one for right-angle viewing and one for direct vision. In cooperation with Leo Buerger of New York, Brown developed in 1908 the Brown-Buerger combination cystoscope, which proved to be very popular well into the century.

Throughout the period from 1905 to 1945, a European instrument maker, Reinhold Wappler, put forth many technical ideas for improvements on existing instruments and for creation of new ones. His contribution to the optical system did much to improve cystoscopic visualization and, in conjunction with Joseph McCarthy, he devised the fore-oblique, or the McCarthy, panendoscope.

The next major advancement in cystoscopy occurred with the development of fiberoptics. This system was actually patented in 1929 but it was not until the work of Hopkins and Capenni in 1954 that fiberoptics with external light sources replaced the distal lamp for illumination of the bladder wall and urethra. Fiberoptics were used not only for illumination but could also be incorporated into a flexible endoscope for transmission of an image through a coherent bundle of glass fibers. Another breakthrough occurred with the development of the rod-lens system for the rigid endoscope, also by Harold H. Hopkins. This system enabled the transmission of light through the endoscope to be increased by a factor of 9 over the standard telescope and also increased the field of view from 40 to 70 degrees [3].

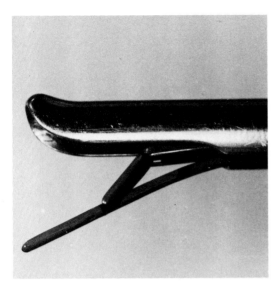

Figure 7-2. *The Albarran lever can deflect a catheter or other flexible instrument passed through the cystourethroscope. It is manually manipulated through a mechanical linkage.*

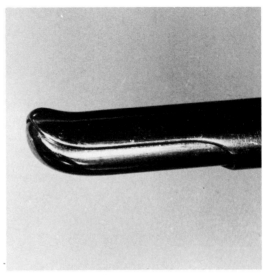

Figure 7-3. *The closed obturator provides a smooth tip for the sheath for tactile passage.*

INSTRUMENTATION

Rigid Cystourethroscopes. Cystourethroscopes are available in many sizes from several different instrument manufacturers, yet basically all of these instruments are quite similar. In general, they consist of three parts: the sheath, the obturator, and the telescope.

The sheath is the outer, most rigid portion of the instrument. It provides an access for irrigation and a channel for working instruments, and, as its major function, serves to protect the changeable telescopes, which are delicate and expensive. The standard design presently available for cystourethroscopes includes both an angled beak at the tip of the instrument and irrigation ports that enter the sheath directly and provide for inflow and egress of irrigation fluid (Fig. 7-1). The working sheath of the cystourethroscope also has a working channel. Many of these instruments have been designed with an oval cross-section to maximize the working channel and the space for the telescope in an instrument of minimal circumference. Access is available through a bridge, which has an angled sidearm usually controlled with a stopcock and a perforated nipple to prevent leakage of fluid when an instrument is in place.

Albarran in 1897 described a lever that passes through the sheath and can be manipulated to deflect a ureteral catheter or other flexible instrument away from the major axis of the sheath (Fig. 7-2). It also has one or two sidearms for the introduction of catheters or instruments, and is particularly useful for directing a ureteral catheter into a ureteral orifice or a flexible instrument toward the dome of the bladder.

Endoscopic instruments are measured by their diameter. Usually the French (Fr.) scale is used. The diameter in millimeters multiplied by 3 is the French size. Cystourethroscopes are available in many sizes, from the short, delicate pediatric instruments (8–12 Fr.) to the larger (24–25 Fr.) instruments capable of accepting a telescope, an Albarran working element, and two working instruments through the same sheath. In practice, the smallest adequate instrument (for adults, 17 or 21 Fr.) is used.

Obturators can be placed into the sheath to provide a blunt, smooth tip for insertion into the urethra. The closed obturator provides a solid intact tip for introduction of the instrument in a tactile, blind fashion (Fig. 7-3). A visual obturator accepts a telescope and fills the space between the telescope and the sheath to provide a smooth surface against the urethra (Fig. 7-4).

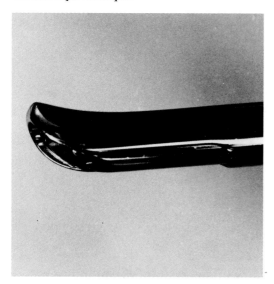

Figure 7-4. *A visual obturator holds the telescope and provides a smooth tip for the sheath for visual passage.*

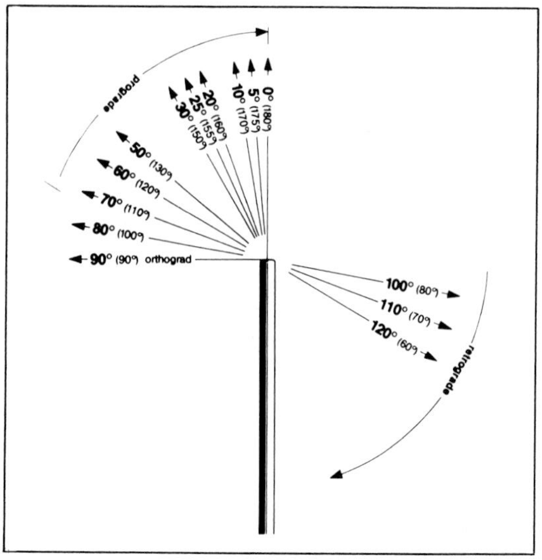

Figure 7-5. *The angle or direction of view of a telescope is indicated by the direction of the center of the visual field relative to the forward axis of the instrument.*

Telescopes have evolved over many years to the accurate, well-illuminated, refined instruments that are available for general use today. The telescope, rather than the sheath, now carries the fiberoptic illuminating system, which extends from the tip of the instrument to the point of attachment of the light bundle just beyond the eyepiece (see Fig. 7-1). The light of the visual image is collected at the objective lens at the tip of the instrument and carried through a rod-lens system to the eyepiece. This system provides a bright, distortion-free image. The angle of view can be varied in the manufacture of the instrument but remains fixed for that instrument. Similarly, the field of view — an arc of 70 degrees in the Hopkins system — can vary.

The angle of the viewing field of the telescope is generally indicated by the difference in degrees between the angle of view and the axis of the instrument (Fig. 7-5). As an example, a telescope lens that is focused to view directly ahead, along the axis of the telescope, is a 0-degree lens. One set at a right angle from the axis of the telescope is a 90-degree or right-angle lens. Retrograde lenses that can best be focused to view the anterior bladder wall and over a large prostate are greater than 90 degrees. Some manufacturers marked older instruments relative to the forward axis, which they considered 180 degrees. This convention is not used for newer instruments.

The telescope is interchangeable within the sheath of the cystoscope. It is held in position by a locking mechanism on the bridge, which in turn is held in position in the sheath. Most telescopes are longer than the corresponding sheath and are extended from the sheath by the bridge. This design allows room for the catheterizing sidearm or the working mechanism of the Albarran bridge. The mechanism for locking the instruments together varies with different manufacturers. With these instruments, the same sheath can be used with a 0-degree lens for urethroscopy and with a 90-degree lens for inspection of the dome of the bladder.

The telescope is by far the most delicate portion of the instrument system. The lenses, including the eyepiece and objective lenses, are glass and consequently breakable. The telescope is sealed against moisture, which will obscure the vision if it enters the system. Although the telescopes are basically sturdy, they can be damaged easily by dropping or by any other sudden blow. They must be handled with care and treated with the respect owed to a fine precision optical instrument.

Lubricant. The outside of the sheath of the instrument should be lubricated to minimize the friction caused by passage into the urethra. Several types of lubricants are available. Most commonly employed is a water-soluble lubricant that is one of the compounds of methylcellulose frequently used in medical instrumentation and digital examination. It is generally nonirritating, will dissolve in urine within the bladder, and will wash from the urethra with the urinary flow. It is packaged in sterile containers.

Other commonly employed lubricants, which we prefer in the otherwise unanesthetized patient, contain anesthetic agents. These are available as 2% xylocaine in sodium carboxymethylcellulose or 0.75% cyclomethycaine sulfate in hydroxypropylmethylcellulose. These materials are optically clear and water soluble, and any that adhere to the lens will wash off with irrigation or with the urine within the bladder. Anesthetic activity is induced by absorption by the urethral mucosa after intraurethral instillation. After the injector cone tip of the tube has been sterilized, it is attached to the tube of anesthetic lubricant and inserted into the meatus. Approximately 15 ml or one-half of the tube's contents is slowly instilled into the male urethra; a smaller volume is used if the patient feels tension in the urethra. A penile clamp is then applied and left in place for 5 to 10 minutes before instrumentation. In the female, 3 to 5 ml of the jelly is instilled into the urethra and left in place 5 to 10 minutes (see Chap. 19).

Non–water-soluble oil or petroleum-based lubricants can also be used. These have the advantage of lasting as a lubricant for long procedures. They have the disadvantages, however, of possibly causing local irritation; lacking solubility in urine or aqueous irrigation solutions; tending to coat the lens, obscuring vision; and possibly softening or dissolving some catheter materials.

Flexible Fiberoptic Cystourethroscopes. Flexible fiberoptic instruments for cystourethroscopy have gained little support and use, perhaps primarily because of the satisfactory instruments already available for cystourethroscopy. In general, the optics and fields of view are superior in the rigid instruments, which also have relatively larger working channels and can be used for numerous procedures. The urologist also has a secure orientation with the rigid instrument. The newer flexible nephroscopes or choledochoscopes, which are also available for cystourethroscopy, provide less accurate visualization, working channels of not more than 5 to 6 Fr., and limited irrigation capacity. The urologist may lose orientation when using the flexible instrument, uncertain of the position of the tip of the instrument and the objective lens. The major advantage of these instruments lies in their flexibility and subsequent comfort to the patient on introduction. They have achieved some use in ureteral catheterization or placement of a ureteral guidewire prior to endourologic percutaneous procedures. With a flexible instrument, cystourethroscopy can be performed with the patient in the supine or prone position, without the need for changing to the lithotomy position. The instrument can also be advanced into the bladder and turned against the back wall of the bladder to enable viewing of the anterior wall including the bladder neck (Fig. 7-6). At present, flexible instruments are not likely to replace rigid cystourethroscopes but have unique capabilities that can be used to supplement the urologist's repertoire.

INDICATIONS AND CONTRAINDICATIONS. Indications for cystourethroscopy include any situation in which (1) information on the static structural anatomy of the urethra or bladder is required, (2) tissue for histologic evaluation is required, or (3) endoscopic access to the upper urinary tract is required. Clearly, evaluation of hematuria, either gross or microscopic, is one of the major indications for cystoscopy. In patients with hematuria, lower urinary tumors (as well as upper tract tumors) must be considered, and the only technique that will adequately evaluate the lower tract directly is cystourethroscopy. After treatment of bladder tumors, patients must be evaluated periodically endoscopically for recurrences. Voiding dysfunction and persistent or recurrent infections, unexplained by radiologic studies, may also be clarified by endoscopic inspection of the urethra and bladder; when the inspection is carried out under topical anesthesia, a rough gauge of bladder tone, capacity, and sensation can be made.

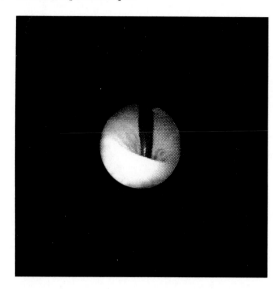

Figure 7-6. *The flexible fiberoptic nephroscope has been used as a cystoscope and passed into the bladder to curve and view the bladder neck in a female. The instrument is seen entering through the bladder neck.*

The major contraindication to cystourethroscopy is the presence or suspicion of a urinary infection. Endoscopy in the presence of acute prostatitis or cystitis may result in severe exacerbation of the infection, frequently with bacteremia or sepsis. When endoscopy is essential despite the coexistence of infection (e.g., the patient with hematuria from bladder neoplasm and cystitis), appropriate antibiotic therapy should first be instituted.

PREOPERATIVE MEASURES

Irrigation. Fluid irrigation through the cystourethroscope is essential to improve visualization in several ways. It distends the lumen to allow viewing of all surfaces, washes debris and blood from the lens, and dilutes blood within the lumen. The choice of irrigating fluid is based on several factors. For simple diagnostic cystoscopy, any standard urologic irrigating solution can be used satisfactorily. A 1-liter container is usually adequate for cystoscopy. Sterile water is frequently used because of its capacity to lyse red blood cells, which permits a slightly clearer field during the presence of bleeding. Saline may provide slightly less irritation to the bladder mucosa. Electrically conductive fluids, however, cannot be used if endoscopic fulguration is necessary (see Chap. 21).

Carbon dioxide has been suggested as an agent for distention of the bladder. When it is used, blood does not disperse throughout the irrigating medium but rather flows along the wall of the bladder and forms clots. Thus, visualization is improved in the presence of bleeding. Urethroscopy with carbon dioxide has gained some support and use by gynecologists.

Anesthesia. Cystourethroscopy can be performed satisfactorily in nearly all women and a vast majority of men with only topical intraurethral anesthesia. This will also suffice for many minor intravesical procedures. The anesthetic techniques appropriate for various, more extensive urologic procedures are discussed in Chapter 20.

TECHNIQUE. Cystourethroscopy combines inspection of the urethra and the bladder. The limitations of earlier instrumentation necessitated two separate procedures for inspection of the urethra and the bladder since each procedure required a different instrument. Instruments that are presently available permit examination of both the urethra and the bladder with the same sheath. The lenses can be changed to provide a full view of all mucosal surfaces.

Inspection of the Meatus. Before attempting to pass any instrument into the urethra, the urethral meatus should be inspected directly for any lesions and for adequacy of the lumen. The meatus should be spread gently, manually, and the lumen inspected. If the meatus is adequate, the procedure can continue with introduction of the instrument. If it appears inadequate, however, the extent of the narrow segment should be determined. Often it is clear if such a narrow area is limited to the meatus itself or to the fossa navicularis. It can then be dilated with a sound or enlarged by meatotomy. If the proximal extent of the narrowing is not obvious, then it should be defined either by urethrogram or urethroscopy with a smaller instrument. In the female, the urethra should be inspected similarly or can be calibrated by passing bougies. It can then be dilated as necessary.

Introduction of the Endoscope. When the meatus is adequate, the tip of the endoscope can be placed into the meatus and advanced into the urethra. The anatomic configuration of the urethra must be recalled and the tip of the instrument should be passed along the ventral aspect of the urethra in the proximal fossa navicularis. To facilitate placement into the urethra and to avoid mucosal trauma, the instrument should have an atraumatic rounded tip. For the cystourethroscope, either the visual or the closed obturator suits this purpose.

Passage of the Cystourethroscope. The cystourethroscope can be passed through the urethra into the bladder either under direct vision or in a blind fashion. Although urologists initially trained in the use of incandescent instruments may find it more familiar to place the cystoscope and obturator directly into the bladder, the atraumatic design of modern cystourethroscopes permits passage under vision.

There are numerous advantages to introduction of the instrument under direct vision. Any obstruction, such as a stricture or foreign body, can be seen; thus it is not necessary to rely on the feel of the instrument passing in the urethra to recognize an impediment. Since it is essential that the urethra be inspected at some time during the procedure, initial inspection during the first passage of the instrument permits examination of the urethral mucosa prior to any minor trauma induced by the instrument itself. Inflammation of the mucosa or neoplastic lesions can be identified readily without traumatic artifact.

In the female, visual introduction is also the preferred technique. Although it offers little advantage for patient comfort, it clarifies the position of the instrument in the urethra, provides a view of the short urethral mucosa, and may allow detection of urethral inflammation or a diverticulum.

The only instance in which it may not be desirable to pass an endoscope into the bladder under direct vision is when a visual obturator is not available. There would then be less chance of mucosal injury by passing the instrument blindly with a closed obturator than by attempting to pass it with a relatively sharp, unprotected sheath and telescope leading the way through the urethra. Overall, visual introduction of the cystourethroscope in patients of either sex offers little disadvantage and should be considered the preferred technique.

BLIND INTRODUCTION. The cystoscope also can be passed directly into the bladder in a blind fashion with the obturator in place. In the male, the penis is held by the urologist's forefinger and thumb and drawn away from the patient's body with enough tension to straighten the urethra as the tip of the cystoscope is passed into the meatus. The cystoscope is then allowed to pass along the urethra. Usually it will pass by itself, essentially falling into the urethra, but in some patients very gentle pressure can be applied to the instrument with the urologist's fingertips to encourage its passage.

As the tip of the instrument reaches the proximal bulbous urethra, the curve of the beak will allow the instrument to turn into the membranous urethra; as the instrument advances farther, the same angulation of the tip will carry it over the bladder neck and into the bladder. When the instrument passes proximally within the posterior urethra, the end of the instrument in the urologist's hand must be lowered to allow the tip to ride into the membranous urethra and over the bladder neck into the bladder.

In the female, the urethral meatus is visualized and the tip of the obturator placed against the meatus and advanced cephalad and slightly anteriorly in a direction approximately toward the umbilicus. The obturator should advance approximately 3 to 4 cm before it is removed and the telescope placed into the sheath. It is not necessary to pass the instrument until resistance is felt since the instrument would then be against the wall of the bladder, with the chance of perforation.

This procedure must be carried out with the greatest gentleness, whether the patient is anesthetized or awake. Forcing the instrument or using it like a lever or pry-bar to get it into the bladder will only result in pain, bleeding, and a false passage. The key factors for successful passage in this fashion are a well-lubricated instrument, an adequate lumen, and an understanding of the anatomic configuration of the urethra.

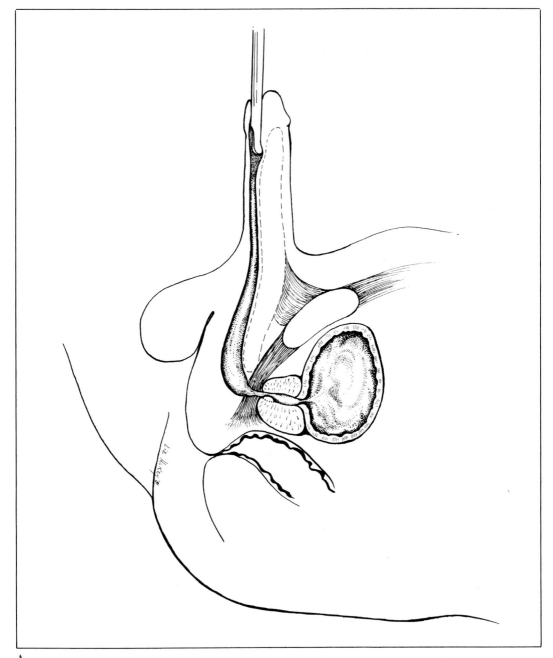

Figure 7-7. *Sagittal views of the male urethra during insertion of a cystourethroscope. The patient is in the dorsal lithotomy position. A. Manual traction on the penis straightens the urethra.*

A

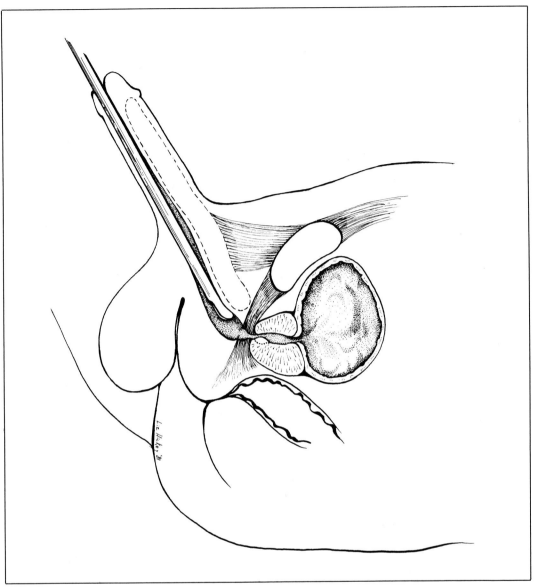

B

Figure 7-7 *(continued). B. The instrument must be lowered as the tip approaches the membranous urethra.*

VISUAL INTRODUCTION AND URETHROSCOPY IN THE MALE.
Under direct vision, the endoscope with either a 0-degree forward viewing lens or a 5- to 30-degree forward viewing lens can be advanced farther from the fossa navicularis into the urethra in the male. The urologist grasps the penis along the corpora cavernosa in one hand and places some traction along the shaft to straighten the urethra (Fig. 7-7A). The instrument is held in the other hand and advanced under direct vision. The entire distal urethra can be inspected in one position (see Fig. 1-2).

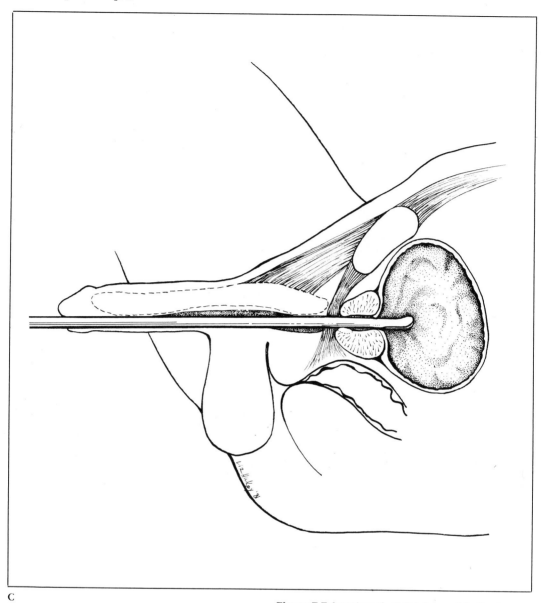

C

Figure 7-7 *(continued). C. It is lowered farther to enter the bladder.*

As the instrument is advanced, note should be made of the various portions of the urethra. The color, vascular pattern, and elasticity of the mucosa are observed. The adequacy of the lumen is also considered. If the lumen is not adequate to accept the instrument, then the mucosa will be damaged and torn or a false passage may be created (Fig. 7-8). To avoid these risks, a smaller instrument should be employed. A second, less desirable technique would be to dilate the urethra with sounds to a caliber at least 2 Fr. units larger than the instrument employed (e.g., 22 Fr. for a 20 Fr. endoscope).

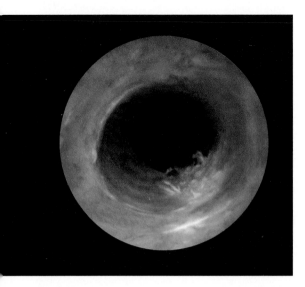

Figure 7-8. *A cystoscope has been passed through a relatively narrow urethra with resultant traumatization of the urethral mucosa.*

As the instrument advances from the pendulous urethra past the penoscrotal junction and enters the bulbous urethra, the angle of the instrument must be changed with lowering of the eyepiece (see Fig. 7-7B). The bulbous urethra can be identified by the larger size and more prominent linear vascular pattern of the lumen, and by the cephalad turn of the lumen (Fig. 7-9). The instrument can then be advanced within the bulbous urethra proximally to the level of the membranous urethra and the sphincter. The eyepiece of the instrument is lowered farther to approach this area directly. The sphincter can usually be readily identified, particularly when local anesthesia is employed. It appears as a shutterlike mechanism with radiation of the mucosal folds and vascular pattern from a small central lumen (see Fig. 1-5). The instrument can be advanced through the sphincter with only gentle, constant pressure.

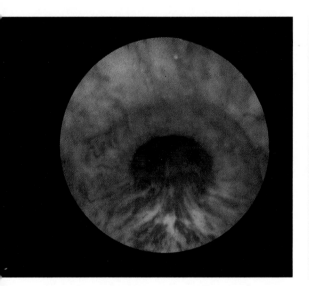

Figure 7-9. *The lumen of the proximal bulbous urethra becomes sharply cephalad as it joins the membranous urethra. Considerable care must be taken to pass instruments at this point in the urethra.*

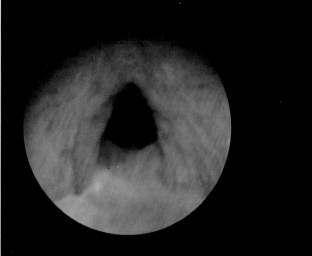

Figure 7-10. *When the 5-degree lens is placed immediately distal to the verumontanum in this 23-year-old male, the entire prostatic urethra and the lumen at the bladder neck can be seen.*

As the tip of the endoscope enters the prostatic urethra, the verumontanum is identified as the major landmark. From this point, the prostatic urethra and the lobes of the prostate can be seen and evaluated (Fig. 7-10). The mucosa, including its color and texture and the presence of any mucosal lesions, should be noted. The size, prominence, and visual obstruction of the prostatic lobes should be noted as well, both with and without the fluid irrigation and with the bladder empty.

Proximally within the prostatic urethra, the bladder neck can be seen. Because of its position, it may present a relative obstacle to passage of the instrument, even under normal conditions. A high bladder neck that forms a prominent lip posteriorly is the most common obstacle encountered. This can be overcome by further depression of the eyepiece and of the instrument to pass the tip into the bladder (see Fig. 7-7C). The adequacy of the bladder neck should be noted, particularly in patients with a history of instrumentation or resection. Bladder neck hypertrophy or true bladder neck contraction with scarring following instrumentation can be noted at this level. The latter may form a small lumen, nearly impassable with the endoscope (see Fig. 8-10). Dilation or treatment by incision, as described in Chapter 8, is required.

VISUAL INTRODUCTION AND URETHROSCOPY IN THE FEMALE. In the female, the tip of the cystourethroscope, with the visual obturator and telescope in place, is positioned at the urethral meatus. It is then advanced under direct vision, usually toward the umbilicus. The central lumen of the urethra should be kept in the center of the field of vision while the instrument is advanced (see Fig. 1-9). The mucosa should be inspected for surface lesions or diverticula.

Irrigation through the instrument will not distend the female urethra but will leak around the instrument. Distention may be achieved by partially occluding the urethra proximally and distally with digital pressure. The forefinger and thumb of one hand can be placed on the instrument during urethroscopy to compress the urethra and the anterior vaginal wall.

In the female, the cystourethroscope is, rarely, inserted inadvertently into the vagina rather than the bladder. Such placement can be minimized by visual insertion of the instrument. Endoscopically, the vagina can be recognized and differentiated from the bladder. The vaginal mucosa is much whiter or paler pink than the bladder (Fig. 7-11). It does not collapse completely with a recognizable posterior wall and does not distend fully with irrigation. The cervix may also be recognized endoscopically. In some pediatric patients, vaginoscopy is an important part of the endoscopic examination (see Chap. 18).

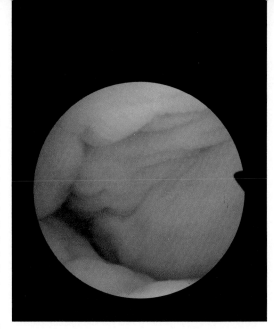

Figure 7-11. *The vaginal mucosa cannot be distended fully with irrigation. The mucosal surface is uniformly pale pink without a prominent vascular pattern.*

Cystoscopy. As the endoscope enters the bladder, the contents can be drained to determine the volume of urine present. Some artifact induced by the irrigant used during urethroscopy may be found but, in the rapid, uncomplicated urethroscopy, will be minimal and nearly insignificant. If vision within the bladder is obscured by bloody urine or clouded by inflammatory debris, repetitive filling and emptying with irrigation fluid through the sheath can clear the field. The bladder is then inspected in a systematic fashion.

The major landmark in the bladder is the bladder neck itself. This is a reference point that cannot be lost or left unrecognized since the instrument passes through it. Another landmark is the bubble of air introduced during instrumentation (Fig. 7-12). It varies in size but is nearly always present and remains at the dome of the bladder with the patient in the dorsal lithotomy position.

The next landmark to be found within the bladder is the interureteric ridge, which is situated posterior to the bladder neck and extends bilaterally to the lateral bladder walls (see Figs. 1-12, 1-13). The ridge varies in its configuration, from less prominent in the female to somewhat more prominent in the male, and may be obscured in the presence of outlet obstruction by the associated trabeculation.

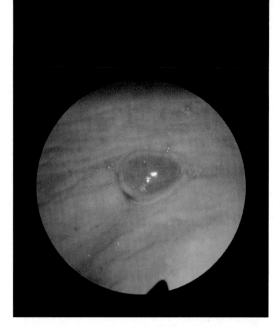

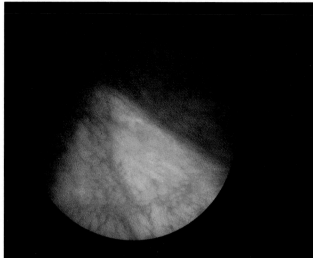

Figure 7-12. *Air introduced into the bladder during instrumentation settles at the dome with the patient in the supine or lithotomy position. There may be multiple bubbles, which may coalesce to form a solitary bubble.*

Figure 7-13. *There is some redundancy and irregularity of mucosa immediately adjacent to this right ureteral orifice with resultant poor visual resolution of the os. There is a paucity of mucosal vessels immediately distal to the orifice (5-degree lens).*

The ureteral orifices can then be identified along the interureteric ridge. They are usually located 1 to 2 cm lateral to the midline bilaterally (see Figs. 1-11, 1-13). A ureteral orifice appears as a slit or a small cleft in the mucosa. There is often some irregularity of the mucosa immediately adjacent to the orifice, giving it an ill-defined, poorly focused appearance. A characteristic vascular pattern is often seen around the orifice (Figs. 7-13, 7-17). Prominent submucosal vessels pass medial, inferior, and lateral to the orifice, leaving a relatively avascular arc immediately distal to the orifice itself. This pattern may be obscured in the presence of mucosal inflammation. The appearance of the orifice varies with the angle of view of the telescope. Each orifice should be inspected with both the forward and lateral viewing lenses (Figs. 7-13 to 7-17, 1-12, 1-15).

If the ureter is obscured by inflammatory changes or an intravesical tumor and must be located for catheterization or limitation of resection, recognition may be enhanced by administering to the patient a dye that is excreted in the urine after intravenous injection. Indigo carmine, which can be seen as a blue liquid streaming from the orifice, has been used for this purpose.

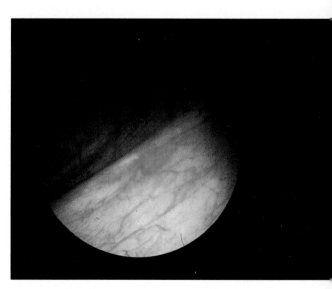

Figure 7-14. *The left ureteral orifice is located typically on the ridge in this female when seen with the 5-degree lens.*

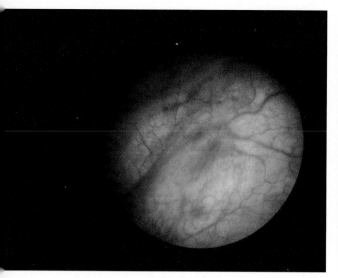

Figure 7-15. *A left orifice with normal mucosal irregularity and a typical mucosal vascular pattern (70-degree lens).*

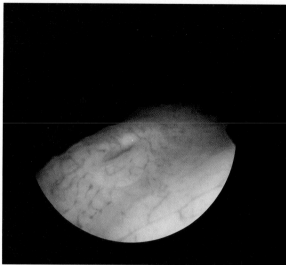

Figure 7-17. *A left ureteral orifice is located prominently but slightly inferiorly on the ureteric ridge, placing it fully within the field of view of the forward viewing 12-degree lens.*

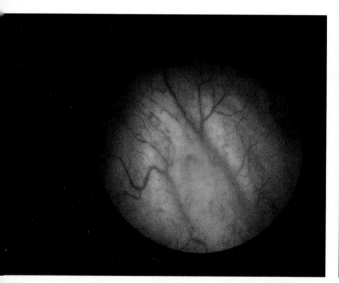

Figure 7-16. *A right orifice shown through the 70-degree lens has normal mucosal irregularity and a typical mucosal vascular pattern.*

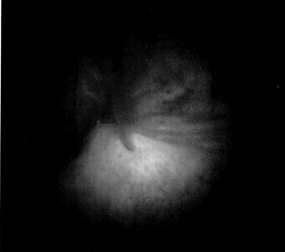

Figure 7-18. *Gross hematuria is apparent as a red stream of urine from this right orifice. In this view it is deflected by the flow of irrigant.*

Each orifice should be observed until urinary efflux can be seen. This will occur with movement of the ureteral musculature on the ridge laterally and an obvious opening of the orifice. The urine can be seen as a darker colored jet of fluid from the orifice and will demonstrate some visual distortion as the fluids of different density mix. The position and configuration of each ureteral orifice should be observed; in addition, once urinary efflux can be seen, it is important to note any hematuria, which appears as an obvious jet of red urine (Fig. 7-18). These points can be viewed with either the forward viewing lens (0–30 degrees) used for urethroscopy or with the 70- to 90-degree lens used for observation of the remainder of the bladder.

After inspection of the trigone, the floor of the bladder immediately posterior to the interureteric ridge (bas-fond) should be noted. Any foreign bodies, including stones and blood clots, are usually located in this most dependent position. The posterior wall of the bladder can usually be observed more easily with a forward viewing lens than with a more angular lens. The remainder of the bladder is then examined in a systematic fashion. It can be examined with a sweeping view of the angular lens (70–90 degrees), moving from the posterior to the anterior surface and then from the floor to the dome of the bladder. Other urologists may prefer to examine the bladder in specific areas such as the posterior wall, or the lower and then the more anterior right or left lateral walls. Using whatever pattern is comfortable, the urologist should inspect the entire bladder systematically to avoid missing any area within the bladder. The anterior wall may be partially obscured by the bladder neck, but it can be brought into view with manual suprapubic compression or can be seen with a retrograde telescope. The mucosa should be observed closely and its color, vascular texture, and configuration, as well as any irregularity, should be noted. The pattern of the underlying musculature is also readily evident, and trabeculation resulting from muscular hypertrophy should also be noted.

At the completion of the procedure, the entire volume of urine and irrigant within the bladder should be drained. Some urologists prefer to instill a solution containing an antibiotic into the bladder at the completion of the procedure to prevent infection. This technique has some support in experimental animal models but has not been confirmed in controlled clinical studies.

The procedure should be recorded in a systematic fashion. This can be done verbally with comment made on each finding or by using a form such as that employed in some institutions. This form provides for easy, reproducible recording of endoscopic findings. The chart of the bladder for mapping the location and size of abnormalities is particularly useful for indicating position (Fig. 7-19).

CYSTOSCOPY THROUGH A SUPRAPUBIC TRACT. Occasionally, the only access to the bladder is through a suprapubic tract. In a well-matured tract of adequate size, the instrument can be passed readily into the bladder. If a small catheter has been in the bladder and the tract is too small for the endoscope, then the tract can be dilated by introducing a guidewire into the bladder and passing dilators over this wire to enlarge the tract, as in dilating a nephrostomy tract. The endoscope can be passed into the bladder with either obturator in place. If the closed obturator is used, then the telescope is replaced into the instrument and the bladder is inspected. The bladder can be distended with irrigating fluid in the usual way, although some leakage may occur along the suprapubic tract around the instrument.

The urologist must reorient himself from this unusual point of view. The landmarks, including the trigone, interureteric ridge, and ureteral orifices are still readily recognizable. In addition, the proximal bladder neck can be seen and remains the major point of reference. Depending on the degree of bladder distention and the patient's neurologic and anesthetic status, the bladder neck may be widely opened or tightly apposed. A urethral catheter passing into the bladder is readily seen entering through the bladder neck (Fig. 7-20).

Because of the position of the instrument, it may be considerably more difficult to catheterize the ureteral orifice in this position. The instrument is approaching the orifice at approximately a 90-degree angle, and any catheter passed through the endoscope is directed against the back wall of the ureteral orifice rather than along the lumen (Fig. 7-21). In this position, therefore, it is essential to use the 70- or 90-degree lens and the Albarran deflecting lever to place a catheter into the ureteral orifice.

FORM 62.29-308-1

THE UNIVERSITY OF CHICAGO HOSPITALS AND CLINICS

CYSTOSCOPIC EXAMINATION

PATIENT NUMBER

Name — First — Last

No. & Street

City & State

PREMEDICATION:

ANESTHESIA:

PROCEDURE:

CLINIC OR FLOOR	DATE

Urine:	Bladder	Rt. Ureter	Lt. Ureter
Microscopic			
Culture			

INSTRUMENTS:

INTRODUCTION:

RESIDUAL URINE:	BLADDER CAPACITY:	TONE:

BLADDER, GENERAL FINDINGS:

TRIGONE AND URETERAL ORIFICES

VESICAL NECK:

PROSTATIC URETHRA:

RETROGRADE STUDIES	CATH. SIZE	CM. INSERTED	REMARKS
RIGHT			
LEFT			

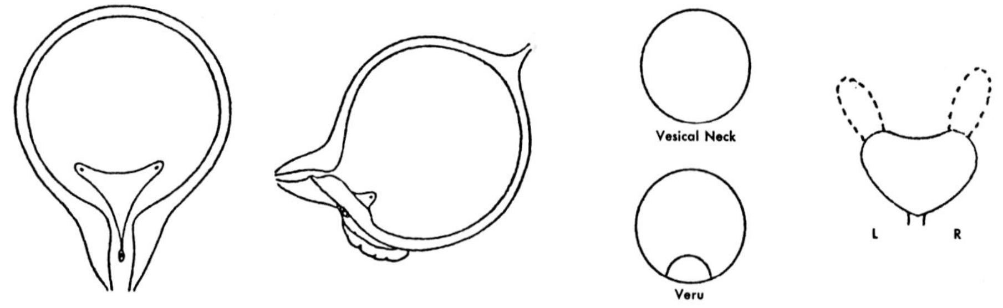

DIAGNOSIS:

ADVICE:

DATE:	SIGNATURE:

Figure 7-19. *A form for recording cystoscopic findings provides a means for complete and reproducible notation.*

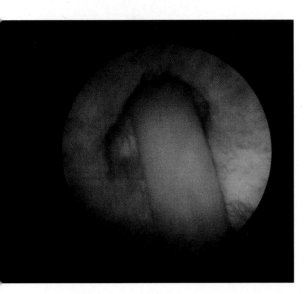

Figure 7-20. *A cystoscope can be placed into the bladder through a suprapubic tract. With a forward viewing lens, the bladder neck is visualized in a 14-year-old boy. A urethral catheter is entering the bladder through the internal urethral meatus. The verumontanum is seen underlying the catheter, and there is minimal prominence of the lateral lobes of the prostate in the young male.*

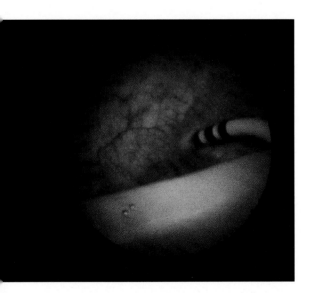

Figure 7-21. *In the same patient, a ureteral catheter has been placed into the left ureteral orifice and is adjacent to the Foley catheter (90-degree lens).*

INTRAVESICAL PROCEDURES. Numerous procedures can be performed with the endoscope within the bladder. A wide range of instruments for each procedure is available from several different manufacturers. Often, several different instruments can perform the same task.

Biopsy. Any mucosal lesions within the bladder that are suspicious for tumors should be biopsied. These include obvious papillary or sessile epithelial tumors and suspicious irregular or erythematous mucosa. Biopsy forceps are available for endoscopic placement into the bladder. These instruments can be divided into two major groups: they are either flexible or rigid. The flexible biopsy forceps are available in sizes from 5 to 9 Fr. The size of the cup and the resultant biopsy are small with the flexible instruments. The major advantage of these forceps, however, is flexibility. They are not limited to working within a straight line but can be passed through an endoscope using the Albarran bridge and the 70- or 90-degree lens to deflect the flexible forceps to observe and biopsy a lesion at an angle away from the instrument. These are particularly useful for lesions at the dome of the bladder.

The tip of the biopsy forceps is passed to the lesion to be sampled under direct vision. The cup is then opened and placed directly against the biopsy site before being closed tightly to include the major point of interest. These forceps generally are not strong enough to cut or bite the tissue sample but must be withdrawn to amputate the tissue. In one forceps design, the tip of the instrument rotates as the instrument is closed to separate the sample from the adjacent tissue.

Samples taken with the flexible biopsy forceps are minute. The 5 Fr. forceps obtains a specimen less than 2 mm in diameter. Since the chance of obtaining a satisfactory biopsy specimen is limited by the size of the forceps, multiple biopsies should be taken. The risk of perforation with these instruments is extremely small; therefore, they can be used safely in females and younger patients. Mucosal biopsy at sites other than the trigone is not painful and local intraurethral anesthesia initially used for endoscopy is sufficient.

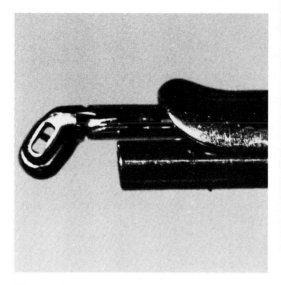

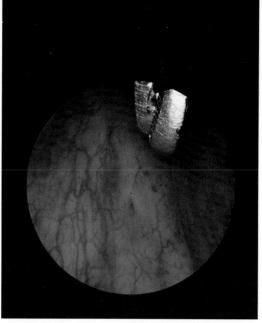

Figure 7-22. *The rigid biopsy forceps protrude from the tip of the cystoscope in view of the forward viewing telescope.*

Figure 7-23. *The rigid biopsy forceps are seen in the upper portion of the field as they approach the left lateral bladder wall posterior to the ureteral orifice seen in the center of the field (12-degree telescope).*

The rigid biopsy forceps provide several advantages. Visibility is generally good with these instruments and, despite their straight design and rigidity, they can reach most areas in the bladder with the possible exceptions of the dome and the anterior wall. More major advantages, however, are the larger size of the tissue sample and the capability of sharply amputating the tissue without crushing it. As an example, the rigid biopsy forceps shown in Figures 7-22 and 7-23 has two basketlike cups that oppose, fitting into or over one another to cut the tissue with a scissorlike mechanism.

These biopsy forceps must be used with caution. The forceps pass through the endoscope's sheath previously placed into the bladder, but the tip of the forceps protrudes beyond the telescope. This design is necessary to allow the forceps to be seen with the forward viewing lens. These forceps also take a larger sample of tissue (up to 6 mm in diameter) and can take a full thickness bite in a thin bladder.

Fulguration. Minor bleeding, such as that resulting from biopsy, can be controlled with endoscopic fulguration. Very small mucosal lesions such as papillomas can be adequately destroyed with fulguration. Numerous electrodes are available for intravesical fulguration. The most common designs are the "ball or acorn" Bugbee types.

The electrode is passed through the working channel of the endoscope and connected with a wire to the electrocautery unit. The patient must be grounded and attached to the unit to complete the circuit. A grounding pad or plate must be in contact with the patient over a wide area to prevent an electrical burn at the contact site. The site of fulguration must be visualized endoscopically. Blood that obscures the vision is irrigated rapidly from the bleeding site and emptied from the bladder. A constant flow instrument such as a resectoscope may facilitate irrigation and visualization in particularly bloody lesions. In other instances, a small blood clot on the mucosal surface may indicate the site of bleeding. The tip of the electrode is then passed to touch the site, and the coagulating current is applied to fulgurate the area. Several applications may be necessary. Satisfactory fulguration can be observed as the tissue turns white or brown with application of the current around the electrode tip. Fairly extensive areas can be fulgurated with repeated application of the electrode and coagulating current. If a larger area must be treated, then the resectoscope loop or the roller electrode should be employed (see Chap. 10).

Ureteral Catheterization. One of the major endoscopic procedures, both in frequency and importance to the patient, is ureteral catheterization. The instruments and techniques involved are discussed in Chapter 13.

Foreign Bodies. Foreign bodies are best removed from the bladder endoscopically using instruments specially designed for this purpose. Usually referred to as "foreign body" or "grasping" forceps, these are available in both flexible and rigid designs. They are usually quite similar to biopsy forceps but have serrations or teeth on their jaws to provide a grasping surface (see Fig. 13-14). The advantages of each design are similar to those noted for biopsy forceps. Because of the irregular edge of the cup, foreign body forceps are generally not suitable for taking specimens of tissue. The specimen will usually pull through the teeth of the forceps since it is not sharply amputated.

The technique of removing a foreign body must vary with the individual finding. As an example, a needle introduced into the bladder can be removed endoscopically by grasping the pointed end first and drawing it through the instrument. Simple inflammatory debris can be irrigated from the bladder by filling and emptying the bladder several times. The size of foreign body removed through the endoscope is limited only by the size of the sheath, the flexibility of the foreign body, or the ability to divide a large specimen into several smaller pieces that can be removed endoscopically.

BLADDER CALCULI. Bladder calculi constitute a major group of foreign bodies requiring removal. The instruments and techniques for these procedures are discussed in Chapter 12.

Intravesical Blood Clots. One of the more common problems confronting the urologist is a patient with hematuria and a large volume of clots within the bladder. The patient may complain of pain from bladder distention or may have continuing hematuria, either of which requires immediate treatment. Blood clots within the bladder usually will not simply flow from the sheath of the endoscope but rather will obstruct the outflow. Smaller clots often will drain easily but usually can be voided just as easily from the bladder. Larger clots or those that have been present and have become organized are firmer and require more active removal. Clots can often be removed by manual irrigation and application of suction pressure directly to the clot with a plunger syringe (Toomey) attached to the endoscope. The lower pressure generated by the Ellik evacuator is often not sufficient for removal of solid clots.

It may also be of value to break the clots into smaller pieces. This can be done with the resectoscope loop without application of the current. The smaller fragments of the clots can then be removed more easily with irrigation.

Particularly firm solid clots develop in patients receiving epsilon-aminocaproic acid (Amicar). This fibrinolysin inhibitor has been useful in preventing continued hemorrhage in several situations, but clots that are already present within the bladder become much more firmly organized and gain a rubbery consistency with inhibition of the urokinase. Although this type of clot can sometimes be removed endoscopically with the techniques described, the rigidity of the clot may preclude endoscopic removal and necessitate cystotomy.

INTRAURETHRAL PROCEDURES. Some procedures can be performed intraurethrally in the same manner described for the bladder. In addition, several unique problems can arise in the urethra itself.

Stricture. The most common abnormality found endoscopically within the urethra is a narrowing or stricture of the urethra. A stricture may be asymptomatic and unexpected at endoscopy. It appears as a narrowing of the lumen, often with some pallor of the fibrous tissue forming the stricture. The endoscope should not be forced against the stricture since doing so will probably create a false passage through the normal urethra rather than dilate the stricture. The stricture can be dilated with a controlled procedure and the appropriate instruments, such as filiforms and followers or Van Buren sounds. If the stricture has a particularly narrow lumen, a filiform can be passed through the cystoscope under direct vision to ensure its placement within the lumen. The endoscope can then be removed and followers used to dilate the stricture in the usual fashion. We prefer, however, to incise the stricture under direct vision with the visual urethrotome to provide an adequate urethral lumen (see Chap. 8).

Foreign Bodies. Foreign bodies (excluding calculi) are more common within the urethra than within the bladder. Removal must be individualized but generally can be aided by endoscopic visualization and removal with grasping forceps.

Tumors. Tumors within the urethra can be biopsied with flexible biopsy or rigid biopsy forceps. An alternative diagnostic technique is brushing for cytologic and histologic samples with techniques similar to those used for upper urinary tract lesions (see Chap. 14).

COMPLICATIONS

Perforation. Passage of any instrument into the urethra may result in injury to the narrow structure. Minor mucosal injury within the urethra (see Fig. 7-8) is common but can be avoided by using a small instrument that the urethra can easily accommodate. Misdirection of the instrument combined with inappropriate force will cause the instrument to pass through normal tissues rather than the lumen, with the resultant creation of a false passage. If the perforation is in the urethra, it may then be impossible to pass the instrument into the bladder. Bleeding may totally obscure the visual field, or it may be impossible to recognize or pass the tip of the instrument into the true lumen. If the instrument is already within the bladder, vision may be obscured by bleeding. If the perforation is on the posterior wall, then urinary leakage into the peritoneal cavity is likely. Perforation at other sites in the bladder are expected to be retroperitoneal. The diagnosis and extent of injury can be confirmed by a cystogram. Treatment includes urinary diversion and drainage by either a urethral catheter or a suprapubic tube, as well as surgical closure of large perforations or those entering the peritoneum.

Infection. Infections may develop after urinary instrumentation. Bacteremia has been reported to occur in as many as 13.3 percent of patients with sterile urine undergoing simple cystoscopy [8] and postoperative bacteriuria has occurred in 2.0 to 6.7 percent of patients [5,7]. Infection is sufficiently rare after routine cystoscopy to warrant avoidance of routine antibiotic prophylaxis. Although such prophylaxis appears to be of value both in experimental models and in clinical series of urologic procedures, the rate of infection is sufficiently low that only those patients who can be identified as being at high risk should be exposed to antibiotics on a prophylactic basis. Patients with an indwelling catheter prior to cystoscopy, however, as well as those with significant outlet obstruction or a large volume of residual urine and particularly debilitated patients may fall into the high risk group, although this identification has not been clarified in clinical studies.

Table 7-1. Endocarditis Prophylaxis for Urinary Endoscopy

1. Patients without history of allergy: (a) aqueous penicillin G, 2 million units IM or IV, or ampicillin 1–2 gm IM or IV, *plus* (b) gentamicin 1.5 mg/kg IM, or streptomycin, 1 gm IM. Doses given 30 min – 1 hr before procedure.

If gentamicin is used, the dose should be repeated every 8 hr for 2 more doses. If streptomycin is used, the same dose should be given every 12 hr for 2 additional doses.

2. Patients with penicillin allergy: (a) vancomycin, 1 gm IV infused over 30 min, *plus* (b) gentamicin 1.5 mg/kg IM, starting 1 hr before procedure.

Both antibiotics should be repeated every 12 hr for 2 more doses.

Source: Adapted from Antibiotic prophylaxis for surgery. *Med. Lett. Drugs Ther.* 21:76, 1979; and E. L. Kaplan, et al., Prevention of bacterial endocarditis. *Circulation* 56:139a, 1977.

ANTIBIOTIC PROPHYLAXIS FOR ENDOCARDITIS. Antibiotic prophylaxis for endocarditis in patients at high risk for developing infections (particularly those with valvular disease) must include coverage for both enterococci and gram-negative organisms. The recommendations of the American Heart Association presently include penicillin or ampicillin and gentamicin administered parenterally preoperatively and continued for a total of three doses (Table 7-1) [4,6].

Stricture Formation. Stricture formation may be a late complication after instrumentation. Although the rate of stricturing after a simple cystoscopy is unknown, it appears to be very low. Strictures are much more frequently seen after long transurethral procedures requiring a larger instrument, such as transurethral resection of the prostate. Even in those cases, the rate of stricture formation is related to the size of the instrument used and the length of the procedure. Strictures may occur after cystoscopy and, based on the evidence obtained from other procedures, it can be recommended that the smallest appropriate instrument be used and that the procedure be as short as possible.

POSTOPERATIVE CARE. Minimal specific medical care is necessary after a simple cystoscopy. Patients must be warned that they may pass small amounts of blood and air per urethra and that they will experience some dysuria during the first several voidings after instrumentation. The need for antibiotic therapy has already been discussed. Generally, postoperative catheterization is neither necessary nor desirable. In some patients with severe bladder outlet obstruction and a large residual volume of urine demonstrated by the endoscopic procedure, catheter drainage may be necessary.

All patients, however, should be warned of the possibility of urinary infection or retention. They should be cautioned regarding the symptoms and the need for medical attention should these conditions develop.

REFERENCES

History of Cystoscopy

1. Hopkins, H. H. The Modern Urological Endoscope. In J. G. Gow and H. H. Hopkins (Eds.). *A Handbook of Urological Endoscopy.* Edinburgh: Churchill Livingstone, 1978. P. 29.
2. Murphy, L. J. T. *The History of Urology.* Springfield, Ill.: Charles C. Thomas, 1972.
3. Nicholson, P. Problems encountered by early endoscopists. *Urology* 19:114, 1982.

INFECTIOUS COMPLICATIONS

4. Antibiotic prophylaxis for surgery. *Med. Lett. Drugs. Ther.* 21:76, 1979.
5. Appell, R. A., Flynn, J. T., Paris, A. M. I., and Blandy, J. P. Occult bacterial colonization of bladder tumors. *J. Urol.* 124:345, 1980.
6. Kaplan, E. L., et al. Prevention of bacterial endocarditis. *Circulation* 56:139a, 1977.
7. Lytton, B. Urinary infection in cystoscopy. *Br. Med. J.* 2:547, 1961.
8. Thompson, P. M., Talbot, R. W., Packham, D. A., and Dulake, C. Transrectal biopsy of the prostate and bacteremia. *Br. J. Surg.* 67:127, 1980.

8

VISUAL INTERNAL URETHROTOMY IN THE TREATMENT OF URETHRAL STRICTURES

Demetrius H. Bagley

Edward S. Lyon

Jeffry L. Huffman

Visual internal urethrotomy (VIU) is the most recent technique in a series of procedures designed for the treatment of urethral stricture. The earliest recorded attempts to treat strictures with graduated dilators date from the sixth century B.C. [1]. The persistence of basically similar techniques, along with a multitude of other procedures subsequently introduced, indicates the lack of routine success and satisfaction with any single procedure. The introduction of visual internal urethrotomy has provided a technique that is relatively simple to perform, has few severe complications, and results in subjective and objective improvement in the majority of patients treated. It should be readily available to the practicing urologist.

DIAGNOSIS OF URETHRAL STRICTURE

Signs and Symptoms. Since a urethral stricture results from contraction of a circumferential scar of the urethra from a previous inflammatory process, trauma or infection, the presenting symptoms are those of lower urinary obstruction. The patient may complain of reduced or intermittent urinary stream or more irritative symptoms such as nocturia, frequency, or urgency. In severe strictures, urinary retention may develop. Congenital strictures produce similar symptoms.

Flow Rate. Determination of the flow rate may detect more subtle changes in the stream than the patient can appreciate [4]. This technique is particularly valuable in detecting recurrent urinary strictures. The patient should be followed at regular intervals with determination of the urinary flow rate. If the flow rate decreases significantly from that obtained immediately after urethrotomy, recurrence of the stricture should be suspected and other diagnostic techniques should be used to define the lumen of the urethra. By generally accepted criteria, a peak flow rate of greater than 15 ml per second has been considered in postoperative series to be an excellent result. A slower rate of 10 ml per second has also been accepted as a satisfactory result if the patient does not have major symptoms.

Since the flow rate is related to the volume of urine passed, a more accurate way to standardize the flow rate for any volume voided is to use a nomogram that relates volume to flow in a standardized population [20]. By using this nomogram, the patient's flow rate can be described in standard deviations relative to a normal population, and thus can be standardized regardless of the volume voided.

Catheterization. The diagnosis of urethral stricture may be suggested by the inability to pass a catheter (16 or 18 Fr.) or an 18 or 20 Fr. sound. Conversely, the diagnosis can be excluded if an instrument of this caliber will pass easily. A sound smaller than 18 Fr. should not be used because of the possibility of perforation of the urethra.

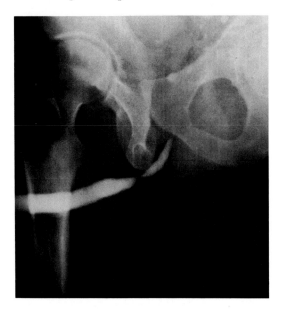

Figure 8-1. *A retrograde urethrogram demonstrates a short stricture of the bulbous urethra.*

Retrograde Urethrography. A retrograde urethrogram can often delineate the full extent of the urethral stricture. The retrograde urethrogram is performed by injection of radioopaque contrast material into the urethra via the urethral meatus. The patient is placed in a sharp (45-degree), oblique position with the hips and knees flexed. This radiographic view demonstrates the urethra in profile while avoiding the overlying bony densities seen on a lateral view. Various catheter tips and clamps have been designed and are commercially available to permit intraurethral administration of contrast without exposure of the physician's hands to the x-ray beam. A 14 Fr. Foley catheter can be used for the introduction of contrast. The tip of the catheter is placed within the urethral meatus. The balloon is located within the fossa navicularis and inflated with 1 to 2 ml of fluid or air to hold the catheter within the urethra and to occlude the lumen. The penis is extended with moderate traction. This technique is comfortable for the patient and convenient for the physician.

The aqueous contrast material employed in the retrograde urethrogram must be suitable for intravenous injection since it frequently enters the paraurethral veins during the study. It should not be mixed with lubricant as a thickening agent. An iodine concentration of 30% provides satisfactory contrast and minimizes sclerosis if it leaks into the periurethral tissue. Minimal pressure should be employed in the intraurethral injection.

An x-ray film should be obtained before and during injection of the contrast to demonstrate the urethral anatomy. A dynamic urethrogram with films taken during the intraurethral instillation of contrast will routinely demonstrate the entire extent of the stricture (Fig. 8-1)[15]. Although fluoroscopy is not essential, its use permits immediate recognition of the site of obstruction and will help delineate the extent of the stricture. It will also demonstrate any contrast flowing intravenously.

Voiding Urethrography. If the retrograde urethrogram does not define the full extent of the urethral stricture, then contrast should be passed into the urethra in an antegrade fashion by voiding urethrogram. If the stricutred area is of adequate caliber, then a fine catheter, such as a no. 8 pediatric feeding tube or a 5 Fr. ureteral catheter, can be passed transurethrally to allow instillation of contrast into the bladder. After removal of the catheter, the patient is asked to void and a voiding urethrogram is performed. This should be done with fluoroscopy but can be performed adequately with individual radiographs taken during voiding. Comparison of the retrograde and antegrade urethrograms will then define the proximal and distal extents of the urethral stricture.

Urethroscopy. Strictures can be visualized with the urethroscope or panendoscope. A severe stricture appears as a sudden narrowing of the urethral lumen with surrounding dense, white, fibrous scarring. No attempt should be made to pass the instrument through such a small densely scarred area since the beak of the instrument may perforate the softer normal urethral mucosa, creating a false passage. Asymptomatic strictures may also be found on urethroscopy. Surprisingly small caliber strictures may be encountered in this way although, more commonly, larger caliber strictures are found in the asymptomatic patient (see Fig. 3-4).

MANAGEMENT OF URETHRAL STRICTURE. Several different types of therapy for urethral strictures have evolved. No single form of treatment will provide routinely successful results in all strictures. Therapy should be individualized to each patient and the characteristics of the stricture in order to provide the best chance of cure. The forms of therapy include (1) dilation, (2) urethroplasty, (3) urethrotomy, and (4) visual internal urethrotomy.

Dilation. The oldest form of treatment is dilation, performed by the passage of successively larger instruments through the narrowed area. Filiforms and followers can be used in dilating most urethral strictures. Filiforms are available in several forms — straight, spiral, or coudé tip. When placed transurethrally, the small tip passes through the small lumen of the stricture into the proximal urethra and bladder. When there are numerous false passages or irregularities of the urethra, several filiforms can be placed into the urethra to fill and obstruct the false passages so that subsequent filiforms can be passed into the actual lumen through the stricture. Once the filiform is passed into the bladder, a follower is attached and also passed through the stricture. Increasingly larger followers can then be passed in a similar fashion. Once a stricture has been dilated, a catheter can be inserted to maintain the lumen and provide urinary drainage.

Van Buren sounds can also be used to dilate strictures. Their use should be limited to either strictures of adequate caliber for passage of the tip of at least the no. 18 sound or longer strictures that have been repeatedly dilated. The tips of smaller sounds may easily perforate the urethral mucosa. An attempt to pass a sound in a very tight stricture such as that shown in Figure 8-5 may also result in a false passage.

Urethral catheters can be used for dilating strictures. Catheters of increasing size may be placed at intervals of 48 to 72 hours until a catheter of adequate size (20–24 Fr.) has been placed transurethrally. This technique can also be used in conjunction with dilation by other instruments. For example, a stricture may dilate easily to only 16 Fr. with filiforms and followers. A catheter of 14 or 16 Fr. may then be placed and subsequently changed to a larger size after 48 to 72 hours.

Urethroplasty. Several forms of urethroplasty have been described for the treatment of severe and recurrent strictures. These include 1- and 2-stage flap urethroplasties and graft procedures. At present, urethroplasty is reserved for patients with severe strictures requiring frequent dilation or those who have failed repeated attempts at urethrotomy. The techniques for urethroplasty will not be discussed.

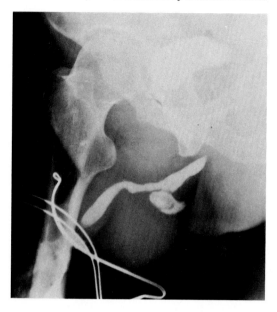

Figure 8-2. *A retrograde urethrogram delineates a urethral diverticulum in a patient after a previous urethroplasty. The filling defect within the diverticulum represents a mass of hair and calculous material.*

The complications of urethroplasty are often symptomatic and can be recognized by urethroscopy. Restricturing of the proximal or distal anastomosis of the urethroplasty is the most frequent complication. A stricture usually presents as a recurrence of voiding symptoms, but it may present as a decrease in the urethral flow rate during follow-up. A significant diverticulum at the site of the urethroplasty may present with postvoid dribbling or urinary infection or following formation of a stone in the diverticulum. A urethrogram will define these lesions (Fig. 8-2). Urethroscopy may reveal the strictured area or the mouth of the diverticulum. If a flap urethroplasty has been used, then hair will grow from the hair-bearing scrotal or perineal skin and may serve as a nidus for intraurethral stone formation (Fig. 8-3).

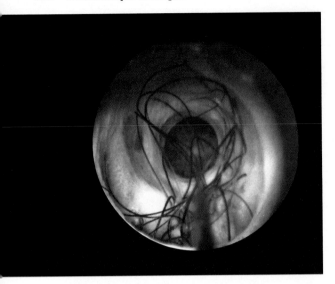

Figure 8-3. *In the same patient, the mouth of the diverticulum can be seen endoscopically with hair passing into the urethral lumen.*

Laser Urethrotomy. Lasers have been used in some short series for incision of strictures, apparently with good results. This technique has the advantage of excellent healing without additional scarring. The instrument is expensive, however, and not generally available. At present it can be considered only a research technique, and its clinical value is not supported by substantial series.

Blind Urethrotomy. Techniques of internal urethrotomy have been employed for treatment of urethral strictures since the midnineteenth century[1]. Although urethrotomy was reported by Paré as early as 1560, recent history dates from the description of urethrotomes by Maisonneuve in 1853 and Otis in 1872. The urethrotome of Maisonneuve consisted of a filiform guide that could be passed through the strictured urethra and to which the urethrotome could be screwed and introduced to cut the stricture from without inward. The design of a blade with a sharp leading edge but a flat outer surface theoretically could minimize damage to the healthy urethra. The Otis urethrotome can be placed into the urethra and the blade adjusted and set to provide an incision to a predetermined caliber.

The major indication for blind urethrotomy has been rapid recurrence of urethral strictures after dilation. Although some authors have reported success in the treatment of strictures with the Otis urethrotome, the frequency of complications has precluded its early routine use in therapy of strictures. Most of the disadvantages of the blind urethrotome have resulted from its application in a blind manner. Damage to the normal urethra and the sphincter with resultant incontinence have occurred[3,9,11].

Treatment of Impassable Strictures. In an emergency situation in which a patient is in acute retention with a stricture that cannot be dilated blindly and an optical urethrotome is not available, a filiform or ureteral catheter can often be passed through the stricture endoscopically under direct vision. The stricture can then be dilated with followers or the ureteral catheter can be left in the bladder for urinary drainage. Alternatively, the bladder can be drained suprapubically by an open or percutaneous technique and the stricture treated in a second procedure.

Visual Internal Urethrotomy. With the development of an optical urethrotome, a more recent technique has been described for urethrotomy under direct vision[19]. Visual internal urethrotomy has eliminated many of the major disadvantages of the blind technique while retaining the advantage of precise incision of the stricture. The depth and extent of incision can be accurately controlled with such precision that even strictures of the proximal bulbous or the membranous urethra near the sphincter can be incised (see Fig. 8-7). This procedure can be controlled accurately to incise only the stricture and may more appropriately be called a "stricturotomy."

The optical urethrotome consists of a mechanism for advancing a knife blade from the sheath into the urethral lumen, a sidearm for introducing a ureteral catheter through the strictured area, and a forward viewing lens (Fig. 8-4). There is also an attachable, split outer sheath, which can be applied over the urethrotome before introduction into the urethra. This permits removal of the internal sheath of the urethrotome on completion of the urethrotomy with maintenance of the lumen by the outer sheath. A urethral catheter as large as 18 Fr. can then be placed through the slotted sheath and the sheath removed over the catheter.

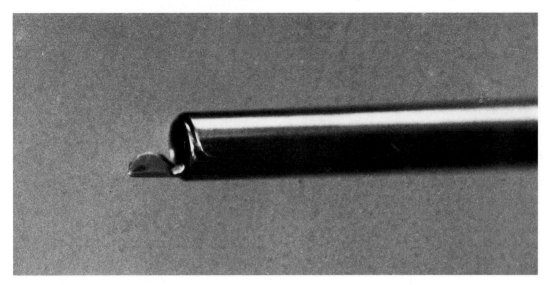

Figure 8-4. *The visual urethrotome has a thumb control for advancing the knife blade, a sidearm to accommodate a ureteral catheter, and an outer split sheath through which a urethral catheter can be passed.*

TECHNIQUE. The assembled urethrotome is inserted into the urethra after lubrication of the instrument and the urethra. It may be difficult to pass the tip of the urethrotome into the urethral meatus under vision since the end is flush and the tip is cylindrical. If so, the obturator may be placed in the instrument and passed, leading the sheath into the urethral meatus. The obturator is then removed, the telescope replaced, and the instrument advanced through the urethra as in diagnostic urethroscopy.

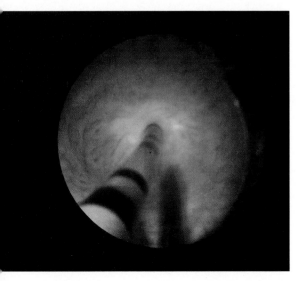

Figure 8-5. *The stricture appears as a small lumen surrounded by pale scar tissue. A 5 Fr. ureteral catheter has been passed through the stricture. The knife of the urethrotome is visible at the 6 o'clock position.*

When the stricture has been visualized, a ureteral catheter can be advanced through the strictured area into the bladder to act as a guide for the incision (Fig. 8-5). Some authors prefer to withdraw the instrument after placing the ureteral catheter into the bladder and then replace the urethrotome into the urethra beside the catheter[13]. Although this movement may afford some increased mobility during the procedure of incision, it requires excessive instrumentation and has not been generally accepted. If a catheter is used as a guide, we prefer to leave it in place through the instrument. One manufacturer has designed an instrument in which a ureteral catheter will pass through the shaft of the knife blade, thus preventing section of the catheter by the blade. In some cases of a small caliber stricture that may not admit the ureteral catheter or a short, well-defined stricture in which creation of a false passage is unlikely, the catheter may not be used, but then there is a risk of creating a false passage.

Next, the stricture is incised. The blade is advanced from the instrument and placed into the lumen of the stricture to incise it at the 12 o'clock or dorsal midline position (Figs. 8-6 to 8-9). Although the urethral incision or stricturotomy can be made at any position, the 12 o'clock position is the safest. If the incision is placed dorsally other than in the midline, the chance is taken of entering the corpora cavernosa. When the incision is placed ventrally, there is a significant risk of passing through the urethra and corpus spongiosum into the subcutaneous tissue or even passing through the skin, thus creating a urethrocutaneous fistula.

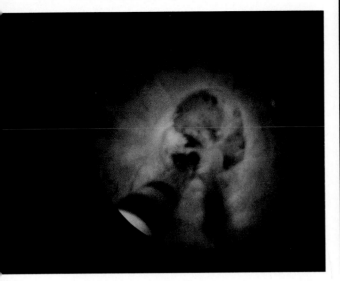

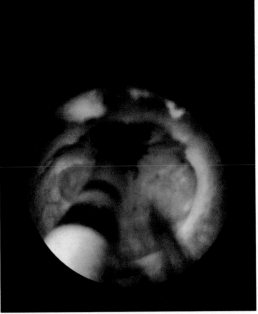

Figure 8-6. *The blade has been advanced alongside the ureteral catheter and the stricture has been incised at the 12 o'clock position. Bands of scar tissue persist at the proximal and distal extent of the incision.*

Figure 8-7. *The stricture has been fully incised. The membranous urethra and the urethral sphincter are evident immediately proximal to the incised area. Note minimal bleeding at the site of incision.*

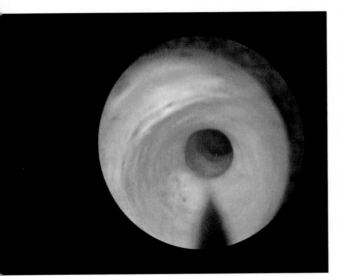

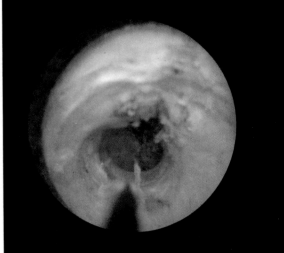

Figure 8-8. *The full extent of a mild stricture can be seen through the urethroscope.*

Figure 8-9. *The stricture has been incised at the 12 o'clock position and is partially open.*

The stricture is incised by applying the sharp edge of the knife blade to the scar tissue to be cut. A new sharp blade is essential for accurate and reliable incision. To cut the stricture, the entire instrument can be moved or the knife blade itself. The incision can be made by rocking the entire instrument in an arclike motion with the fulcrum at approximately the midpoint of the instrument while withdrawing the instrument for the length of the incision. The knife blade remains applied to the stricture in the midline ventrally while the entire instrument is moved. Although the procedure is viewed endoscopically, the field of view is limited because the instrument is turned with the telescope facing the wall of the urethra at an acute angle. The area of the stricture and incision is again inspected after the cut has been made to assess the extent and adequacy of the stricturotomy. If a portion of the stricture is still obvious or if individual restricting fibrous bands remain, then the procedure can be repeated to incise the remaining portion of the stricture. Only when the lumen is open and will accept the instrument, and all restrictive bands have been divided, is the incision complete.

An alternative operative technique is to divide the fibers of the stricture with repetitive, back and forth movements of the blade and its shaft, using the thumb control to advance and withdraw the blade. As the stricture is incised, the bands of scar retract laterally and the urethrotome and knife are advanced to complete the incision of the stricture with successive repetitions. In the case of a long stricture, this technique may allow more variation in the depth of the incision.

The incision should extend through the full thickness of the scar tissue forming the stricture into the underlying pink, vascularized tissue at the depths of the stricture (Figs. 8-7 to 8-9). This procedure causes only minimal bleeding, which can usually be controlled by placing a urethral catheter. Fulguration should be avoided to prevent further tissue necrosis and scarring.

We recommend incision of the stricture only to the level of well-vascularized, normal-appearing tissue and to a depth that will provide a lumen to admit the instrument. Although incision to a fixed, larger diameter (e.g., 30 Fr.) has occasionally been recommended, it does not appear to be necessary and, in some cases, may lead to extravasation of irrigant and cause harm[16]. The incision also should extend proximally and distally into any normal-appearing mucosa involved in the stricture process, which usually will not distend fully.

After incision of the stricture, the urethrotome can be advanced through the proximal urethra into the bladder. There is little danger of inadvertent damage to the urethra since the blade is retracted within the sheath of the urethrotome. The inner sheath and the working element with the telescope are then removed, leaving the slotted outer sheath in place to maintain a channel through the recently incised urethra. A Foley catheter as large as 18 Fr. can be inserted through the slotted sheath into the bladder and the sheath removed over the catheter.

TREATMENT OF MULTIPLE STRICTURES. Multiple strictures present particular problems for treatment. It may be difficult to pass a filiform or a small ureteral catheter through two strictures. Although the instrument may traverse the first stricture easily, it may be misdirected by that stricture and not pass the second obstruction. Treatment of strictures by visual internal urethrotomy may be difficult since incision of the first stricture may cause sufficient bleeding to obscure vision of the second stricture. In the normal urethra, the irrigating fluid will flow from the instrument proximally within the urethra to the bladder but a small caliber stricture proximal to another stricture may partially obstruct the flow of the irrigating fluid. This problem can be overcome by intermittently allowing the outflow of fluid through the instrument or by using a constant flow urethrotome. Irrigation can also be instilled through a ureteral catheter passed inside the working side channel, and subsequently drained through the irrigation channel of the instrument.

106

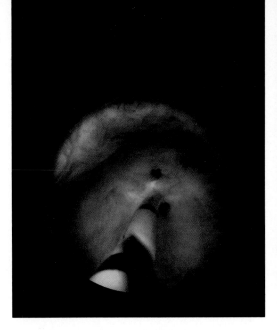

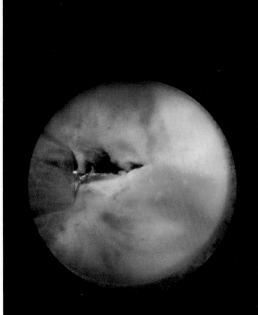

Figure 8-10. *A very stenotic bladder neck contracture is shown with a 5 Fr. ureteral catheter for comparison.*

Figure 8-11. *The initial incision is made laterally.*

TREATMENT OF BLADDER NECK CONTRACTURE. Bladder neck contractures may develop after bladder neck procedures, particularly prostatectomy. The symptoms are those of bladder outlet obstruction and usually cannot be distinguished from those of urethral stricture. The diagnosis can be confirmed as outlined above for stricture (Fig. 8-10; see also Chap. 4).

Just as for stricture, treatment consists of incision with a cold knife blade. For bladder neck contracture, however, incision should be made bilaterally, usually at the 3 and 9 o'clock positions (Fig. 8-11). If the bladder neck does not open fully, then a third incision can be made at the 12 o'clock position. Each incision is carried deep enough to free the circular cicatrix. The mucosa of the bladder proximally and the prostate distally can be seen to separate with the incision, allowing the full thickness of the incision to be appreciated (Figs. 8-12, 8-13). Catheterization and postoperative care are similar to the procedures previously outlined for urethral stricture.

The results of incision for bladder neck contracture have uniformly been good. Recurrences after this therapy have been rare and can be treated with a second procedure as necessary.

ANTIBIOTIC THERAPY. The urine must be cultured and any infection treated appropriately prior to urethrotomy. Even when the urine is sterile, we prefer to begin patients on antibiotics, prophylactically, prior to the procedure, and continue them postoperatively for a short period following removal of the catheter. The urine will then be free of bacteria and no extravasation of infected urine into the paraurethral tissue through the site of the incision will occur when the patient voids.

ANESTHESIA. Internal urethrotomy can be performed under general, spinal, or even local anesthesia (see Chap. 20). Local anesthesia with the intraurethral administration of 10 ml of 2% lidocaine jelly is satisfactory for VIU in many patients. General or spinal anesthesia should be considered in patients who are particularly anxious, in those with long and dense strictures, and in children. When the procedure is performed under local anesthesia, the patient can be discharged the same day or even be treated as an outpatient. A catheter is left intraurethrally and the patient instructed to return or to remove it personally in 2 days.

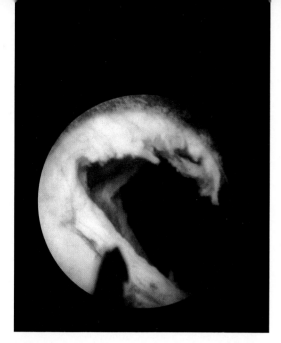

Figure 8-12. *The prostatic urethral mucosa and bladder mucosa can both be seen after a full thickness incision.*

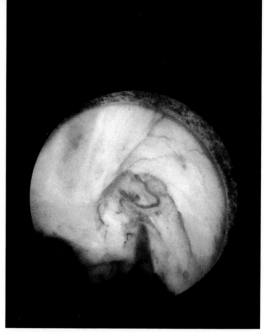

Figure 8-13. *The glistening yellow of the perivesical fat is evident at the depth of the incision (center of field).*

PERIOD OF CATHETERIZATION. The optimal period for catheterization following visual internal urethrotomy remains controversial. Recommendations have ranged from 6 weeks to 1 to 2 days to even no catheterization. From the accumulated series, catheterization at these different periods appears to result in similar success rates. Catheterization for 6 weeks is recommended to permit full reepithelialization of the urethra. A lesser period is recommended to avoid urethral inflammation and resultant strictures in other sites within the urethra. We have chosen to leave a catheter within the urethra until all bleeding from the urethrotomy ceases and coagulum is allowed to form over the site of incision, about 1 to 3 days.

HYDRAULIC DILATION. Hydraulic dilation of the urethra has been recommended by some authors. Following urethrotomy, the patient voids with manual compression of the urethra at the glans of the penis to dilate the entire urethra with the pressure of the urine. Theoretically, the urethra will be dilated and "bridging over" of the incised area with scar tissue will be minimized. Other urologists have objected to this technique because of the possibility of extravasation of urine through the area of incision into the paraurethral tissues. Although some authors have advocated the injection of steroids into the strictured area or dilation with catheters lubricated with steroid creams, these techniques have generally not been accepted and little evidence exists of their value.

COMPLICATIONS. The complications of visual internal urethrotomy have been relatively infrequent and mild. In the reported series, immediate postoperative complications have affected 2 to 15 percent of patients. Complications have included sepsis, hemorrhage, penile edema, and epididymitis (Table 8-1). In one series[16] impotence occurred in 4 of 179 patients (2.2%). Impotence resolved gradually over 6 to 12 months in 2 of the patients but remained unchanged for more than 1 and 4 years in the other 2 patients. The patients experiencing impotence in that series were characterized by long, dense strictures requiring relatively extensive incisions, and they each experienced massive penile edema postoperatively.

Table 8-1. Complications of VIU
(combined series of 1,376 patients)

Complication	Patients (%)
Hemorrhage	2.3
Sepsis	2.7
Penile edema	1.9
Hematoma	0.5
Epididymitis	0.2
Impotence	0.2
Other	2.4
Total	10.2

Table 8-2. Series of Visual Internal Urethrotomy for Urethral Stricture

Series	Year	No. Patients	Complications (%)	Satisfactory Results (%)	
				After Single Urethrotomy	Overall
Lipsky[13]	1977	32	9.3	53	83
Matouschek[14]	1978	518	11.0	66.8	79.3
Gaches[6]	1979	197	8.4	51.8	81
Renders[17]	1979	44	11.4		75
Sachnoff[18]	1980	75	9.0	71	71
Walther[22]	1980	60	2.0	83	93 (6 mo)
Fourcade[5]	1981	123	15.4		76 (5 yr)
Smith[21]	1981	39	13.0		95 (2 yr)
Bekirov[2]	1982	128	5.5	70	85
Gibod[7]	1982	160	7.5		56 (6 mo), 43 (1 yr), 25 (2 yr)
Total		1,376			

Notably absent from the list of complications in the published literature is incontinence. The accuracy afforded by visual control of the incision permits sparing of the sphincter in most cases. If, however, following a transurethral resection of the prostate (TURP) the presence of a stricture masks a sphincter injury, stricture release may uncover preexisting incontinence.

RESULTS. The results of visual internal urethrotomy for treatment of urethral strictures with a single or, in some cases, also a secondary procedure have been very good. The success rates have ranged from 52 to 83 percent with a single procedure and from 56 to 88 percent overall (Table 8-2). Although the criteria for the grading of satisfactory results have varied, there is general agreement that unsatisfactory results occur with recurrent strictures requiring either more than two urethrotomies or further treatment such as urethroplasty. Many reports have used urinary flow rate as an indication of an adequate urethral lumen. A flow rate greater than 10 or 15 ml per second has been accepted as a good result. Most failures are evident within 6 to 9 months but recurrent strictures may develop several years after treatment.

The success rate with visual internal urethrotomy can be related to several factors in the techniques of treatment or the character of the stricture. A period of catheterization lasting less than 1 week appears to be associated with better voiding results than catheterization for more than 1 week. In several series, better results were seen with short, single strictures than with long or multiple strictures. The success rate appears to be similar with strictures of inflammatory, iatrogenic, or traumatic origin. The pattern of the strictures has been similar in most series (Table 8-3). Failure is more frequent in anterior urethral strictures than in bulbous strictures, but cure rates approaching 100 percent are routinely reported with bladder neck contractures.

Table 8-3. Etiology of Strictures Treated by VIU in 1,376 Patients

Etiology	Patients (%)
Infection	24.8
Trauma	
Iatrogenic	43.4
External	7.9
Congenital	2.9
Other	0.2
Unknown	20.7

VISUAL URETHROTOMY FOR OBLITERATED URETHRA.

Severe strictures with total obliteration of the urethral lumen may develop after urethral trauma. These lesions are not life threatening when urinary drainage has been provided proximally by suprapubic drainage, but reestablishment of urethral continuity can offer normal urinary and sexual function. Although reconstruction can be accomplished by urethroplasty, continuity can also be reestablished endoscopically.

In some patients, a very fine opening in the urethra may remain, although it may be functionally nonexistent. The opening can be defined by injecting methylene blue into the bladder through a suprapubic puncture or catheter and then manually pressing on the bladder. The urethral opening can then be seen cystoscopically and the incision made at the 12 o'clock position.

The length of the obliterated segment can be defined by placing radiographic contrast medium within the proximal and distal portions of urethral lumen. A retrograde urethrogram will outline the distal lumen of the urethra. Contrast placed into the bladder with the patient attempting to void will define the proximal urethra. Alternatively, an endoscope placed through the suprapubic tract into the bladder can be used to place a small catheter, such as a ureteral catheter, through the bladder neck into the proximal urethra for instillation of contrast.

To use the endoscopic approach, access must be available to the proximal and distal margins of the obliterated lumen. A metal sound or a lighted instrument should be passed through the suprapubic tract and bladder into the urethra and then advanced to the level of obstruction. A light, such as a fiberoptic light bundle or a flexible nephroscope, is preferable since the light shining through the tissue will serve as a guide during advance of the urethrotome. The flexible nephroscope has the additional advantage of visual placement through the bladder into the urethra.

Distally, the urethrotome is placed through the urethral meatus into the urethra and advanced to the point of obstruction (Fig. 8-14). The scar tissue obliterating the urethral lumen is then incised along the tract toward the point of light to a depth sufficient to permit advancement of the urethrotome. When the proximal lumen of the urethra is entered, the sound or nephroscope is removed and the urethrotome can be advanced into the bladder.

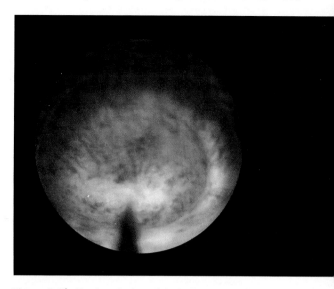

Figure 8-14. *Total occlusion of the bulbous urethra is evident in this male after previous urethral trauma.*

A urethral catheter is then placed through the sheath of the instrument and left through the urethra for at least 6 weeks prior to its removal. In these patients with total loss of continuity of the urethra, full reepithelialization of the incised segment should occur while the catheter is in place. We prefer to maintain suprapubic drainage during this time until satisfactory voiding has been established through the urethra.

There is a high risk of reformation of the stricture and, therefore, the patient must be followed very closely, both symptomatically and with determination of urinary flow rates. A second (or even more) urethrotomy or dilation may be necessary to maintain the urethral lumen. Several authors have described their experience with this procedure in relatively few patients. It appears to be as successful a technique as urethroplasty[12], and one that deserves further evaluation.

USE OF INTERNAL URETHROTOMY.

The excellent results reported with visual internal urethrotomy for treatment of urethral stricture, as well as the low complication rate, combine as major advantages supporting this technique. Visual internal urethrotomy should be considered for the primary treatment of urethral strictures as well as for recurrences developing after dilation or urethroplasty.

REFERENCES

1. Attwater, H. L. The history of urethral strictures. *Br. J. Urol.* 14:39, 1942.
2. Bekirov, H. M., Tein, A. B., Reid, R. E., and Freed, S. Z. Internal urethrotomy under direct vision in men. *J. Urol.* 128:37, 1982.
3. Carlton, F. E., Scardino, P. L., and Quattlebaum, R. B. Treatment of urethral strictures with internal urethrotomy and 6 weeks of Silastic catheter drainage. *J. Urol.* 111:191, 1974.
4. Cole, A. T., Peterson, D. D., Biddle, W. S., and Fried, F. A. Uroflowmetry: A useful technique in the management of urethral strictures. *J. Urol.* 112:483, 1974.
5. Fourcade, R. O., et al. Endoscopic internal urethrotomy for treatment of urethral strictures. *Urology* 18:33, 1981.
6. Gaches, C. G. C., et al. The role of selective internal urethrotomy in the management of urethral stricture: A multi-centre evaluation. *Br. J. Urol.* 51:579, 1979.
7. Gibod, L. B., and LePortz, B. Endoscopic urethrotomy: Does it live up to its promises? *J. Urol.* 127:433, 1982.
8. Katz, A. S., and Waterhouse, K. Treatment of urethral strictures in men by internal urethrotomy. A study of 61 patients. *J. Urol.* 105:807, 1971.
9. Kinder, P. W., and Rous, S. N. The treatment of urethral stricture disease by internal urethrotomy: A clinical review. *J. Urol.* 121:45, 1979.
10. Kircheim, D., Tremann, J. A., and Ansell, J. A. Transurethral urethrotomy under vision. *J. Urol.* 119:496, 1978.
11. Konnak, J. W., and Kogan, B. A. Otis internal urethrotomy in the treatment of urethral stricture disease. *J. Urol.* 124:356, 1980.
12. Lieberman, S. F., and Barry, J. M. Retreat from transpubic urethroplasty for obliterated membranous urethral strictures. *J. Urol.* 128:379, 1982.
13. Lipsky, H., and Hubmer, G. Direct vision urethrotomy in the management of urethral strictures. *Br. J. Urol.* 49:725, 1977.
14. Matouschek, E. Internal urethrotomy of urethral stricture under vision—A five year report. *Urol. Res.* 6:147, 1978.
15. McCallum, R. W., and Colapinto, V. The role of urethrography in urethral disease. I. Accurate radiological localization of the membranous urethra and distal sphincters in normal male subjects. *J. Urol.* 122:607, 1979.
16. McDermott, D. W., Bates, R. J., Heney, N. M., and Althausen, A. Erectile impotence as complication of direct vision cold knife urethrotomy. *Urology* 18:476, 1981.
17. Renders, G., DeNobel, J., Debruyne, F., Delaene, K., and Moonen, W. Cold knife optical urethrotomy. *Urology* 15:475, 1979.
18. Sacknoff, E. J., and Kerr, W. S. Direct vision cold knife urethrotomy. *J. Urol.* 123:492, 1980.
19. Sacse, H. Die transurethral schorfe Schlitzung der Haunuohrenstriktur unter Sicht. *M.M.W.* 116:2147, 1974.
20. Siroky, M. B., Olsson, C. A., and Krane, R. J. The flow nomogram. II. Clinical correlation. *J. Urol.* 123:208, 1980.
21. Smith, P. J. B., Dunn, M., and Roberts, J. B. M. Surgical management of urethral stricture in the male. *Urology* 18:582, 1981.
22. Walther, P. C., Parsons, C. L., and Schmidt, J. D. Direct vision internal urethrotomy in the management of urethral strictures. *J. Urol.* 123:497, 1980.

9
TRANSURETHRAL RESECTION OF THE PROSTATE

Edward S. Lyon

Jeffry L. Huffman

Demetrius H. Bagley

Of all the procedures carried out by urologic surgeons, transurethral resection of the prostate (TURP) typifies their specialty and sets them apart from other surgeons. The procedure, almost more than any other, is the focus of considerable time, thought, and discussion, not only by the urologic trainee but by the practicing urologist as well. The drive for perfection of transurethral prostatectomy, perhaps more than any other endoscopic technique, remains a lifelong goal for all practicing urologists.

THE BENIGN PROSTATIC HYPERTROPHY PROBLEM. Vesical outlet obstruction, with consequent choking of the urinary stream, develops as a problem of advancing years. The symptom complex of prostatism may develop slowly, almost unnoticed by the individual until he is required by the urging from his bladder to arise during the night on one or more occasions. In response to the increased outlet resistance at the bladder neck, the bladder wall musculature becomes thicker and more powerful to accomplish its task. After bladder filling, the spontaneous contraction of the now more powerful bladder creates pressures that the individual finds difficult to suppress, thereby inducing an unnatural sense of urgency to void. As the prostate continues to enlarge, bladder emptying becomes less complete, and the resultant residual volume of urine necessitates more frequent trips to urinate. As the increasing symptoms become less tolerable to the patient, he may seek remedy for his malady. On the other hand, the symptoms may ameliorate spontaneously for a period, convincing the patient that he can avoid seeking attention for the problem. The development of superimposed infection, a bladder stone, or acute urinary retention may be the event for which he finally demands medical attention.

One of the more serious consequences of benign prostatic hypertrophy (BPH) is obstructive uropathy with upper tract deterioration. This condition may develop asymptomatically and be unnoticed by the patient. In addition, it may not be obvious on physical examination. Often discovered only through determination of blood urea nitrogen or serum creatinine, or perhaps through an excretory urogram, the possibility of renal deterioration demands that some determination of renal function be made when the urologist initially evaluates the patient with BPH.

Although there is little need for further justification of surgical correction of bladder neck obstruction when these secondary conditions arise, indications for prostatic surgery are not so well defined in other, less extreme, circumstances. In the absence of objective indications of bladder neck obstruction, such as bladder trabeculation, development of a residual volume of urine, or reduced caliber and flow of the urinary stream, the urologist must be careful to avoid unwarranted surgical intervention since the symptoms may not be the result of obstruction alone but rather the manifestation of an inflammatory or neurologic disorder. Indication for surgery early in the course of prostatic enlargement may be mainly the patient's own intolerance of his symptoms. All urologists must develop their own criteria for selecting patients to undergo transurethral resection for BPH.

While there are relatively few contraindications for prostatic surgery, the benefits to be achieved from the procedure must be compared to the hazards and consequences of the operation. Any condition that would create a hazard for surgery or anesthesia must be thoroughly evaluated and corrected since the urgent need to relieve obstruction can be bypassed with catheter drainage. With the bladder decompressed, pre-existing medical conditions compromising a surgical procedure can undergo appropriate treatment before embarking on the operation. Individuals who are completely bedridden, have a relatively brief life expectancy, or are mentally unable to benefit from the procedure, may be managed best with catheter drainage.

PROSTATECTOMY

Preoperative Evaluation. A decision to correct bladder neck obstruction surgically must be preceded by a detailed evaluation of the urinary tract. Many different studies have been employed both to evaluate the prostate directly and to search for secondary effects. Unfortunately, many of these tests have degenerated into routine preoperative studies without scientific justification of their merit or cost effectiveness as screening tests. Perhaps the most obvious and readily accepted procedure is direct digital palpation of the prostate on rectal examination. This single examination affords such valuable information that prostatectomy without it, such as in the patient after proctectomy, is a risk-laden undertaking fraught with dangerous complications. Manual examination of the prostate allows estimation of the size, configuration, and consistency of the gland as well as the condition of the rectum and any coincidental masses. In a study of tests differentiating carcinoma of the prostate, Guinan and coworkers[2] found digital examination of the prostate to be the most valuable test in recognizing the presence and extent of the tumor.

Urinalysis is another study that is essential for the preoperative evaluation. It is a major screening test for urinary infection as well as a sensitive index for systemic diseases such as diabetes mellitus or primary renal disorders.

Determination of the urinary flow rate will quantitate the quality of the patient's urinary stream. Further urodynamic testing can be reserved for those patients in whom it is specifically indicated.

Laboratory studies, such as the blood urea nitrogen and serum creatinine, are useful as noted above for indicating the presence of significant renal deterioration. The serum acid phosphatase may indicate the spread of carcinoma beyond the prostatic capsule and will rarely be elevated in the patient with a normal prostatic examination.

The value of the intravenous pyelogram as a routine preoperative study before prostatectomy has been questioned[1]. When used prospectively, it does not appear to be cost efficient in detecting either severe upper tract damage or neoplasms. Nevertheless, many individual urologists have found it of value in indicating early obstructive changes and for estimating residual urinary volume. In occasional patients, renal tumors may be discovered, and it is difficult to evaluate questions of cost effectiveness in these individual patients[3]. The study also gives an indication of the status of the upper tract should the rare instance of damage to the ureteral orifice be encountered postoperatively.

Cystoscopy is an essential part of the preoperative evaluation. When there is a high expectation of prostatectomy, the cystoscopy may be deferred until the time of the anesthetic immediately prior to the procedure, thus saving the patient the distress of a preoperative examination. On the other hand, when the possibility of surgery is low, preliminary cystoscopy may be helpful in determining whether to avoid or to proceed with the operation. One must remember that the reason for the operation is not that the prostate is enlarged but rather that the prostate is causing a problem for the patient that deserves remedy. The urologist cannot determine by looking at the prostate endoscopically whether or not the individual can urinate adequately through the lumen being visualized. Some prostates appear cystoscopically to have only minimal enlargement but may cause intolerable symptoms, while others may be extremely large without causing incapacitating symptoms or objective evidence of significant obstruction. Cystoscopy is most useful for determining the presence of associated factors such as trabeculation, bladder calculi, or urothelial neoplasms.

Route. All surgeons must determine, based on their experience and ease with the procedure, their own methods of approaching any particular gland surgically. In general, the smaller the prostate gland, the harder it is to remove in an open procedure and the more amenable it is to a transurethral operation. Conversely, the larger the gland, the easier an open surgical procedure becomes while the transurethral approach increases in difficulty. Preliminary cystoscopy is valuable in evaluating the size of the gland and thus assisting in a decision on the surgical approach. Currently it is estimated that approximately 90 percent of the prostatectomies performed for BPH are done transurethrally.

Instrumentation. Forerunners of the current-day resectoscopes appeared in the middle and late 1920s. Several developments occurred during this period to mark the beginning of transurethral resection of the prostate. Stern[8] developed a movable wire loop that could be kept under observation during its excursion through cystoscopic instruments. It could be used to trim away obstructing prostatic tissue with a radio frequency current.

McCarthy[6] attempted to overcome the resulting bleeding by application of a different current. It was not until Davis, however, in collaboration with Liebel-Flarsheim Company, modified the system to combine a radio frequency cutting current with an effective coagulation current that the Davis Bovie generator was developed. Davis then developed the technique of prostatic resection and control of bleeding by coagulation, thus defining the operative approach and demonstrating the effectiveness and safety of the procedure. By the late 1930s it became clear that transurethral resection of the prostate was developing into an important technique for the relief of prostatic obstruction.

In the ensuing 50 years the basic idea of the movable loop with a cutting and coagulation current has remained the same. Many improvements in the mechanics, optics, illumination, and electrical generators have evolved, however, making the modern-day instrument far easier and safer to use. The mechanism utilizing a rack and pinion gear developed by Stern is still preferred by many urologists today. The Stern instrument requires two hands for operation. One hand is required to move the pinion gear while the other hand holds the instrument proper.

In addition, there are many other types of working elements from which the modern-day urologist can select his preference. A variety of single-handed instruments using either a thumb or finger action to move the loop have been developed by Iglesias, Baumrocker, and others.

A more recent variation in the instrument has been the development of the continuous irrigation system[5]. The standard, intermittent one-way flow has been replaced by a continuous two-way flow so that the working element can remain in the sheath and the operator can maintain good visibility without the need to empty the bladder. Thus, the resection can be continued for longer uninterrupted periods. The instrument contains two channels in the two concentric sheaths in order that the irrigant can flow into one channel and exit from the other. The outflow may be assisted by a pump or other suction device to ensure exit of the fluid with minimal intravesical pressure.

Early reports utilizing continuous flow resectoscopes stressed the impressively low volume of fluid absorbed systemically and the blood loss. In these studies, however, there was no control group of comparable resections with conventional instruments. In a controlled study, Flechner and Williams[4] compared 36 randomized patients who had undergone prostatectomies with either the continuous flow resectoscope or the conventional resectoscope. They found no statistically significant differences in blood loss, resection rate, or irrigant absorption between the two groups. Those authors, however, anecdotally noted the value of the continuous flow resectoscope in maintaining a constant volume in the bladder during resection of urothelial tumors. In that study the same residents were the resectionists in both groups. In the hands of an experienced resectionist, the rate of bladder filling and the need to empty the bladder frequently may be a more significant factor since the actual resection may be considerably faster.

We prefer the continuous flow resectoscope and appreciate the ability to maintain the position of the instrument when there is bleeding within the prostatic fossa and there is no need to empty the bladder. Preference for one or the other instrument remains a very personal choice of the individual surgeon.

An alternative technique to obtain continuous flow during prostatic resection has also been described by placing a catheter suprapubically into the bladder. At the initiation of the procedure, the bladder is filled and distended with irrigating fluid and a suprapubic catheter is passed through a percutaneous trocar puncture into the bladder. The catheter allows drainage of fluid from the bladder during the resection. With this procedure, which has been described in detail by Reuter[7], there is a unidirectional flow from the resectoscope through the prostate and bladder and out the catheter. Thus, any blood and chips are washed away from the instrument. Although difficulty with obstruction of the outflow port of the earlier catheters with prostatic chips arose, more recent designs with multiple drainage holes have overcome this difficulty. This technique provides the same advantages of continuous flow while maintaining a low intravesical pressure. It necessitates, however, an additional invasive procedure with its own risks.

Electrosurgery. Electrosurgical units provide two essential functions for endoscopic surgery: cutting and hemostasis. These units generate bipolar, high-frequency electrical currents that perform the function of cutting or coagulation at a radius of approximately 3 mm from the resectoscope loop[11] and then pass harmlessly through the patient. Most units function at frequencies well above those that stimulate neuromuscular responses and, provided that a conductive grounding plate is used to complete the electrical circuit, the patient is not harmed from unwanted muscular convulsion or thermoelectric burns.

Three forms of electrical currents provide the desired effects necessary for transurethral electroresection. These currents—cutting, coagulating, and blended—differ in wave patterns and frequency, and thus produce varied effects on tissue.

The *cutting current* is a continuous, high-frequency wave that is undamped with repeating equal amplitude oscillations[11]. Its effect is dissolution of tissue with little or no coagulation. The effect is maximized with a more powerful current and with tissue that has a high content of water. A fine caliber loop provides more concentrated current for efficient cutting whereas a large caliber loop or one encrusted by tissue will disperse the current and impede cutting. Although using powerful cutting currents with a rapid cutting stroke allows efficient cutting with less tissue destruction, using a level high enough to cause arcing or flaming should be avoided.

The *coagulating current* has a slower wave frequency than the cutting current and is highly damped or impeded with recurring oscillations of progressively decreasing amplitude. The newer solid state electrosurgical units use blocking oscillations to provide this type of wave whereas older models used a spark gap.

The current produced coagulates by dessicating tissue, which causes shrinkage and retraction of blood vessels. Whereas the thermal build-up with the cutting current is negligible, the heat produced by coagulation can be very destructive to tissues[10]. It is essential to use the lowest effective setting for coagulation and not prolong its application. Prolonged coagulation or using high coagulating currents leads to charring of the tissues (black coagulation) instead of surgical hemostasis with limited tissue destruction (white coagulation)[10].

The third current form is the *blended current,* which combines the wave properties of the cutting and coagulating currents to allow cutting with effective hemostasis. It is especially useful when resecting vascular tissue such as bladder carcinoma to allow some hemostasis during the initial cutting stroke. The proportions of each current can be adjusted, allowing the urologist to obtain the desired effect according to what is visualized endoscopically. Usually a minimal level of coagulating current is added so that the cutting effect is not diminished by dessicating the tissue.

The use of electrical currents during transurethral surgery may lead to unintentional thermoelectric burns to the patient, urologist, or other operating room personnel. Fortunately, presently used solid state units with advanced electronics have built-in safeguards to minimize these complications.

For a high-frequency electrical current to pass harmlessly through the patient once released by the active electrode (resectoscope loop), the electrical circuit must be completed by a grounding plate properly attached to the patient and to the electrosurgical unit. This plate must make contact with a wide area of skin that is not insulated by hair or other nonconducting materials. Plates that have poor skin contact may allow current flow through a limited skin area, resulting in electrical burns. Water-soluble conductive gels help to enhance conductivity and diminish heat build-up at the site of the grounding plate.

Patient grounding plates with faulty connections to the electrosurgical units may force current to leave the patient by alternative routes, such as the urologist, anesthesia equipment, electrocardiograph leads, thermocouple probes, or any metal contacts, once again leading to thermoelectrical burns. Most electrosurgical units presently used have built-in safeguards that do not allow the current generator to operate if the ground plate is not attached or the electrode is faulty.

The irrigation fluid must be nonconductive so that the current will pass through the small area of tissue at the tip of the electrode rather than dissipate in a large volume of conductive solution within the bladder. If the instrument does not cut the tissue at the beginning or suddenly during the resection, in addition to determining that the resectoscope is properly connected to an activated electrosurgical unit, the surgeon should be alert to the possibility that a conductive solution, such as saline, has been introduced into the system.

Other injuries occur when the resectoscope loop is activated accidentally during its removal and placement while still within the metal sheath. This may lead to urethral or meatal burns. Stray electrical currents may also involve the urologist since he or she is well grounded by the operating room floor. Suggestions to limit these occurrences include better insulation of the resectoscope loops, thicker nonconductive gloves, and nonconductive operating chairs for transurethral surgery[9].

Technique. No topic at urologic meetings inspires more participation, interest, and variety than the techniques of transurethral resection of the prostate. Each urologist has developed his or her own perfections to, or idiosyncrasies regarding, the techniques. In this discussion, we must rely heavily on our individual preferences, but we attempt to indicate those points at which there is considerable variation in technique.

In order to resect a modest-sized gland, the urologist must first select an instrument. In general, it is best to use the smallest instrument that will do the job. While one of the authors prefers to use a 24 Fr. resectoscope, another prefers the slightly larger resection capability of the 26 Fr. instrument for most resections. The still larger 28 Fr. instrument, which can be reserved for larger adenomas, offers even greater capability. The instrument and urethra should both be lubricated liberally. A film of sterile petroleum jelly can be applied to an insulated sheath to provide lubrication for a longer period, while a conductive lubricant should be used on a conductive, metal sheath.

The adequacy of the urethral lumen should be determined by passing sounds prior to any attempt to pass the resectoscope itself. We prefer to dilate the urethra with Van Buren sounds to a lumen two French sizes larger than the resectoscope. If the urethra does not accept the selected sounds, then internal urethrotomy or perineal urethrostomy should be considered to provide an adequate lumen or to bypass the distal urethra. The resectoscope should not be passed transurethrally for the procedure if the lumen does not readily accept the instrument since such trauma, coupled with the resultant edema in the urethra, will frequently result in a stricture.

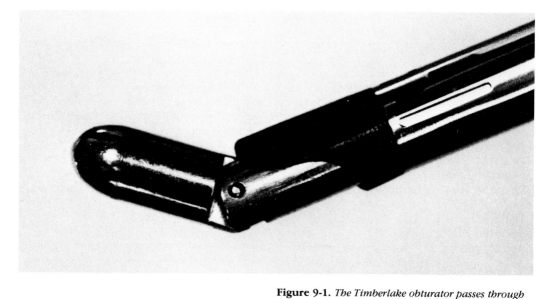

Figure 9-1. *The Timberlake obturator passes through the resectoscope sheath to fill the lumen and provide an angled tip to help guide the instrument into the bladder.*

Accurate placement of the instrument can be accomplished best with the use of a visual obturator to introduce the instrument under direct vision. As noted in Chapter 7, whenever a procedure is undertaken for visualization of the prostate or bladder, the urethra must be inspected, preferably when the instrument is initially introduced. As the tip of the endoscope passes through the prostatic urethra, the urologist can assess the length of the gland accurately for the first time. By positioning the telescope at the verumontanum—the distal landmark of the prostate—and then passing it proximally to the vesical neck, the length of prostatic urethra requiring resection can be accurately measured.

Alternatively, the resectoscope can be placed transurethrally into the bladder using only tactile control. An obturator should be in place to fill the lumen of the sheath during passage (Fig. 9-1). The telescope is placed into the sheath after it reaches the bladder. The prostate and bladder are then inspected as noted.

After the instrument enters the bladder, the lumen is inspected to locate the landmarks and the configuration of the prostate. The visual obturator and forward viewing telescope are removed and a right-angle telescope is substituted as necessary to allow thorough inspection of the interior of the bladder. At this point, it is necessary to determine if a coexisting bladder tumor, which should be treated first, is present. It is also important to determine the relative positions of the ureteral orifices with regard to the vesical neck as well as any intravesical extension of the prostate.

It is essential in planning a resection to identify the presence or absence of significant median lobe enlargement, intravesical lateral lobe enlargement, and the relative positions of the ureteral orifices. For the inexperienced resectionist, median lobe enlargement may appear as lateral lobe hypertrophy if the instrument passes to one of the sides of the median lobe rather than over the top of the lobe (see Figs. 4-7, 4-8). The entire anatomic configuration of the prostate should be appreciated to prevent miscalculation of gland size in relationship to the bladder.

Once the orifices have been located and the intravesical prostatic enlargement determined, it is important to identify the distal extent of the prostate in the region of the verumontanum (see Figs. 4-6, 4-9). This configuration should be committed to memory since the resectionist will use the verumontanum many times during the resection as a landmark to avoid injury to the urethral sphincter, located just distal to the verumontanum. It may be helpful to mark the level of the verumontanum on the lateral and anterior surfaces of the mucosa with coagulation current so that the distal extent of the prostate can be recognized without turning the instrument back to the 6 o'clock position while resecting laterally and anteriorly at the apex of the gland.

Resection. Several nationally respected resection-ists, when gathered for a panel discussion on the techniques of transurethral resection of the prostate, opened their respective statements with the following lines.

Speaker 1: "I always begin my resection at the 12 o'clock position with a long bold cut and then proceed down on one lobe or the other at the capsular plane."

Speaker 2: "I never start at 12 o'clock—it seems as though every time I resect at 12 o'clock, I get into bad bleeding. I save that until the last."

Speaker 3: "I like to begin with a median lobe first and then proceed to the larger of the two lateral lobes leaving the roof until last."

All of these experts get good results from their resections because all strive for the same end point, even though they take different routes to achieve it. Their diversity of approach demonstrates that more than one way is available to remove the prostate successfully with a resectoscope.

The aim of the procedure is to remove as much adenoma as possible while preserving the true prostate, bladder neck, and sphincter. The resection should be carried to the level of the capsule, or true prostate, at each level. At that point, bleeding can be controlled, voiding function will be optimized, and the possibility of regrowth will be minimized.

MEDIAN LOBE. If the median lobe is enlarged, we think that there are good reasons to resect that lobe first (Fig. 9-2). Since the resection involving the median lobe is necessarily carried out within the bladder rather than the prostatic urethra, clarity of the irrigation fluid within the bladder is crucial to visualize the intravesical landmarks. If one has resected elsewhere in the prostate initially and generated significant bleeding, then vision within the bladder may be sufficiently restricted to make resection of the median lobe less than ideal.

The median lobe is best approached by having sufficient irrigant in the bladder to keep the wall away from the resecting loop. The continuous flow instrument can be used in this situation, just as in the resection of bladder tumors, to maintain a nearly constant volume within the bladder. The resection is then begun laterally at the top of the median lobe by placing the loop on the intravesical side and pulling the lobe toward the instrument slightly before engaging the cutting current. Thus, the resectionist can ensure that the loop is not against the bladder wall while the current is activated. A series of cuts across the top of the median

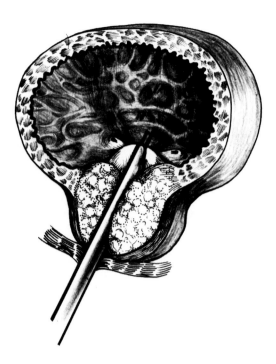

Figure 9-2. *The resectoscope has been passed transurethrally into the bladder, which is partially distended with irrigant. There is some prominence of the median lobe but the orifices are visible.*

lobe is then made, with care taken not to leave any significant bleeders even though the same area will be resected again in the next series of cuts. The median lobe should be removed in pieces from its anterior surface to the bladder neck. Any attempt to amputate the median lobe at its base may result in loss of a large mass of adenoma into the bladder with subsequent difficulty in retrieval.

This is also the time to adjust the cutting current so that the loop cuts sharply through the adenoma without fouling the wire. The minimal current that will cut without fouling the loop should be used since an excessively high cutting current will make the adenoma easier to resect but will also facilitate resection of the bladder wall, prostatic capsule, and urethral sphincter. Since the adenoma is the easiest of these tissues to cut, the use of a minimal setting will allow one to recognize when the loop is held against either the muscular fibers of the bladder or the prostatic capsule. This differential cutting can help to identify these structures and thus to avoid extensive damage.

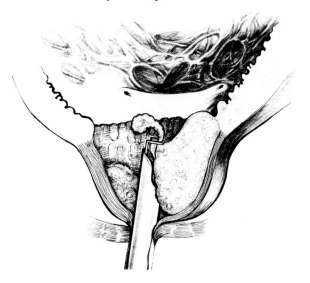

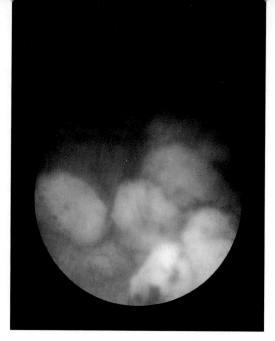

Figure 9-3. *The median lobe and the proximal portion of the right lateral lobe have been resected. The resection continues with the proximal portion of the left lateral lobe.*

Figure 9-4. *Within the bladder, numerous chips of prostatic adenoma are partially obscured by blood within the irrigant.*

As the resection approaches the base of the median lobe, the urologist must remain alert for fibers of the bladder wall musculature (Fig. 9-3), the identification of which signifies complete resection. The position of the ureteral orifices must also be known in order to avoid injury during this portion of the resection. Before leaving the area of the median lobe, thorough inspection for the completeness of the resection and control of bleeding must precede the next step in TURP, resection of the lateral lobe.

As prostatic chips begin to accumulate on the bladder floor, the inexperienced resectionist may identify them as prostate to be resected and, therefore, inadvertently begin to resect the posterior bladder wall (Fig. 9-4). Obviously, this must be consciously avoided.

LATERAL LOBES. The lateral lobes of the prostate are approached after complete resection of the median lobe with accurate hemostasis. Although resectionists strongly disagree as to exactly which part of the vesical neck to approach first, there is almost universal agreement that the resection should begin at the vesical neck rather than at the apex of the prostate.

One of the authors prefers to begin the resection at either the 1 or 11 o'clock position, resecting the larger of the two lateral lobes first. Another of the authors prefers to begin at the 5 or 7 o'clock position to control the major vascular supply early. If there is significant intravesical extension of the adenoma, this must be resected initially by angling the instrument toward the side of the lobe being resected and catching the intravesical extension of the gland with a loop to be certain that one does not resect the bladder wall (Figs. 9-4, 9-5, 9-6). Resection is continued at that site to determine when the intravesical extension has been completely removed and to identify the junction of the bladder wall and the base of the prostate. When resecting at the 5 and 7 o'clock positions along the bladder neck, considerable care must be taken to identify the ureteral orifice prior to each looping of the intravesical extension since the adenoma may extend intravesically to a point superior to the location of the orifice. The remainder of the intravesical prostatic tissue on that same side can then be resected without trying to make long strokes along the full length of the prostatic urethra. Rather, the resecting strokes can be limited to the length of the bladder neck.

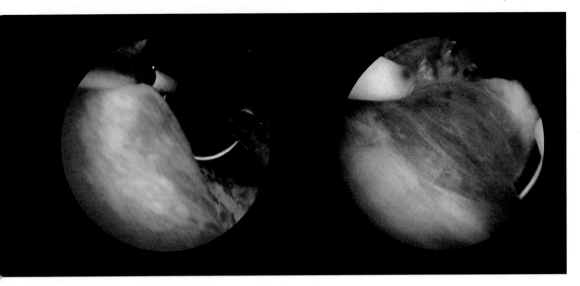

Figure 9-5. A, B. *A full chip of the adenoma is taken using the full depth of the resectoscope loop.*

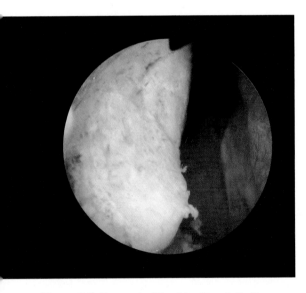

Figure 9-6. *Removal of the chip of prostatic tissue reveals the typical fluffy white appearance of the benign prostatic adenoma.*

Resection of tissue at the bladder neck accomplishes several aims: (1) By allowing the opening of the vesical neck area, the tissue blocking the vesical neck can be removed, which permits the prostatic chips to fall freely into the bladder. (2) It enables the resectionist to identify with some security the edge of the bladder wall and the junction with the prostate itself. (3) The surgeon can resect across the vascular channels that supply much of the rest of the adenoma. Although there are major arterial vessels in this area, they can usually be seen and accurately fulgurated with the electrocautery loop, which thus allows resection of much of the remainder of the adenoma with only modest bleeding.

No further resection of bladder neck tissue is necessary once the initial resection shows that the fluffy, opaque, white adenomatous tissue has been removed, leaving the vesical neck fibers exposed (Fig. 9-7). Contracture of the vesical neck after prostatic resection has been thought to result from overextensive resection and fulguration at the bladder neck. Manipulation should be limited to that necessary to provide an adequate lumen with removal of the adenoma.

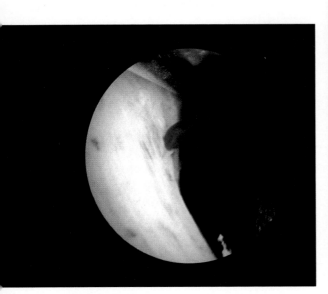

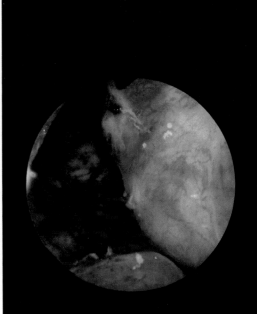

Figure 9-7. *Resection within the proximal prostatic fossa has been carried to the level of the prostatic capsule. The radially arranged fibers of the bladder neck and the capsule are evident. There is a venous bleeder at the bladder neck.*

Figure 9-8. *After resection of the right lobe of the prostate, the verumontanum is evident at the 6 o'clock position and the unresected lobe remains. There is minimal bleeding within the prostatic fossa.*

Once the resectionist is satisfied that the intra-vesical extension of the adenoma has been removed with adequate hemostasis, the main body of lateral lobes within the prostatic urethra can be approached. The remainder of the lateral lobe is resected by withdrawing the instrument to a point near the verumontanum, extending the loop past the bulk of the adenoma, and taking long, sweeping bites through the lobe. The strokes at first are passed in a straight line but, as the resection approaches the prostatic capsule, the loop must be brought toward the operator while the instrument is angulated to the side. The excursion of the loop thus forms a curved arc, such as would be used to remove the meat from the inside of a coconut.

On completion of the resection in one area, it is evident that the consistently fluffy, opaque, white adenomatous tissue changes abruptly into mottled white and blotchy fibrous material. This tissue, which sometimes has a slightly glassy appearance, identifies the prostatic capsule. No further resection of that tissue should be made because of the possibility of perforation through the capsule, which may also be identified by fat or darkness beyond. It is not unusual to identify a thin place in the prostatic capsule either by observing a small area of fat directly or identifying translucent edematous adventitial tissue in a small area. This is indicative of a small capsular perforation, and the resection can be continued at those areas where adenoma remains.

If a large perforation is made, then the urologist must consider its location and significance to judge whether the procedure should be terminated at that point. The major concern is whether there is a wide open channel through which large volumes of fluid can exit during the remainder of the resection, or whether the location is near the base of the prostate posteriorly where fluid could collect and raise the bladder floor behind the trigone, thus creating considerable difficulty in recognizing the vesical outlet.

In resecting the lateral lobe, occasionally it appears that the resection is nearly complete when the prostatic capsule contracts slightly and forces a mass of adenoma that had not been recognized previously into the operative fluid. Clearly, more resection of that tissue is then indicated. More adenoma may be delivered into the lumen with a finger placed in the rectum. When one lateral lobe has been completely resected, a similar procedure is performed on the opposite side (Fig. 9-8).

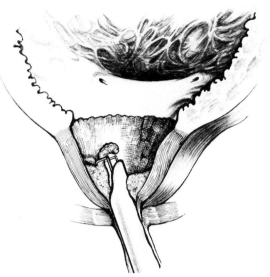

Figure 9-9. *After resection of the median lobe and the proximal portions of both lateral lobes, the residual tissue at the apex of the prostate is carefully resected to the level of the verumontanum.*

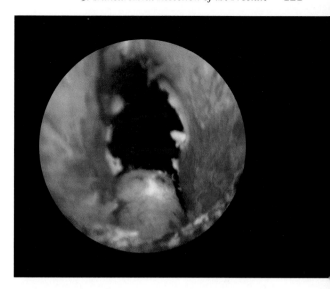

Figure 9-10. *The resection has been completed bilaterally to the level of the verumontanum, and the prostatic fossa is visually open. The sphincter remains intact.*

Areas of inspissated prostatic fluid or purulent material are often opened during prostatic resection. When encountered, they should be widely unroofed to allow permanent drainage. They can be recognized as thick, yellow white, semiliquid material that slowly oozes into the lumen. If the flow ceases and the orifice or site cannot be recognized, often more can be expressed with prostatic compression from a finger in the rectum.

Calculi are frequently found in the substance of the prostate during resection. They are most common in patients with a history of prostatic inflammation and can be found compressed with the capsule by the adenoma.

During the resection of a lateral lobe, it is advantageous to leave a cushion of adenomatous tissue near the verumontanum to allow continuation of the resection at a fairly rapid rate. Leaving this apical tissue allows for a margin of safety by ensuring that the sphincter is well away from the cutting loop, thus allowing the urologist to take multiple bites without looking back to the verumontanum for identification of its location (Fig. 9-9). The apical tissue that has been left is then resected at the conclusion of the surgery. This part of the procedure is frequently the most delicate. The mucosa over the apical tissue has many vessels running in a parallel fashion just under the surface, which may cause troublesome bleeding during this stage of the resection (see Figs. 4-2, 4-6, 4-7, 4-9). It is also very important to avoid resecting the verumontanum since this landmark is crucial in identifying the distal margin of resection (Fig. 9-10).

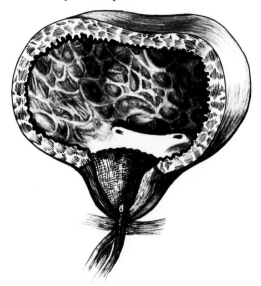

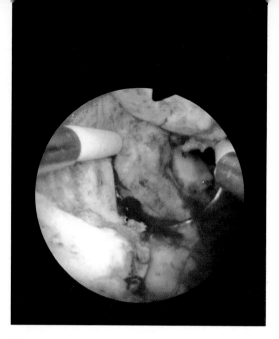

Figure 9-11. *The transurethral resection of benign prostatic hypertrophy has been completed when the adenomatous tissue has been removed to the level of the capsule throughout the prostatic fossa from the bladder neck to the level of the verumontanum.*

Figure 9-12. *A vein at the depth of the resection is actively bleeding. The loop is positioned at the bleeding site. The previously resected bladder neck is visible in the background.*

Rarely, the apical tissue that appears to extend somewhat beyond the verumontanum can be approached best by reverse cutting with the loop. With this technique, the loop is placed against the adenomatous tissue at the apex and the cut is made in the direction toward the bladder rather than toward the operator. Only very short excursions of the loop must be employed to remove the most distal portion of the apical tissue that appears to come close to the external sphincter. This technique must be used with the utmost care and is rarely indicated.

At this point, as the urologist positions the tip of the instrument near the verumontanum and looks into the bladder, instead of seeing adenomatous tissue meeting and obstructing the prostatic urethra, he or she sees either no tissue, total darkness, or, in the case of a smaller gland, the vesical neck tissue with shaggy edges, which has the appearance of a wide open channel (Figs. 9-10, 9-11). The resectionist feels somewhat like the artist near the completion of a painting. There is always another place to take a small stroke or another piece of shaggy tissue that could be removed. There is always some point of decision in determining the completion of the resection. It is not as definite as putting in the last stitch at an open operation.

Hemostasis. Since transurethral resection is a visual procedure, it is essential to maintain adequate hemostasis to allow clear visibility and to maintain the procedure's safety and accuracy. The urologist can cut the tissue desired under direct vision and leave intact the tissues recognized as important structures. Obviously, if vision is lost due to poor hemostasis, it is impossible to do a safe, accurate procedure. Not every bleeding vessel must be coagulated, however. Frequently, the resection will continue in an area with a bleeder, and it would be a waste of time to coagulate each site as it appears. Rather, one should coagulate bleeders at the base of the resected area before leaving that region to resect in another area (Figs. 9-12, 9-13). We find that it is frequently helpful to reduce the water pressure by turning the inflow stopcock partially off. The subsequent slow flow of irrigant and low pressure maintain visibility while the bleeders are allowed to appear. It is often easier to recognize successfully the relatively slow bleeding sites.

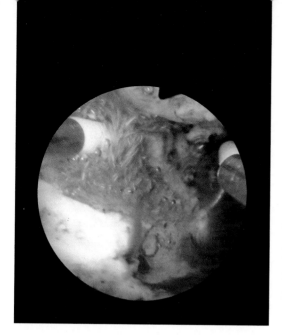

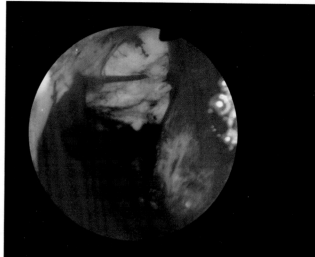

Figure 9-13. *Application of the coagulation current electrocauterizes tissue at the site of bleeding but results in bubbles within the irrigation fluid.*

Figure 9-14. *An arterial bleeder forms a well-defined stream of blood within the irrigant, which becomes diffuse as it bounces from the side of the prostatic fossa. Such forceful arterial bleeding may not have an obvious site and is described as "ricochet" bleeding.*

Occasionally, with the irrigant flowing at a full rate and the operator searching for bleeders, the entire field fills with swirling blood. It may be difficult to identify the source of the bleeding. By turning the volume of inflow down, the stream of the bleeding can be followed to its base and successfully coagulated. Sometimes bleeding will appear to come from one spot in the prostate despite repeated attempts to coagulate the region thoroughly. In such a situation, coagulation may fail to stop the bleeding because the blood is actually shooting across from the opposite wall of the prostate and ricocheting off, not originating from, the region (Fig. 9-14).

Removal of Resected Tissue. The chips of prostatic tissue that have been resected fall back into the bladder during the procedure (see Fig. 9-4). As the bladder is intermittently emptied during the procedure, particularly with the conventional resectoscope, chips will often be drained with the irrigation fluid. With the continuous flow instrument, since the bladder empties less frequently, more of the fragments remain on the floor of the bladder after completion of the procedure. Removal during the procedure can be facilitated by placing the tip of the resectoscope into the bladder along the floor as the chips collect; thus, when the telescope and working element are removed, the chips will be washed from the bladder. The tip of the instrument can be passed across the vesical floor as the irrigant drains.

The fragments can be actively irrigated from the bladder, usually with the Ellik evacuator. This instrument consists of a rubber bulb and a glass or plastic chamber partially subdivided by a narrow waist. The evacuator should be completely filled with irrigating fluid before it is attached to the resectoscope sheath. The bladder should be allowed to fill partially with irrigant to provide some volume within the vesical lumen. In this way, the bladder wall is held away from the instrument and is not drawn into the end of the sheath obstructing it. The bulb of the evacuator is compressed to force fluid into the bladder and allowed to expand to draw it back into the evacuator. The tip of the resectoscope sheath should be maneuvered to prevent suction of the bladder mucosa into the lumen. As fluid returns to the evacuator, the chips will fall into the lower chamber and remain there as the bulb is again compressed to repeat the procedure.

A Toomey syringe can be used for irrigation as an alternative technique. Although this instrument lacks the Ellik evacuator's second chamber to trap the fragments, it can actively remove fragments along with irrigant. After the evacuator or syringe stops drawing chips and evacuation appears complete, the telescope should be replaced into the resectoscope sheath to reinspect the bladder to determine that no residual fragments remain to obstruct the catheter or the urethra.

COMPLICATIONS DURING TRANSURETHRAL RESECTION

Blood Loss. Individual bleeding vessels are inevitably opened during routine prostatic resection, and can be thoroughly coagulated as the resection reaches the prostatic capsule in each area (see Fig. 9-7). The amount of blood lost can be related to the volume of adenoma resected, the technique employed, and any complicating factors (Table 9-1).

In addition, however, resection may open a large venous sinus that pours massive amounts of blood into the operative field. These sinuses are most frequent along the roof of the prostatic urethra near the vesical neck. Hence, if one looks for bleeding only laterally or posteriorly, an anterior source may not be discovered. The resectionist must consciously look at the roof with low irrigation pressure to identify the source of bleeding. Attempts to coagulate a small sinus may be successful by fulgurating circumferentially adjacent to the site of bleeding.

When a large sinus is bleeding, fulguration is usually not possible and large amounts of blood may be lost during repeated futile attempts. Frequently the sinus keeps bleeding until the procedure is terminated and a Foley catheter, with its balloon inflated, is pulled down against the vesical neck and kept on traction. This is usually quite adequate to compress the venous sinus and to stop the bleeding.

If the venous sinus is entered early during the resection, it may be necessary to terminate the resection, place a catheter on traction to secure hemostasis, and then to continue the resection at another sitting. Usually the best hemostasis can be obtained by resecting the adenoma fully to the capsule and then fulgurating individual bleeding sites. By using a high irrigation pressure, the visual field can usually be cleared of blood. The resectionist must remember, however, that irrigant can enter the venous sinus, and although a high pressure prevents the acute bleeding, it causes another complication, absorption of a large volume of irrigant.

Excessive Fluid Absorption. Large volumes of irrigation fluid may be absorbed intravascularly during transurethral resection. Intraoperatively, the resectionist may not note any unusual circumstances but the anesthesiologist may recognize a transient rise in blood pressure as fluid is added to the circulating volume. As greater volumes of fluid are absorbed, hyponatremia and edema develop. The blood pressure subsequently falls and the patient may become disoriented and confused in a full-blown clinical picture known as the *transurethral (TUR) syndrome.* This syndrome was recognized early in the history of transurethral resection of the prostate, but has become less common as the responsible factors were recognized. It is caused by the absorption of hyponatremic irrigant, which is associated with prolonged resection time, a large volume of adenoma, and, most specifically, the use of a high water pressure. The irrigating pressure must never be greater than 60 cm of water, and a lower pressure can further eliminate the intravascular absorption of irrigant[32]. Additionally, the resectionist should make a conscious effort to identify open venous sinuses through which large volumes of fluid can be absorbed at relatively lower pressures.

When using the constant flow resectoscope, low intravesical pressure is just as important. Although an accurate monitoring system is available, pressure can also be monitored clinically. The posterior wall of the bladder can usually be seen during the resection if it is partially collapsed. If it is maintained in that position, the resectionist can be confident that the intravesical pressure is in a reasonable range.

Treatment of the dilutional hyponatremia consists of administration of hypertonic sodium chloride solution in combination with diuretics. Fluid overload causes a great risk in elderly individuals, particularly those with a history of congestive heart failure, and must be actively treated should these patients require resuscitation.

Table 9-1. Blood Loss During Transurethral Resection of the Prostate

Series	Year	No. Patients	Average Wt. Resected (gm)	Resection Time (min)	Blood Loss (ml/gm)
Frank and Lloyd[12]	1959	29	10.5	38	9.3
Geist and Haglund[13]	1962	43	33.4	52	7.2
Madsen, et al.[16]	1964	20	11.3	40	15.0
Robson and Sales[18]	1966	76	17.9	NS	15.4
Perkins and Miller[18]	1969	110	11.6	64	22.2
Greene[14]	1971	144	32	NS	9.5
MacKenzie, et al.[15]	1979	62	47.6	32.3	1.9b
Flechner and Williamsa[4]	1982	20	18	50	11.9b
Flechner and Williamsa[4]	1982	16	26	61	10.9

aComparative study.
bContinuous flow resectoscope.

NS = not studied.

Perforation. It is not unusual to see thin areas or even small perforations in the prostatic capsule during transurethral resection. Thin areas can be recognized as patches with definite thinning of the capsular fibers through which veins or fat can be seen. With true perforation, the periprostatic fat may be seen adherent to the capsule. In general, the resection can be continued with extreme care if thinning or the most minor perforations are recognized. The instruments should not be directed toward the thinned area or perforation and a very low irrigation pressure (<30 mm of water) should be maintained. A more serious perforation, also referred to as a "free perforation," classically occurs at the vesicoprostatic junction. A large defect can be seen, and often irrigation fluid can be observed flowing in and out of it. Although some authors have advocated open surgical repair of such perforations, experience with visual incision of bladder neck contractures, which often extends into the perivesical tissue, would suggest that catheter drainage alone may be sufficient (see Figs. 8-12, 8-13). Fortunately, free perforations are rare and can usually be avoided by carefully monitoring the depth of resection at the bladder neck with continuous visual control.

Unrecognized perforations can be most troublesome. Major perforations, particularly those occurring at the vesical neck, may allow egress of large volumes of irrigant, which may collect subtrigonally and cause the bladder to elevate. If this develops, it may be difficult to pass the resectoscope into the bladder or to pass a urethral catheter into proper position within the bladder. The instrument can be advanced into the bladder by angulating it rather markedly anteriorly to pass over the posterior lip of the bladder wall, which has been pushed anteriorly toward the pubis. Similarly, when placing a Foley catheter in this situation, a stylet may be useful to ascertain passage of the instrument anteriorly. Excessive force in passing the catheter should never be employed since the instrument may then pass posterior to the bladder. Perforation should be considered in patients with symptoms of fluid overload and in those with abdominal symptoms and signs. Cystography is employed to determine the integrity of the bladder.

Bladder Explosions. Intravesical explosions during transurethral resections are usually evidenced only by popping sounds from within the bladder. Rarely, more severe explosions resulting in vesical injury have been noted. Gases liberated during electrosurgery contain hydrogen in high concentration derived from the electrolysis of intracellular water (Fig. 9-13)[33]. With the addition of oxygen from the air, a potentially explosive mixture results. Although this dangerous mixture of gases can be avoided by preventing the inflow of air, doing so is usually quite difficult. It is safer to empty the gas bubbles frequently by draining the bladder and compressing it suprapubically.

EARLY POSTOPERATIVE COMPLICATIONS

Intraluminal Bleeding. A certain amount of bleeding can be considered normal. This can be managed in one of two ways. Many urologists now prefer to use continuous bladder irrigation through a three-way Foley catheter to dilute any blood and immediately wash it from the bladder before potentially obstructive clots can be formed. On the other hand, a catheter can be placed transurethrally for drainage alone and irrigated manually to maintain free drainage. This technique, however, demands constant monitoring and presents a greater risk of obstruction of the catheter. Many other resectionists have developed habits of meticulous hemostasis and may prefer to avoid the risk of bacterial contamination with either continuous or intermittent irrigation. They may place a catheter for drainage and irrigate only in those instances when it becomes obstructed.

If the bladder fills with clots and irrigation becomes impossible, it is sometimes best to reinstrument the patient, evacuate the clots, and inspect the prostatic fossa for bleeding sites that can be coagulated. Drainage is then reestablished through a Foley catheter. In rare circumstances, an open surgical procedure may be necessary to pack the prostatic fossa if adequate hemostasis cannot be obtained by reinstrumentation.

Acute Epididymitis. The use of antibacterial agents to treat preexisting urinary tract infections prior to transurethral procedures, together with preventive measures to avoid contamination of the urine or prolonged use of a catheter, will greatly reduce the chance of postoperative epididymitis. Earlier attempts to prevent epididymitis by ligation of the vas deferens have not proved efficacious in controlled studies. If epididymitis develops, the causative organism can usually be recovered from the urine and appropriate antibacterial therapy should be instituted.

Incontinence. After removal of the drainage catheter following transurethral resection of the prostate, many patients have urgency and relatively poor control of bladder emptying for the first day or two. These complications may result from irritation of the bladder and lowering of the voiding pressure. Most patients experience only mild urgency incontinence. This condition should not be confused with true incontinence, which results from the loss of sphincteric action.

Incontinence resulting from damage to the sphincteric mechanism may take one of several forms, and can be considered as a spectrum of dysfunction. The most severe form, or total incontinence, is manifest early as constant leakage of urine through the urethra. In this situation, there is essentially no active or passive obstruction to the passage of urine. Thus, any urine passes through the urethra before accumulating within the bladder. Total incontinence is perhaps the greatest disaster of transurethral resection of the prostate. Although artificial sphincters are available for surgical implantation, there is no simple, satisfactory treatment for this complication.

Less severe sphincteric damage will result in stress urinary incontinence. In this case, the patient's residual sphincteric action is adequate to retain urine under normal conditions but can be overcome with increasing intraabdominal pressure in situations of stress such as coughing or strenuous physical activity. In these patients some additional benefit may be gained from administration of an alpha-sympathomimetic agent to increase the posterior urethral tone.

Disturbances of Sexual Function. Impotence, or the inability to obtain an erection, is a very rare complication of transurethral resection of the prostate. The nerves responsible for erection course along the lateral aspect of the true prostate and therefore are beyond the extent of the usual resection. Psychogenic factors should also be considered in these patients[31].

Lack of ejaculation, or less forceful ejaculation, is a more common result of transurethral resection of the prostate. It should be discussed with the patient as a frequent side effect of the procedure, although it does not uniformly develop. A possible explanation for its occurrence may be that the semen passes into the bladder rather than through the urethra following resection of the bladder neck, but some patients with an adequate resection continue to have normal antegrade ejaculation.

LATE COMPLICATIONS

Hemorrhage. Late hemorrhage may occur 1 or more weeks after the patient has returned to his home following resection of the prostate. The patient may be able to relate it to physical activity but more often he notes the acute onset of gross hematuria without recognizable precipitating factors. He may notice only mild blood tinging of the urine, or the more severe gross hematuria with formation of clots and urethral obstruction known as *clot retention*. In the latter case, the patient will have to return for reinstrumentation and evacuation of the clots. The bleeding will often clear spontaneously; if active bleeding continues, however, several days of catheter drainage or even reinstrumentation for inspection of the prostatic fossa may be necessary. This late hemorrhage presumably occurs because of sloughing of necrotic coagulated tissue within the prostatic fossa.

Urethral Stricture. The most common late complication after transurethral prostatectomy is urethral stricture. The reported incidence has varied from 4 to 29 percent. The initiating factor appears to be circumferential injury to the urethra during the procedure. The size of the resectoscope or the catheter used postoperatively, the length of resection, and possibly the presence of infection have been related to stricture formation. In a prospective series, Hart and Fowler[29] could not demonstrate any relationship between urethral stricture formation and the material or size of the urethral catheter or the presence of organisms in the urine and urethra.

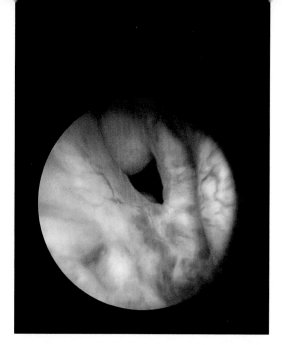

Figure 9-15. *A bladder neck contracture has developed after previous prostatic resection.*

The size of the resectoscope remains the most important factor. It has been suggested that the urethra can be enlarged to accommodate the instrument by dilation[30] or by internal urethrotomy[27,28]. The distal urethra can be bypassed entirely by placing the resectoscope through a perineal urethrostomy[28]. Both internal urethrotomy and perineal urethrostomy have been shown to result in significantly fewer urethral studies in controlled studies[27,28]. The safest policy remains to use the smallest instrument practical for the procedure and to avoid unnecessary delays that could prolong the procedure. We generally dilate the urethra with sounds to a lumen two French sizes larger than the resectoscope and reserve urethrotomy or perineal urethrostomy for specific patients in whom the urethra is small.

Bladder Neck Contracture. Circumferential contraction of scarring at the bladder neck may result in a significant contracture obstructing the outflow of urine (Fig. 9-15). Contracture has been considered to develop after excessive resection and, possibly more importantly, extensive fulguration of the residual tissue and muscular fibers at the bladder neck. Electrosurgical manipulation of the bladder neck should be limited to resection of the adenoma and fulguration to only actively bleeding vessels. Treatment has included dilation, resection of the contracture with the injection of steroids, and visual incision, which has resulted in excellent cure rates (see Chap. 8).

CARCINOMA OF THE PROSTATE. Transurethral resection cannot provide curative treatment of carcinomas of the prostate classified above stage A since these neoplasms usually arise in the peripheral posterior prostate, an area that resection generally will not even sample. Transurethral resection, however, can be employed as a palliative procedure to relieve obstruction from the intraluminal extension of the neoplasm.

Although carcinoma of the prostate often cannot be distinguished from benign prostatic hypertrophy, there are many patients with extensive local tumor growth that, in addition to obstructing the lumen rigidly, fixes the prostatic urethra and hinders movement of the resectoscope. The verumontanum may be distorted or even obscured by the tumor and the external sphincter is often involved. The risk of incontinence is considerably higher after resection of a neoplasm of the prostate, more frequently as a result of tumor infiltration of the sphincter and the membranous urethra than of direct damage to the sphincter.

Although the resection can be initiated in the same fashion as that for BPH, an attempt to carry the resection to the capsule may easily result in perforation since infiltration of the tumor will blur the usual border between adenoma and capsule. Since the rigid tumor does not collapse into the lumen as seen with benign prostatic tissue, a channel cut through the rigid neoplastic tissue will remain open and provide an adequate channel for urinary passage. It is not essential and, in fact, is risky to attempt to resect the entire tumor and clear the fossa to the prostatic capsule. The postoperative care of patients with neoplasms of the prostate treated with transurethral resection is the same as that described for benign disease.

Infection. There is some risk of infection whenever the urinary tract is violated by instrumentation. Although bacteriuria is relatively uncommon after simple cystoscopy, occurring in approximately 5 percent of patients, the rate increases to between 10 and 40 percent after transurethral resection of the prostate (Table 9-2). Many patients are asymptomatic and the infection is discovered only when the urine is cultured. Sepsis is even less common, occurring in 18 of 1,604 patients followed after transurethral resection of the prostate[25]. In 11 of the 18 patients, sepsis developed after resection had been performed in the presence of urinary infection without appropriate treatment. In the remaining 7 patients, the urine was infected and the patient became septic at the time of removal of the catheter.

Table 9-2. Bacteriuria Following
Transurethral Resection of the Prostate

Series	Year	No. Patients	Bacteriuria (%)
McGuire[24]	1974	57	22.8
Gonzales, et al.[22]	1976	59	40.8 (1 day)
Gibbons, et al.[20]	1978	45	11.1
Appell, et al.[19]	1980	80	11.2
Nielsen, et al.[26]	1981	53	26.4 (3 days) 42.0 (7 days)
Holl and Rous[23]	1982	40	12.5
Goldwasser, et al.[21]	1983	25	32.0

The hope of preventing infection after resection of the prostate has resulted in considerable interest in the prophylactic administration of antibiotics. Numerous studies have examined the value of antibiotic administration before or after transurethral resection of the prostate, but the results have been quite variable. Nielsen's group[26] found that the administration of cefoxitin begun preoperatively and continued postoperatively until after removal of the urinary catheter resulted in a significant decrease in bacteriuria 7 days after the procedure. Goldwasser and co-workers[21] found that sulfamethoxazole-trimethoprim given in either of 2 regimens (preoperatively and postoperatively for 10 days, or 2 doses, 1 preoperatively and 1 postoperatively) resulted in a significant decrease in postoperative bacteriuria.

At the present time, it is clear that any patient with infected urine should be treated with the appropriate antimicrobial agent prior to endoscopic manipulation. We do not employ antibiotic prophylaxis routinely in prostatectomy patients with sterile urine, but reserve it for high-risk patients, the elderly, or those with concomitant systemic disease. The urine should be cultured preoperatively and prior to catheter removal so that any patient with infected urine can be treated with appropriate antibiotics. In addition, any patient with valvular heart disease or a prosthetic vascular device should be given antibiotics prophylactically prior to and after the procedure. The recommended schedule includes ampicillin (or vancomycin in patients allergic to penicillin) and an aminoglycoside (see Chap. 7).

REFERENCES

Preoperative Evaluation

1. Bauer, D. L., Garrison, R. W., and McRoberts, J. W. The health and cost complications of routine excretory urography before transurethral prostatectomy. *J. Urol.* 123:386, 1980.
2. Guinan, P., Bush, I., Ray, V., Vieth, R., and Bhatti, R. The accuracy of the rectal examination in the diagnosis of prostate cancer. *N. Engl. J. Med.* 303:499, 1980.
3. Pinck, B. D., Corrigan, M. J., and Jasper, P. Preprostatectomy excretory urography: Does it merit the expense? *J. Urol.* 123:390, 1980.

Instruments

4. Flechner, S. M., and Williams, R. D. Continuous flow and conventional resectoscope methods in transurethral prostatectomy: Comparative study. *J. Urol.* 127:257, 1982.
5. Iglesias, J. J., Sporer, A., Gellman, A. C., and Seebode, J. J. New Iglesias resectoscope with continuous irrigation, simultaneous suction and low intravesical pressure. *J. Urol.* 114:929, 1975.
6. McCarthy, J. F. A new apparatus for endoscopic plastic surgery of the prostate, diathermia, and excision of vesical growths. *J. Urol.* 26:695, 1931.
7. Reuter, H. J., and Jones, L. W. Physiologic low pressure irrigation for transurethral suprapubic torcar drainage. *J. Urol.* 111:210, 1974.
8. Stern, M. Resections of obstructions at the vesical orifice. *J.A.M.A.* 87:1726, 1926.

Electrosurgery

9. Goodman, G. R. Electrosurgery burns and the urologist. *J. Urol.* 116:218, 1976.
10. Mitchell, J. P., and Lumb, G. N. The principles of surgical diathermy and its limitations. *Br. J. Surg.* 50:314, 1962.
11. Weyrauch, H. M. *Surgery of the Prostate.* Philadelphia: Saunders, 1959.

Blood Loss

12. Frank, R. M., and Lloyd, F. A. A clinical study on the effectiveness of adrenosem in transurethral resection. *J. Urol.* 82:243, 1959.
13. Geist, R. W., and Haglund, R. V. Failure of intravenous injections of estrogen (Premarin) to decrease loss of blood during transurethral prostatic resection. *J. Urol.* 87:593, 1962.
14. Greene, L. F. Use of hemostatic bag after transurethral prostatic resection. *J. Urol.* 106:915, 1971.
15. MacKenzie, A. R., Levine, N., and Scheinman, H. Z. Operative blood loss in transurethral prostatectomy. *J. Urol.* 122:47, 1979.
16. Madsen, P. O., Kaveggia, L., and Atassi, S. A. The effect of estrogens (Premarin) and regional hypothermia on blood loss during transurethral prostatectomy. *J. Urol.* 92:314, 1964.
17. Perkins, J. B., and Miller, H. C. Blood loss during transurethral prostatectomy. *J. Urol.* 101:93, 1969.
18. Robson, C. J., and Sales, J. L. The effect of local hypothermia on blood loss during transurethral resection of the prostate. *J. Urol.* 95:393, 1966.

Infections

19. Appell, R. A., Flynn, J. T., Paris, A. M. I., and Blandy, J. P. Occult bacterial colonization of bladder tumors. *J. Urol.* 124:345, 1980.
20. Gibbons, R. P., Stark, R. A., Corres, R. J., Jr., Cummings, K. B., and Mason, J. T. The prophylactic use or misuse of antibiotics in transurethral prostatectomy. *J. Urol.* 119:381, 1978.
21. Goldwasser, B., et al. Prophylactic antimicrobial treatment in transurethral prostatectomy: How long should it be instituted? *Urology* 22:136, 1983.
22. Gonzales, R., Wright, R., and Blackard, C. E. Prophylactic antibiotics in transurethral prostatectomy. *J. Urol.* 116:203, 1976.
23. Holl, W. H., and Rous, S. N. Is antibiotic prophylaxis worthwhile in patients with transurethral resection of the prostate? *Urology* 19:43, 1982.
24. McGuire, E. J. Antibacterial prophylaxis in prostatectomy patients. *J. Urol.* 111:794, 1974.
25. Murphy, D. M., Falkiner, F. R., Carr, M., Cafferkey, M. T., and Gillespie, W. A. Septicemia after transurethral prostatectomy. *Urology* 22:133, 1983.
26. Nielsen, O. S., Maigaard, S., Frimodt-Moller, N., and Madsen, P. O. Prophylactic antibiotics in transurethral prostatectomy. *J. Urol.* 126:60, 1981.

Strictures

27. Bailey, J. J., and Shearer, J. R. The role of internal urethrotomy in the prevention of urethral stricture following transurethral resection of the prostate. *Br. J. Urol.* 51:28, 1979.
28. Bissada, N. K. Transurethral resection of prostate via perineal urethrostomy: Follow-up report. *Urology* 10:39, 1977.
29. Hart, A. J. L., and Fowler, J. W. Incidence of urethral strictures after transurethral resection of prostate: Effects of urinary infection, urethral flora and catheter material and size. *Urology* 18:588, 1981.
30. Lentz, H. C., Melbust, W. K., Forest, J. D., and Melchior, S. Urethral strictures following transurethral prostatectomy. Review of 2,223 resections. *J. Urol.* 117:194, 1977.

Other Techniques and Complications

31. Madorsky, M. L., Ashamalla, M. G., Schussler, I., Lyons, H. R., and Miller, G. H. Post-prostatectomy impotence. *J. Urol.* 115:401, 1976.
32. Madsen, P. O., and Naber, K. The importance of the pressure in the prostatic fossa and absorption of irrigation fluid during transurethral resection of the prostate. *J. Urol.* 109:446, 1973.
33. Ning, T. C., Atkins, D. M., and Murphy, R. C. Bladder explosions during transurethral surgery. *J. Urol.* 114:536, 1975.

10
TRANSURETHRAL RESECTION OF BLADDER TUMORS

Demetrius H. Bagley

Edward S. Lyon

Jeffry L. Huffman

Endoscopic inspection and resection remain the major techniques for diagnosis and treatment of bladder tumors. Although some bladder tumors can be detected radiographically on cystogram or excretory urogram, most early neoplasms can be detected only by direct endoscopic inspection of the bladder. Therefore, any patient suspected of having a bladder tumor, whether because of an episode of gross hematuria or because of a previous bladder tumor, must be examined by cystoscopy. The procedure permits the identification not only of the presence of a tumor within the bladder but also of the number and location of the lesion, together with a preliminary estimation of tumor grade and stage. Biopsy and resection of the tumor and its base for full pathologic examination will provide information on the grade and stage of the tumor and will allow design of appropriate treatment.

BIMANUAL EXAMINATION. Every patient undergoing endoscopic evaluation and treatment of a bladder tumor must be evaluated with a bimanual examination. After suitable anesthesia has been administered but before the perineum has been prepared and draped, the examination should be performed. After a thorough rectal examination has been completed, the urologist's second hand is placed on the lower abdomen, and the pelvic organs, particularly the bladder, are palpated between the two hands. Particular note must be made of any bladder mass, induration of the bladder wall, or thickening within the area of the bladder. Low-grade, low-stage tumors are usually not palpable while infiltrating lesions, which are more solid and larger, can be felt with the examining hands. Larger nodal masses may also be palpated in this way. The bimanual examination is an essential part of the evaluation of a bladder tumor. It must be performed in every patient before the physical characteristics have been altered by resection of the tumor, through either removal of a tumor mass or development of an inflammatory reaction.

ENDOSCOPIC INSPECTION. Endoscopic inspection remains the most valuable procedure for the diagnosis of bladder tumors. The techniques employed are those described in Chapter 7. Several aspects, however, should be stressed. The urethra must be inspected to detect any associated intraurethral lesions. We, therefore, prefer to introduce the cystourethroscope under direct vision, and thus to view the uninstrumented urethra initially. As the instrument enters the bladder, the usual landmarks such as the bladder neck, ureteral orifices, and intraureteric ridge are noted. Obvious bladder tumors and suspicious mucosal areas are then identified and located with respect to the standard landmarks. It is often helpful for future reference to locate any lesions on a map of the bladder, such as that described in Chapter 7.

The endoscopic appearance of the tumor will also offer some indication of the stage and grade of the tumor. Small papillary lesions are usually low grade and low stage while solid-appearing sessile tumors are more likely to be higher grade and higher stage. Tumors attached to the mucosa by a small stalk usually are not invasive and thus are lower stage. Conversely, tumors that have spread along the bladder wall forming a firm, nondistensible region are quite likely invasive lesions involving the musculature of the bladder.

BIOPSY. In every patient undergoing evaluation for urothelial cancer, biopsies of the tumor and the tumor base, as well as any suspicious lesions within the bladder, should be taken. Every effort should be made to obtain tissue with minimal crushing or thermal artifact. Muscular invasion and the depth of invasion can be determined only by obtaining samples from the bladder wall.

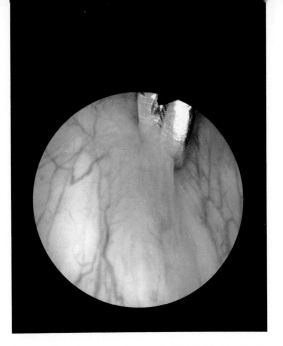

Figure 10-1. *A low-grade superficial bladder tumor is biopsied with the rigid biopsy forceps.*

Adequate biopsies can be obtained with several different instruments. Cup biopsy forceps provide a satisfactory specimen of tissue with minimal crushing artifact and without electrocoagulation of the tissue. These forceps are available in a rigid design with a true double cup configuration or a basket design that does not entirely surround the specimen. Flexible forceps are also available. These are usually of the double cup or clam shell design and can be obtained in sizes from 5 to 10 Fr. The rigid instrument (Fig. 10-1) provides a larger piece of tissue (up to 5–6 mm) than the flexible instrument, which has greater maneuverability. Flexible forceps are almost essential for biopsy of lesions located on the anterior wall or dome of the bladder. The forceps should cut the tissue to provide a clean margin of the biopsy specimen without crushing it. Other urologists prefer to grasp the specimen with forceps but to tear it from the bladder with an adjacent piece of mucosa instead of cutting it with the edge of the biopsy forceps. In this way, they can obtain a larger piece of tissue. Although the rigid biopsy forceps can take a full thickness biopsy of a relatively thin bladder (Fig. 10-2), they are relatively safer to use and less frequently cause perforation than the resectoscope loop. These forceps should be used with care in biopsying the bladder. Foreign body or grasping forceps, which have toothed or serrated jaws, will not obtain a uniformly satisfactory specimen since the tissue will pull through the teeth.

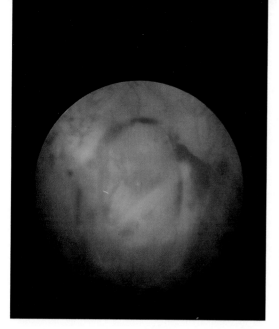

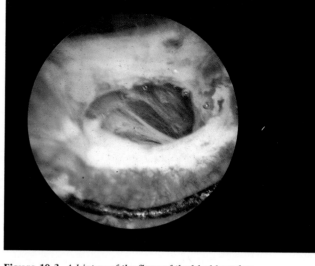

Figure 10-2. *The rigid biopsy forceps can perforate the bladder by taking a full thickness sample of the bladder wall. The typical yellow, glistening fat is evident at the depth of this biopsy site. The muscular fibers of the bladder wall are also evident.*

Figure 10-3. *A biopsy of the floor of the bladder taken with the resectoscope extends through the full thickness of the bladder wall. Perivesical connective tissue is visible at the depth of the biopsy site. Erythematous mucosa is evident superiorly and inferiorly.*

Some endoscopists prefer to use a resectoscope with a cutting loop for biopsy of bladder tumors. The potential disadvantages of this technique are a higher risk of perforation of the bladder (Fig. 10-3) and distortion of the tissue on histologic examination caused by electrocoagulation. The specimen obtained with the resectoscope may fall from the loop into the bladder and be difficult to retrieve. Although it may be adherent to the cutting loop and be removed easily from the bladder, it more frequently is adherent when the current is too high, and the coagulation artifact will usually be present. We prefer to reserve this technique for larger or more solid-appearing tumors and specifically to avoid it when taking selected site biopsies.

Alternatively, a sample can be taken with the resectoscope loop without use of the cutting or coagulation current. As the loop is drawn across a soft friable tumor, tissue will be drawn toward the resectoscope sheath. As it is trapped between the loop and the sheath, the tissue can be torn from the base and removed for histologic study. Samples of the muscular layers can then be taken utilizing the cutting current and the resectoscope loop.

Samples of tissue should be taken from the bulky portion of the tumor, from the base of the tumor, and from the muscular layer of the bladder wall to assess the presence of muscular invasion by the tumor. Any of the forceps or resectoscope loops can obtain adequate samples of each portion of the tumor. With a small flexible biopsy forceps, it may be necessary to take several samples to obtain adequate material. The rigid biopsy forceps can obtain a larger sample of tissue while the resectoscope loop can often obtain a sample of tumor and the bladder wall with a single sampling.

In the patient initially presenting with a bladder tumor or the patient being evaluated for cystectomy or partial cystectomy, additional biopsies should be taken of any erythematous or otherwise suspicious mucosa; normal-appearing urothelium should also be biopsied at random or selected sites. Random or selected site biopsies can be taken on the opposite wall of the bladder or at other distant sites that are grossly normal. Common sites include the midposterior wall and the area lateral to each orifice. It may be possible to detect carcinoma in situ in these otherwise normal-appearing areas of the bladder.

PREOPERATIVE MEASURES

Positioning the Patient. The dorsal lithotomy position is generally the most satisfactory and the most frequently used for transurethral resection of bladder tumors. Biopsy and resection with rigid instruments of tumors located at the dome of the bladder can be facilitated by positioning the patient so that the dome is in a more dependent position. The bubble will rise to the least dependent portion, which will then be the floor of the bladder. To achieve this orientation of the bladder, the patient can be placed in the "jack-knife" position similar to that used for hemorrhoidectomy or sigmoidoscopy. This is convenient in the female but may be more difficult for urethral instrumentation in the male. Therefore, in the male, the lateral position can be used to bring the dome into a more accessible position. With this orientation, the bubble will rise to the opposite lateral wall, leaving the dome covered with fluid and readily accessible to the rigid resectoscope.

Other manipulations will also render lesions in difficult positions more accessible. By using the dorsal lithotomy position in a patient with a posterior wall tumor, the posterior wall can be brought toward the bladder neck by partially emptying the bladder. The back wall is then available for biopsy or resection. The dome can be delivered more closely to the resectoscope by manually applying pressure to the lower abdomen and suprapubic area. This maneuver is more successful in the anesthetized patient but can be used any time.

Irrigation Fluid. Any nonconductive irrigating fluid can be used for transurethral resection of bladder tumors. Since usually little of the fluid is absorbed, an isoosmotic solution such as that necessary for transurethral resection of the prostate is not essential. For large bulky tumors, an isoosmotic, nonconductive solution such as 1.5% glycine should be used. Water is usually employed for smaller tumors and has the theoretic advantage that it may lyse tumor cells, thus preventing their implantation and growth. This effect, however, has not been documented either clinically or in an animal model.

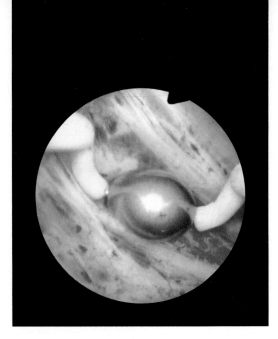

Figure 10-4. *A roller ball is used to fulgurate the muscle of the bladder wall at the base after resection of a superficial tumor.*

Instruments. The same resectoscope used for resection of the prostate can be used for bladder tumors. Modifications of the instrument, however, have proved useful for resection within the bladder. A longer beak on the instrument, described as a "bladder beak," extends over the area of excursion of the resectoscope loop and keeps redundant tumor or bladder mucosa from falling into the path of the resectoscope loop from the side opposite the loop itself. This modification has many advantages when the bladder is partially distended with fluid, as often is the case for bladder tumor resection.

The constant flow resectoscope is particularly useful for resecting tumors within the bladder. The constant flow of irrigant clears any blood within the bladder to provide a clear visual field. The inflow and outflow rates can be adjusted so that a constant volume of fluid is maintained within the bladder. Thus, the bladder remains at a constant volume and the walls of the bladder are stationery without the change of position caused by frequent filling and emptying.

In addition to the standard resectoscope loop, the roller ball is often useful for rapid fulguration of large areas of mucosa or the resected base of a wide-spread tumor (Figs. 10-4, 10-5). Adherence of tumor to the larger surface of the roller ball is more prominent than with the resectoscope loop.

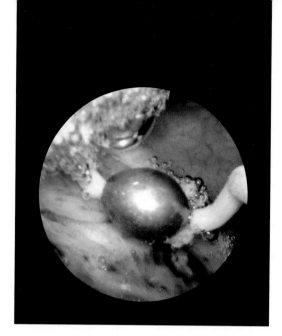

Figure 10-5. *Coagulation is extended beyond the margin of resection into normal-appearing mucosa.*

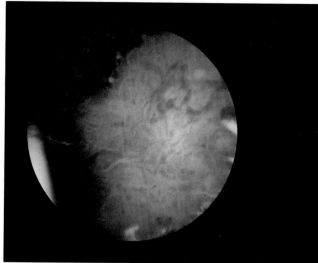

Figure 10-6. *A low-grade, low-stage transitional cell carcinoma is located on the left lateral bladder wall. The resectoscope loop is seen approaching the tumor, which is also shown in Figs. 10-7 and 10-8.*

TECHNIQUE

Small Tumors. The entire treatment of low-grade, low-stage bladder tumors can be performed endoscopically. The technique for treatment of these tumors varies according to the size of the lesion. Small tumors (<1 cm in diameter) should be biopsied to provide tissue for histologic diagnosis (see Fig. 5-24). Frequently, the biopsy will remove the entire tumor and the base can then be fulgurated with a Bugbee electrode or the resectoscope loop. When several similar tumors are present, it may be acceptable to fulgurate the others without biopsy. In every case, however, tissue should be obtained by biopsy from the largest or most solid-appearing tumor for histologic evaluation. The intent must be to biopsy the worst-appearing portion of the bladder to determine the highest grade or stage of the lesion present in the bladder.

Medium Tumors. With medium-sized tumors (1–4 cm) resection is usually necessary. A biopsy should be obtained with forceps to prevent the artifacts noted. Alternatively, of course, a biopsy can be taken with the resectoscope loop. The biopsy should include a portion of the bulk of the tumor, the base, and the junction of the tumor with the bladder itself. The depth should be sufficient to obtain a specimen of the bladder muscle.

The lesion can then be resected with a resectoscope utilizing the standard loop electrode (Fig. 10-6). Application of the current for resection must be done only when the loop is being drawn toward the sheath to minimize the possibility of perforation (Fig. 10-7). Either the pure cutting current or a blend of cutting and coagulation current can be used if the electrocautery instrument is so equipped. Particularly with these tumors, the constant flow resectoscope is useful to maintain a constant volume in the bladder and to maintain the tumor in its stationary position.

Resection can be started at the edge of the tumor in the most accessible portion. The resection is continued stepwise to include the bulky papillomatous portion and the stalk, and then the base of the tumor. Following resection of the tumor itself, the base should be reresected to obtain a sample of the muscular wall of the bladder to be sent as a separate specimen for examination for invasive tumor. Hemostasis can be maintained by fulguration of bleeding areas with either the loop electrode or, if a larger area has been resected, the roller ball (Fig. 10-8).

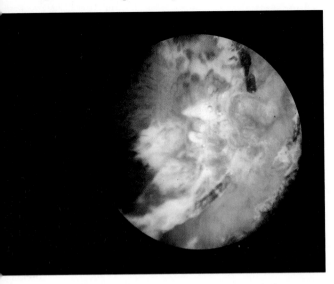

Figure 10-7. *As the loop is drawn through the tumor, the urologist judges the depth of the cut under direct vision. Hemostasis is maintained by fulguration of bleeding sites.*

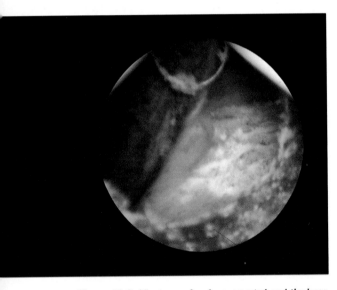

Figure 10-8. *The tumor has been resected and the base fulgurated lateral to the left ureteral orifice.*

Large Tumors. Large tumors (>4 cm in diameter) provide particular problems for transurethral resection. Although these tumors are rarely impossible to resect, they frequently present many technical difficulties. Three approaches have been advocated for the endoscopic treatment of large bladder tumors. Barnes[3] has suggested early resection of the base of the tumor. The resection is started 1 cm lateral to the obvious tumor in normal bladder mucosa and carried toward the base of the tumor to resect the stalk. The surrounding normal-appearing mucosa is resected circumferentially around the base. The amputated tumor mass is then removed through the resectoscope sheath. These low-grade, bulky tumors are quite soft and friable and can be irrigated from the bladder through a sheath with a Toomey syringe or Ellick evacuator. In attempting to use this technique, it is often difficult to locate the base of the tumor accurately since the papillary fronds and bleeding from the cut surface of the bladder may obscure the resectionist's vision.

The second technique begins the resection in any accessible portion of the tumor, as described for medium tumors. Often a large portion of the papillary part of the tumor must be resected before the base of the lesion can be identified. Considerable bleeding may be encountered during resection of very bulky papillary tumors. Although pure cutting current can be used and causes minimal fouling of the electrocautery loop, a blend of cutting and coagulation current may decrease the bleeding.

A third technique employs pure coagulation and pure cutting currents and has proved satisfactory in resection of bulky papillary tumors. During the initial portion of the excursion of the loop, the coagulation current is applied to coagulate the fronds of the tumor and draw them toward the resectoscope. Just before completion of the excursion, the cutting current is applied and the segment of tumor that is caught within the loop and has been fulgurated at its base is amputated. This technique demands coordination of the operator's foot controlling the two pedals but minimizes bleeding. Very large tumors as well as those considered medium sized can be resected in this way with very little blood loss.

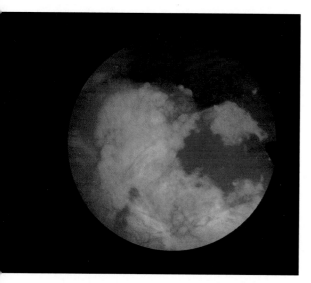

Figure 10-9. *A sessile bladder tumor located at the inferior right bladder neck (7 o'clock position).*

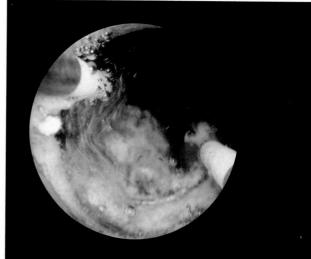

Figure 10-10. *The tumor shown in Fig. 10-9 is resected as several chips, and the base is fulgurated.*

High-Grade Solid Tumors. Immediately on inspecting the bladder that contains a solid massive tumor (Figs. 10-9, 5-29, 5-32), the urologist knows that he or she is dealing with an aggressive, high-grade, and probably high-stage tumor. For an accurate histologic diagnosis, tumor tissue must be examined. Resection of the tumor at its junction with the bladder wall will provide this tissue (Fig. 10-10). Although the urologist may find it impossible to resect the entire tumor, the resection should be carried to the base of the junction of the tumor and the bladder wall to gain a sample of the bladder muscle for histologic examination (see Fig. 5-30).

Transitional cell bladder tumors, which do not extend beyond the lamina propria (T1 or less), are theoretically amenable to local therapy by transurethral resection. Those with microscopic invasion of the superficial muscle of the bladder are also potentially curable locally by transurethral resection. More radical therapy should be considered if the individual patient is complicated by a history of previous tumors, by severely limited bladder capacity, or by the presence of either multiple tumors or associated carcinoma in situ. More deeply invasive tumors (T3 or T4) have such a limited choice of local control with conservative transurethral therapy that early radical therapy must be considered with definitive irradiation, surgery, or a combination of these modalities[14].

SPECIAL CATEGORIES OF TUMORS

Large Patches of Low-Grade Tumors. Papillary tumors may appear as individual or multiple papillary lesions with a "mulberry" appearance or as large patchy lesions (see Fig. 5-24). Grossly it may be difficult to distinguish these lesions from inflammatory reactions of the mucosa (see Figs. 5-9 to 5-12). In these cases it is advantageous to obtain multiple biopsies of the lesion with careful mapping of the areas from which the biopsies are taken and also to take selected biopsies of the normal-appearing mucosa. If the lesion proves on histologic examination to be a tumor, then the entire area may be more easily fulgurated than resected. A roller ball electrode (see Fig. 10-4) is advantageous when used to fulgurate large areas of mucosa. As the ball is moved back and forth over the involved surface, the coagulating current is applied and the tissue within the excursion of the electrode is fulgurated.

Tumors at the Ureteral Orifice. Tumors are often located near the ureteral orifice. The position of the orifice and the submucosal tunnel should be carefully noted and considered in the resection of tumors. The orifice may be obscured by the presence of a large tumor or of numerous confluent smaller lesions. The orifice can be visualized after intravenous administration of indigo carmine, which will be excreted in the urine within 5 to 15 minutes. The site of efflux can then be identified as the orifice. Endoscopic vision may be obscured by the blue urine following this technique, which should be reserved for cases in which the orifice is obscured. Resection with a cutting current can be carried across the ureteral orifice with minimal risk of subsequent scarring and obstruction. Fulguration of the orifice with a coagulation current, however, will almost certainly lead to scarring and possible obstruction of the orifice. Tumors actually within or extending from the ureteral orifice require ureteroscopic evaluation, treatment, and follow-up (see Chap. 15).

Simultaneous Resection of Bladder Tumor and Prostate. There has been considerable controversy regarding the appropriate timing of resections of both the prostate and a simultaneously occurring bladder tumor. In experimental tumor systems, transitional cell tumors can implant on damaged urothelium and, theoretically, a similar situation should occur clinically during resection of bladder tumors. Although these theoretic disadvantages of simultaneous prostatectomy in tumor resection exist, in two controlled series there was no evidence for any increased implantation of tumors in the prostatic fossa with simultaneous treatment[9,11,13]. Although simultaneous resection is an accepted procedure, we do not advocate it as a routine plan of therapy but prefer to resect the bladder tumor first and, as a subsequent operation, resect the prostate.

Open Fulguration. In the vast majority of patients, any lesions within the bladder can be reached endoscopically. In rare instances, it may be necessary to perform an open surgical procedure to expose the bladder for treatment of a tumor that cannot be reached transurethrally. If this rare situation develops, a partial cystectomy may be the best choice of procedure. Occasionally, an additional tumor may be found within the bladder at the time of the procedure, and it could be excised and the base fulgurated. Rarely, a bladder tumor that was missed on cystostomy prior to another procedure, such as open prostatectomy, may require removal. In any case, after an open surgical procedure on the bladder, subsequent endoscopic procedures will be much more difficult because of the fixation of the dome of the bladder to the anterior abdominal wall. Therefore, every effort should be made to avoid opening the bladder for treatment of urothelial tumors, except for the single definitive treatment of a tumor by partial cystectomy. The risk of implantation of tumors outside the bladder is too great to consider open electroresection of bladder tumors in any but the most extenuating circumstances.

Carcinoma In Situ. Carcinoma in situ (CIS), which is limited to the bladder and not associated with papillary or solid lesions, is usually treated initially after diagnosis by biopsy with transurethral resection and fulguration of recognizable lesions to the extent possible. More extensive lesions may require adjuvant intravesical therapy with a chemotherapeutic or immunotherapeutic agent[10].

COMPLICATIONS. The complications most frequently encountered in resection of bladder tumors are infection, reflux, bleeding, and perforation (Table 10-1). Careful resection and thorough inspection of the bladder after resection will minimize the possibility of complications.

Infection. Urinary infections are relatively common following transurethral resection of bladder tumors. In 3 reported series, the rate has been 19.4, 24, and 38.9 percent[1,5,8]. These values are higher than the incidence usually reported for transurethral resection of the prostate. Appell and co-workers[1] found that a high association existed between the presence of bacteria within the resected tumor and a subsequent urinary infection. Goldwasser's group[8] could not confirm these findings but observed that only 3.4 percent of tumor cultures were positive. Regardless of the source of the infecting organism, the rate of infection was significant in all three series.

Table 10-1. Complications of Transurethral Resection of Bladder Tumors

Series	Complication	Patients (%)
Appell, et al.[1]; Dick, et al.[5]; Goldwasser, et al.[8]	Infection	19.4, 24.0, 38.9
Freed[7]	Reflux	19
Dick, et al.[5]	Hemorrhage (requiring transfusion)	13
Dick, et al.[5]	Perforation	5
Dick, et al.[5]	Postoperative mortality	1.3

At present there is no information regarding the value of antibiotic prophylaxis of infection after transurethral resection of bladder tumors. The majority of infections are cystitis; systemic, life-threatening infections are much less common. The urologist, however, should be alert to the possibility of infection and follow the patient closely with urine cultures and utilize antimicrobial agents when indicated.

Vesicoureteral Reflux. Vesicoureteral reflux after transurethral resection of bladder tumors has been documented to occur in 19 percent of patients in 1 series[7]. Although most of the patients remained asymptomatic and without loss of renal function, renal deterioration did occur in 2 patients. Reflux apparently results from scarring of the trigone following tumor resection and fulguration. Certainly it might be expected with a tumor located at the orifice necessitating resection of the orifice and distal intravesical ureter, but reflux may also develop after resection of more distant tumors. The reasonable approach is to treat the intravesical tumor appropriately and deal as necessary with any complication of reflux that may occur.

Hematuria. Hematuria following transurethral resection of the bladder is extremely common. Bleeding may vary according to the extent of resection; for example, it may be insignificant after resection of a small papillary tumor but pronounced after resection of a high-grade lesion extending into the bladder wall. Hemorrhage requiring transfusion developed in 13 percent of patients in the series of Dick and associates[5]. The chance of postoperative bleeding can be minimized by fulguration of the entire resected area and meticulous hemostasis intraoperatively. Continued hemostasis during the resection will maintain full visibility during the procedure and allow the resectionist to fulgurate bleeding sites accurately and to resect to the desired depth. The use of simple catheter drainage or constant bladder irrigation postoperatively remains the choice of the individual surgeon. There is still a risk of perforation through the area of resection if the catheter becomes obstructed with blood clot and, therefore, great care must be exerted to maintain a patent drainage system.

Perforation. Various degrees of perforation of the bladder may occur and were detected in 5 percent of patients in the series of Dick's group[5]. Perforations pose the immediate problem of urinary leakage and a potentially serious threat of dissemination of neoplastic cells into the perivesical tissues. Small or minor perforations extending through the full thickness of the muscular wall of the bladder may result even with a forceps biopsy and certainly may be made with a resectoscope (see Figs. 10-2, 10-3). A minor perforation that extends only through the retroperitoneal portion of the bladder can be treated by transurethral catheter drainage for a few (2–4) days. The patient may experience some local pelvic discomfort and a febrile reaction is not uncommon, although serious sequelae are rare.

A more serious perforation is that which results from a full thickness cut with a resectoscope loop on the posterior wall of the bladder extending intraperitoneally. This perforation can be recognized endoscopically by inspection of the area and occasionally by visualization of loops of bowel at the depth of the perforation. In some cases, the rapid loss of irrigation fluid into the peritoneal cavity will be the first indication of perforation. The diagnosis can be confirmed with a cystogram, which will usually demonstrate leakage of the contrast into the peritoneal cavity.

Full thickness perforation extending intraperitoneally must be treated surgically. The abdomen should be explored to determine any damage to the bowel. The perforation should be closed in three layers and the bladder drained with a urethral catheter. Some urologists advocate segmental resection of the site of the tumor and perforation. Since the bladder contains, or has recently contained, a tumor, every attempt should be made to use a large transurethral catheter and to avoid a suprapubic drainage catheter to prevent further contamination of the perivesical area with urine containing tumor cells.

Unrecognized perforations should be considered in any patient who develops abdominal pain, tenderness, or distention in the postoperative period after transurethral resection of the bladder lesion. The diagnosis can be made most accurately by cystography. Operative drainage of any urinoma, repair of the perforation, and catheter drainage of the bladder should then be performed.

Obturator Spasm. The obturator nerve courses immediately adjacent to the inferolateral bladder wall and bladder neck as well as the lateral extent of the prostate. During transurethral resection in these areas, the electric current can directly stimulate the nerve and thus cause contraction of the adductor muscles. This produces a violent medial adduction of the leg, which may result in inadvertent bladder perforation. Since this action results from direct stimulation of the nerve, it can be eliminated only by blocking the nerve conduction distal to the point of stimulation. This can be accomplished by neuromuscular blockade with agents such as curare or succinylcholine. These agents can be used only with general anesthesia and mechanical support of the patient's respiration. When spinal anesthesia is used, the obturator nerve can be blocked by injecting a local anesthetic to infiltrate the area of the obturator nerve as it passes through the obturator canal [2].

SURVEILLANCE AFTER THERAPY. The urologist must be constantly alert to the possibility of recurrent bladder tumors after treatment of the first lesion. Whether these are recurrent tumors at the same site, implants at other locations, or entirely new lesions expressing the multicentricity of transitional cell neoplasms remains a theoretic consideration, but the problem confronting both patient and urologist is the diagnosis and treatment of the new lesions. Since the patient remains at high risk of developing bladder tumors, endoscopic surveillance of the bladder mucosa should be maintained. The bladder should be inspected by cystourethroscopy at intervals of 3 to 4 months. This interval has become accepted as a reasonable period to allow any inflammatory reaction to subside and to permit recurrent tumors to become recognizable without growing to a large, unmanageable size. After the patient has been tumor-free for 2 years, the period between endoscopies can be lengthened to 6 months or longer. The importance of endoscopic surveillance after a tumor-free interval of 4 to 5 years is less certain, but the patient must still be considered at risk, and yearly endoscopy is a conservative program to detect new lesions.

ADJUVANT THERAPY. The high incidence of tumor recurrence after endoscopic therapy has stimulated considerable interest in adjuvant therapy. The risk of recurrence varies with the grade, size, and number of the initial tumors. The chance of developing a subsequent invasive tumor is approximately 4 percent after a Ta lesion but increases to nearly 30 percent after a T1 lesion. Data from the National Bladder Cancer Collaborative Group indicate that among a group of 259 patients documented to be tumor-free after endoscopic resection, only 65 percent remained disease-free after 1 year and only 52 percent were tumor-free after 2 years [4]. The theories regarding management of tumor recurrence, which include the possibility of reimplantation of live tumor cells at the time of endoscopic resection or development of new tumors in urothelium suffering from preneoplastic field changes, support the concept of total intravesical therapy, possibly at the time of endoscopic resection. Several forms of therapy have been attempted, each with various advantages.

Intravesical Balloon. Blandy[6] has advocated the use of the Helmstein intravesical balloon for eradication of the bulk of large or multiple papillary tumors prior to resection of the stalk and base. With this technique, a large balloon on the tip of the catheter is inserted into the bladder under constant epidural anesthesia and inflated with saline to a pressure that is 10 mm Hg greater than the patient's diastolic blood pressure. The pressure is maintained at that level for 6 hours by adding saline to the balloon as necessary. Thus, ischemic necrosis of the papillary portion of the tumor is obtained. Papillary tumors may be selectively affected because of angulation of blood vessels passing through the stalk. Although considerable necrotic debris may be passed in the urine over the following 2 to 4 weeks, subsequent endoscopic inspection of the bladder will show minimal residual tumor at the bases of the lesions, which then can be easily resected. This technique has been useful primarily for otherwise unresectable tumors but does not appear to be effective in regard to the otherwise uninvolved mucosa.

Interstitial Radiation. Although external beam radiation has not been indicated for definitive or adjunctive therapy of superficial bladder cancer and recently has been questioned as an adjuvant for extirpative therapy of invasive lesions, interstitial radiation has been examined in superficial bladder cancer with impressive results. Implantation of radium, radioactive gold, and tantalum have shown excellent patient survival and tumor eradication. These techniques have produced sufficiently high response rates to indicate the value of further studies[13].

Intravesical Chemotherapy. Intravesical administration of chemotherapeutic agents has been suggested in patients with multiple recurrent bladder tumors. When administered postoperatively, thiotepa, mitomicin C, and doxorubicin hydrochloride (Adriamycin) have increased the number of patients who remained tumor-free postoperatively[13]. It has been suggested that many of the recurrences seen after resection of bladder tumors actually represent implantation of tumors dispersed at the time of resection. Strong support for this theory is the observation that many recurrences take place at the dome of the bladder wall but that very few primary tumors occur in that location. This has led to the suggestion that chemotherapeutic agents should be instilled into the bladder immediately after resection of the tumor rather than later in the postoperative period.

Complications of intravesical chemotherapy have included granulocytopenia and vesical irritation but these do not appear to be increased by immediate postoperative instillation. The ultimate role of intravesical chemotherapy in the treatment of bladder tumors remains to be demonstrated.

Intravesical Bacillus Calmette-Guérin. Initial studies utilizing bacillus Calmette-Guérin (BCG) as a nonspecific immunostimulant have produced excellent results in preventing bladder tumor recurrence. In three different studies examining the role of intravesical BCG in preventing recurrence of superficial bladder tumors, there has been a significant decrease in the recurrences in the immunotherapy group[13].

Favorable results were also seen when intravesical BCG was used in conjunction with intradermal BCG for the treatment of diffuse flat carcinoma in situ. There was marked decrease in the incidence of positive bladder biopsy in patients treated with the immunotherapy when compared with a control group treated by transurethral resection alone. The patients also noted a marked relief of irritative urinary symptoms. Similar results have been obtained in a shorter series utilizing intravesical BCG alone without systemic administration[10].

There are numerous variables to be considered in the use of BCG for immunotherapy. These include the specific strain and viability of the BCG employed and the timing and route of administration. The optimal conditions for BCG immunotherapy have not yet been determined.

Laser Therapy of Bladder Tumors. Lasers have also been used for the endoscopic treatment of bladder tumors[12]. The term *laser* represents *l*ight *a*mplification of *s*timulated *e*mission of *r*adiation. Several types of instruments, which vary in their functional capabilities, are available. The carbon dioxide and argon instruments give little tissue penetration and have not been used widely for endoscopic urologic procedures. The neodymium-YAG laser causes a deep coagulation injury, which may extend through the full thickness of the bladder wall. It has proved to be of greater value in the bladder.

The laser beam is transmitted by a quartz glass fiber passed through a rigid or flexible endoscope and directed to the target tissue. The length of exposure and the power (watts) are accurately regulated to calculate the dosage of energy (joules) applied to the lesion.

Entire small bladder tumors can be coagulated by several applications of laser radiation with exposures lasting only a few seconds. Larger tumors can be eradicated more efficiently by first resecting the bulky portion of the tumor with the standard electroresectoscope and then coagulating the base with the laser. Since the laser coagulates tissue, it provides hemostasis as well and allows operation in a bloodless field.

The major advantages of laser treatment of bladder tumors include the lack of bleeding and subsequent accuracy, the usual elimination of a need for a catheter postoperatively, and the patient's comfort. Among the disadvantages, there is some danger of injury to bowel overlying the posterior wall of the bladder because of forward scatter from treatment of a lesion in that area. The instrument is expensive and no convincing evidence as yet exists that treatment of bladder tumors endoscopically with a laser provides any greater success than conventional therapy.

REFERENCES

1. Appell, R., Flynn, J. T., Paris, A. M. I., and Blandy, J. P. Occult bacterial colonization of bladder tumors. *J. Urol.* 124:345; 1980.
2. Augspurger, R. R., and Donohue, R. E. Prevention of obturator nerve stimulation during transurethral surgery. *J. Urol.* 123:170, 1980.
3. Barnes, R. Cited in S. Silber, *Transurethral Resection.* New York: Appleton-Century-Crofts, 1977. P. 177.
4. Cutler, S. J., Heney, N. M., and Friedell, G. H. L. Longitudinal Study of Patients With Bladder Cancer: Factors Associated With Disease Recurrence and Regression. In W. M. Bonney and G. R. Prout, Jr. (Eds.), *Bladder Cancer* (AAU monograph). Baltimore: Williams & Wilkins, 1982. Pp. 35–46.
5. Dick, A., Barnes, R., Hadley, H., Bergman, R. T., and Ninan, C. A. Complications of transurethral resection of bladder tumors: Prevention, recognition and treatment. *J. Urol.* 124:810, 1980.
6. England, H. R., Rigby, C., Shepheard, B. G. F., Tresidder, G. C., and Blandy, J. P. Evaluation of Helmstein's distention method for carcinoma of the bladder. *Br. J. Urol.* 45:593, 1973.
7. Freed, S. Z. Vesicoureteral reflux following transurethral resection of bladder tumors. *J. Urol.* 116:184, 1976.
8. Goldwasser, B., Bogokowsky, B., Nativ, O., Sidi, A. A., and Mony, M. Urinary infections following transurethral resection of bladder tumors—Rate and source. *J. Urol.* 129:1123, 1983.
9. Greene, L. F., and Yalowitz, P. A. The advisability of concomitant transurethral excision of vesical neoplasm and prostatic hyperplasia. *J. Urol.* 107:445, 1972.
10. Herr, H. Carcinoma in-situ of the bladder. *Semin. Urol.* 1:15, 1983.
11. Laor, E., Grabstald, H., and Whitmore, W. F. The influence of simultaneous resection of bladder tumors and prostate on the occurrence of prostatic urethral tumors. *J. Urol.* 126:171, 1981.
12. Smith, J. A., and Dixon, J. A. Laser photoradiation in urologic surgery. *J. Urol.* 131:631, 1984.
13. Soloway, M. S. Surgery and intravesical chemotherapy in the management of superficial bladder cancer. *Semin. Urol.* 1:22, 1983.
14. Whitmore, W. F. Management of invasive bladder neoplasms. *Semin. Urol.* 1:34, 1983.

11
CHROMOCYSTOSCOPY AND MICROSCOPIC CYSTOSCOPY

W. B. Gill

Jeffry L. Huffman

Edward S. Lyon

Demetrius H. Bagley

In vivo detection of malignant or premalignant bladder urothelium has become increasingly important with the realization that carcinoma in situ and sessile tumors, which tend to be high grade and potentially invasive, are frequently difficult to recognize by ordinary cystoscopy. Several methods employing selective chemical markers of abnormal urothelium have been developed for the in vivo detection of malignant urothelium. These selective in vivo chemical methods, which result in "colored" urothelial surfaces, are designated as *chromocystoscopy*. This chapter reviews the in vivo methods currently available for the clinical detection of uroepithelial neoplasms and other abnormal urothelium (Table 11-1), including the chromocystoscopic techniques of (1) tetracycline fluorescent chromocystoscopy, (2) hematoporphyrin derivative fluorescent chromocystoscopy, (3) intravesical ionic dye (methylene blue) ordinary light chromocystoscopy, and (4) microscopic chromocystoscopy (in vivo urothelial histology with cellular resolution).

TETRACYCLINE ULTRAVIOLET FLUORESCENT CHROMOCYSTOSCOPY. Tetracycline fluorescent cystoscopy was the first development in chromocystoscopy. Following Rall's report[12] in 1957 of the appearance and persistence of fluorescent material in tumor tissue after tetracycline administration, Whitmore, Bush, and Esquivel[14] in 1964 described "tetracycline ultraviolet fluorescence in bladder carcinoma" and the development of an "ultraviolet-light endoscope." A 200-watt (W) mercury arc lamp with quartz optics provided high-energy peaks at wavelengths of 366 and 403 nanometers (nM), which excited tetracycline to fluoresce at a wavelength of 520 nM, which emitted a golden yellow color readily detected by employing a yellow filter in the cystoscope to eliminate other scattered radiation in the visible range. Whitmore and Bush[13] reported that 70 of 86 patients (81%) showed tetracycline ultraviolet fluorescence of their bladder tumors following oral tetracycline for 2 to 6 days.

Table 11-1. Methods for In Situ Mapping of Bladder Cancer (In Vivo Detection of Malignant Urothelial Surfaces)

A. Natural cystoscopic appearance of areas of frank tumor, ulceration, inflammation
B. Random (selected site) biopsy of normal-appearing bladder surfaces
C. Chromocystoscopy (in vivo chemical markers of abnormal urothelium)
1. Tetracycline fluorescence chromocystoscopy
2. Hematoporphyrin derivative fluorescence chromocystoscopy
3. Intravesical ionic dye binding with ordinary light chromocystoscopy
4. Microscopic chromocystoscopy (in vivo urothelial histology with cellular resolution)

Microscopic tetracycline ultraviolet fluorescence was reported successful by Barlow and co-workers[1] in 7 of 29 patients with bladder tumors; fluorescence of calcium salt encrustations of 5 of these tumors yielded especially strong results. Barlow's group also reviewed the proposed sites for tetracycline localization: inflammatory tissue, macrophages, mitochondria, peptides, protein-bound complexes, depolymerized mucopolysaccharides, chondroitin sulfate, and beta-lipoproteins in the presence of calcium ions. Tetracycline fluorescence cystoscopy for in situ mapping of bladder cancer has not gained wide popularity, which is probably due to the high expense of endoscopic equipment and the variable reported rates of false positives and false negatives.

HEMATOPORPHYRIN DERIVATIVE FLUORESCENT CHROMOCYSTOSCOPY. The use of a hematoporphyrin derivative (HpD) in tumor detection dates back to the 1961 report of Lipson, Baldes, and Olsen[11]. It was not until 1976, however, that Kelly and Snell[10] reported the use of hematoporphyrin derivatives in the diagnosis and phototherapy of carcinoma of the bladder. Benson and his associates at the Mayo Clinic[2] have been instrumental in further development of hematoporphyrin derivatives for detection and localization of in situ carcinoma of the bladder.

Hematoporphyrin derivatives are prepared by treatment of commercial grade hematoporphyrin with a mixture of sulfuric and acetic acids. HpD is a complex mixture of porphyrins, including mono- and diacetates of hematoporphyrin. HpD is usually given intravenously 2 to 48 hours before examination of the bladder. Fluorescence of HpD requires excitation at 400 to 410 nM, and special optical filters and electronics have been developed by the Mayo group for detecting the salmon red emission at about 630 nM.

At the Mayo Clinic, 16 patients undergoing cystectomy have been treated with intravenous HpD 2 to 48 hours before surgery[2]. Fluorescent mapping under violet–near ultraviolet light of the cystectomy specimens showed perfect correlation with semi-step sectioning histology of either transitional cell carcinoma, carcinoma in situ, or severe dysplasia. Regenerating mucosa surrounding recent biopsy sites gave faint fluorescence.

The current endoscopic equipment for HpD fluorescence provides simultaneous viewing with normal white light through the conventional endoscope and special optical filters and electronics for detecting HpD fluorescence at 630 nM with conversion to an audio signal. Although that system does not provide direct visualization of fluorescence, the Mayo group is investigating the possibility of direct fluorescent visualization with rigid endoscopes[2].

INTRAVESICAL IONIC DYE CHROMOCYSTOSCOPY WITH METHYLENE BLUE. Urothelial injury has been found to result in crystal adhesion only to abnormal urothelium in experimental animals[7]. During further studies we found that several ionic histochemical dyes (cationic methylene blue, toluidine blue, alcian blue, anionic Evans blue, Congo red, and trypan blue) would bind in vivo only to injured urothelium but not to normal urothelium in rats and guinea pigs[6]. An additional observation by our group has been the frequent finding of microscopic crystals of stone salts or gross crystalline masses adherent to the surfaces of human bladder tumors[4].

With these correlations in mind of crystal and dye adherence only to injured urothelium in animals and crystal adherence to abnormal urothelium of bladder tumors in humans, we postulated that bladder tumors might have abnormal urothelial surfaces, which would result in the in vivo binding of intravesical ionic dyes to the surfaces of bladder tumors but not to normal urothelium. Methylene blue was chosen because of its availability for human use and our previous animal experience with its selective staining of only injured urothelium. The cationic structure of methylene blue is:

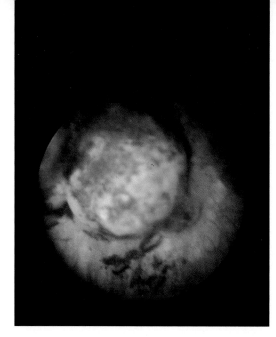

Figure 11-1. *Standard foroblique cystoscopic view of a papillary bladder tumor stained by methylene blue in 0.9% saline with unstained normal urothelium in the background (note fragment of tumor surface washed off by endoscopic irrigation).*

Table 11-2. In Vivo Intravesical Methylene Blue Staining of Human Bladder (Transitional Cell) Carcinomas

Procedure	No. Patients	Positive Methylene Blue Stain (no. patients)
Total cystectomy	12	12
Partial cystectomy	1	1
Endoscopic treatment	39	35
Total	52	48 (92%)

Intravesical instillations of methylene blue resulted in selective surface staining of bladder tumors in vivo without staining of the background of normal urothelium in 48 of 52 patients (Table 11-2). The endoscopic appearance of methylene blue–stained tumor is shown in Figure 11-1. Cup forceps biopsies of in vivo methylene blue–stained papillary tumors usually demonstrate multiple fronds of tumor with areas of deeper staining tumor nuclei and lighter staining cytoplasm. Although both cationic methylene blue and anionic Evans blue dyes are taken up by mouse bladder tumors as well as human bladder tumors, binding to tumor nuclei is more intense with cationic dyes than with anionic dyes.

We found that the blue staining of tumor surfaces varied from complete, uniform gross coverage to patchy mottled coverage. The intensity of the staining and extent of surface coverage was related to at least three observed variables: (1) Vigorous endoscopic irrigation could wash off small patches of stained surfaces and leave a mottled appearance. (2) Under microscopic examination of frozen section or polarized light stereomicroscopy of the surfaces of unsectioned biopsy specimens, crystalline masses of calcium oxalate or uric acid were seen to adhere to the surfaces between the dye-stained areas. (3) Higher-grade tumors usually bound to the dye more extensively than lower-grade tumors.

Specificity of in vivo staining was probably related to the normal permeability, which would allow the ionic dyes to gain access to the normally protected underlying urothelial cells[8], of tumor surfaces or areas mechanically scraped through Foley catheterization or cystoscopy. Semi-step sectioning of cystectomy specimens showed good correlation between in vivo dye binding and histologic tumor demonstration of frank carcinoma, carcinoma in situ, or dysplasia. Areas of hyperplasia, bacterial cystitis, and radiation cystitis did not bind to methylene blue. The 4 patients whose tumors did not bind to methylene blue had previously received chemotherapy, which might account for the false-negative results.

In vivo staining was accomplished by instilling 0.1% methylene blue in saline (0.9% NaCl) intravesically via a Foley catheter[3]. The methylene blue solution ran in under gravity with no more than 20 cm of water pressure to a maximum of 400 ml. Usually the bladders held volumes of less than 400 ml under 20-cm water pressure. After 5 minutes of in vivo staining, the methylene blue solution was drained and the bladder was lavaged 3 times by "gravity fill" and drainage with 90 ml of 0.9% saline.

Endoscopy was then immediately carried out with either a cystoscope or a resectoscope. Endoscopic photography was performed with an Olympus 35-mm camera, an automatic flash exposure photographic unit, and high-speed (ASA 400) Ektachrome film (see chap. 19)[9]. Biopsies were accomplished with either cystoscopic rigid cup biopsy forceps or transurethral electrosection loops. Biopsy specimens were placed into either formalin (10% phosphate–buffered formal saline) for permanent hematoxylin and eosin histologic sections or cold saline for frozen sections. Biopsies were taken from both stained and unstained areas. Twelve patients undergoing total cystectomy were also stained in vivo by intravesical instillation of 0.1% methylene blue just before the start of surgery. The bladders were opened and photographed and sectioned for both frozen and formalin-fixed permanent sections after completion of the cystectomies.

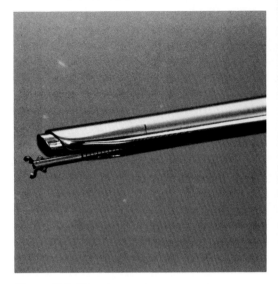

Figure 11-2. *The microscopic cystoscope has an examining sheath and a working sheath, which will accept small flexible-biopsy forceps.*

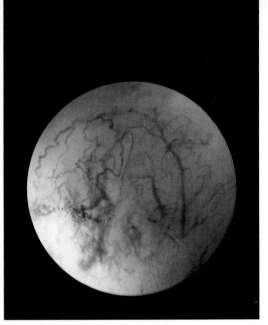

Figure 11-3. *View of bullous edema cystitis through a microscopic cystoscope shows a peripheral vascular pattern in an arc extending from the base, approximately 20× original magnification (stained cells in a linear pattern are the result of cystoscope trauma prior to instillation of methylene blue in 0.9% NaCl).*

In vivo intravesical staining with methylene blue has proved a simple and safe procedure employing regular endoscopic equipment that has facilitated endoscopic localization for biopsy and fulguration-resection of transitional cell carcinomas. The nature of the solvent with respect to the effects of pH, ionic strength, osmolality, and glycosaminoglycans on ionic dye binding in vivo to tumor urothelium is currently under investigation. The in vivo ligand binding to abnormal urothelial surfaces as demonstrated by these studies with ionic dyes may give further insights into the roles of abnormal urothelial surface electrochemistry in the pathogenesis and therapy of uroepithelial neoplasia.

MICROSCOPIC CHROMOCYSTOSCOPY (IN VIVO UROTHELIAL SURFACE HISTOLOGY). By combining magnification cystoscopy and microscopic cystoscopy with intravesical ionic dye chromocystoscopy, we have been able to develop in vivo urothelial surface histology with resolution of cytologic detail [5].

Magnification cystoscopy can be accomplished with magnification lenses for endoscopic photography. Fixed magnification lenses up to 200 mm and zoom lenses from 1.4 to 2× magnification enable the cystoscopist to view the cystoscopic ocular image readily through the camera screen. Magnification cystoscopy when combined with intravesical dye chromocystoscopy gives detectable resolution of nuclear staining of human bladder tumors (approximately 10× total magnification).

Microscopic cystoscopy has recently become available with the development of microscopic colposcopes and hysteroscopes. The contact microscopic endoscope of Karl Storz Instruments has two lens systems controlled by a push-button switch in the handle for either 60× or 150× magnification, which can be increased by up to a factor of 1.4 with a zoom camera lens and screen (Fig. 11-2). Without contact with the urothelium, these two lens systems, which can be focused, give either 1× or 20× magnification for panoramic viewing of the bladder surfaces. Microscopic chromocystoscopy, the combination of microscopic cystoscopy with intravesical ionic dye chromocystoscopy, results in both in vivo urothelial surface histology and resolution of subcellular details.

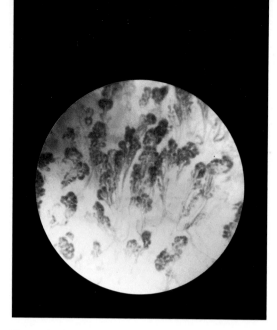

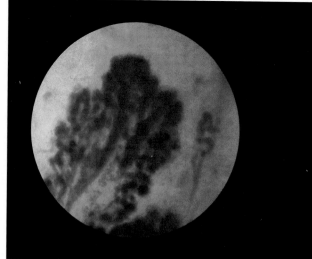

Figure 11-4. *Papillary tumor vasculature is character-ized by a dense arborization with terminal tufting (ap-proximately 20× original magnification through the microscopic cystoscope).*

Figure 11-5. *Higher magnification (approximately 150× through microscopic cystoscope) of papillary tu-mor shown in Fig. 11-3. (Note terminal tufting from a central vascular stalk.)*

Staining of urothelial surface cells for micro-scopic chromocystoscopy can be done in two different ways. Differential staining of tumor or other abnormal urothelium without dye binding to normal urothelium is performed with 0.1% (2.67 mM) methylene blue in distilled water for 15 to 20 minutes since the penetration and binding of ionic dyes is an inverse function of the ionic strength of the solvent. Microscopic chromocystos-copy has been performed on the following disease entities: (1) uroepithelial (transitional cell) carci-nomas, grades 1 to 3; (2) chronic cystitis with "bul-lous edema"; (3) Hunner's chronic interstitial cystitis; (4) flat carinoma in situ; and (5) normal urothelium. The bladders were all viewed with the microscopic cystoscope before and after sequential staining with methylene blue in 0.9% NaCl, 0.45% NaCl, and water.

Vascular patterns were determined initially by microscopic cystoscopy before methylene blue staining. Differences are readily seen between the typical vascular patterns of normal urothelium and those of the hyperplastic urothelium of bullous edema cystitis (Fig. 11-3) and uroepithelial carci-noma, papillary grade 2 (Figs. 11-4, 11-5). The tumor vasculature is characterized by a dense ar-borization with terminal tufting from a central vascular stalk. Bullae of hyperplastic, cystitis uro-thelium show a peripheral vascular pattern in an arc extending from the base. Both of these abnor-mal patterns contrast with the straighter, less dense vasculature of normal urothelium.

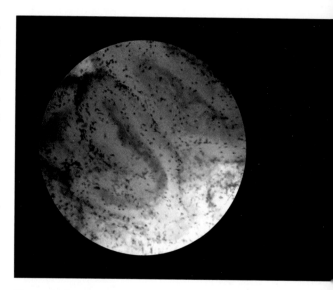

Figure 11-6. *Microscopic chromocystoscopy of a papil-lary bladder tumor stained with methylene blue (note papillary tumor with vascular cores and overlying stained tumor cells at 60× original magnification).*

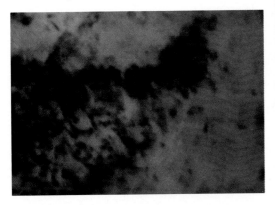

Figure 11-7. *Microscopic chromocystoscopy of tumor shown in Fig. 11-4 at 150× original magnification (note deeply stained, somewhat irregular tumor nuclei).*

Selective tumor-staining patterns with methylene blue in 0.9% NaCl without staining of normal urothelium are shown of papillary grade 2 carcinomas in Figures 11-6 and 11-7. Note the selective staining of the papillary tumors and the vascular stalk covered with uroepithelial tumor cells, which together comprise the papillary tumor unit.

Cytologic detail is resolvable with the highest magnification (150×), as shown in Figure 11-7. Note the large, irregular, heavily stained tumor nuclei as seen through the microscopic cystoscope. With improved lighting for photography, endoscopic photographs should approach the clarity seen directly through the microscopic cystoscope (Fig. 11-8).

Generalized staining of normal urothelial surface cells was accomplished by methylene blue in water after previous selective staining of tumor and abnormal urothelium by methylene blue in high ionic strength sodium chloride solutions. The cytologic resolution of normal urothelial surface cells showed relatively round, regular nuclei and abundant cytoplasm.

These efforts demonstrate the feasibility of performing in vivo urothelial surface histology with resolution of cellular detail. The in vivo patterns noted of tumor vasculature, differential tumor susceptibility of staining in higher ionic strength solvents, and tumor histological and cellular detail have aided in interpretation of the location and extent of these lesions. The microscopic cystoscope marks a significant addition to the urologist's endoscopic armamentarium.

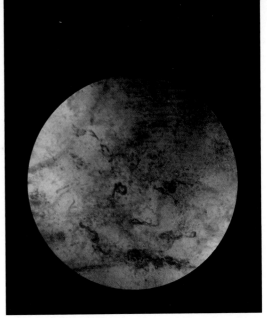

Figure 11-8. *Flat carcinoma in situ seen through the microscopic cystoscope (low-power contact) after methylene blue staining exhibits diffuse cellular uptake with pleomorphic nuclei and hypervascularity with tortuous vessels.*

With more experience and refinement of the procedure, we believe that in vivo urothelial histology by microscopic chromocystoscopy should enhance the ability of the urologist to diagnose and treat diseases of abnormal urothelium, both malignant and benign. Also, further studies of in vivo ligand binding to abnormal urothelial surfaces, as demonstrated by these studies with a cationic dye, may give further insights into the roles of abnormal urothelial surface electrochemistry in the pathogenesis, diagnosis, and therapy of uroepithelial neoplasms.

REFERENCES

1. Barlow, K. A., Maurice, B. A., Chir, M., and Atkins, P. Ultraviolet fluorescence of bladder tumors following oral administration of tetracycline compounds. *Cancer* 19:1013, 1966.

2. Benson, R. C., et al. Detection and localization of *in situ* carcinoma of the bladder with hematoporphyrin derivative. *Mayo Clin. Proc.* 57:548, 1982.

3. Gill, W. B., et al. Selective surface staining of bladder tumors by intravesical methylene blue with enhanced endoscopic identification. *Cancer* 53(12):2724, 1984.

4. Gill, W. B., Huffman, J. L., and Lyon, E. S. Stone crystals adherent to the urothelial surfaces of human bladder tumors. *Proc. North Cen. Sec. Am. Urol. Assoc.* 56:25, 1982.

5. Gill, W., Huffman, J., Lyon, E., and Bagley, D. In vivo urothelial surface histology by microscopic chromocystoscopy. *J. Urol.* 130:669, 1983.

6. Gill, W. B., Jones, K. W., and Schoenberg, H. W. Deleterious effects of certain intravesical urological solutions on the urothelium of rat bladders. *Proc. Am. Urol. Assoc.* 76(78):111, 1981.

7. Gill, W. B., Ruggiero, K. J., and Straus, F. H., II. Crystallization studies in urothelial-lined living test tube (the catheterized female rat bladder). *Invest. Urol.* 17:257, 1979.

8. Hicks, R. M., Ketterer, B., and Warren, R. C. The ultrastructure and chemistry of the luminal plasma membrane of the mammalian urinary bladder: A structure with low permeability to water and ions. *Phil. Trans. Royal Soc.* B 268:23, 1974.

9. Huffman, J. L., Bagley, D. H., and Lyon, E. S. Endoscopic photography of the urinary tract. *Proc. Am. Urol. Assoc.* 77(478):197, 1982.

10. Kelly, J. F., and Snell, N. E. Hematoprophyrin derivative: A possible aid in the diagnosis and therapy of carcinoma of the bladder. *J. Urol.* 115:150, 1976.

11. Lipson, R. L., Baldes, E. J., and Olsen, A. M. The use of a derivative of hematoporphyrin in tumor detection. *J. Nat. Cancer Inst.* 26:1, 1961.

12. Rall, D. P., Loo, T. L., Land, M., and Kelly, M. G. Appearance and persistence of fluorescent material in tumor tissue after tetracycline administration. *J. Nat. Cancer Inst.* 19:70, 1957.

13. Whitmore, W. F., and Bush, I. M. Ultraviolet cystoscopy. *J.A.M.A.* 203:153, 1968.

14. Whitmore, W. F., Jr., Bush, I. M., and Esquivel, E. Tetracycline ultraviolet fluorescence in bladder carcinoma. *Cancer* 12:1528, 1964.

12

ENDOSCOPIC TREATMENT OF BLADDER CALCULI

Demetrius H. Bagley

Jeffry L. Huffman

Edward S. Lyon

Bladder calculi have occurred and been documented as a medical and surgical problem for centuries. The treatment of bladder calculi was one of the earliest specialized surgical procedures, with the development of these techniques forming a major portion of the history of surgery[9,13]. Although the trend throughout history has been toward a lower incidence of calculi as nutrition and medical care improve, stone disease in the bladder remains a therapeutic problem confronted by urologists.

PREDISPOSING FACTORS. There are numerous conditions predisposing to formation of calculi within the bladder. The prevalence of bladder calculi is related to the prevalence of these underlying factors. Crystals are formed in the urine within the bladder and as the outflow obstruction prevents their ready passage through the urethra, larger calculi are formed. Superimposition of infection, particularly with urea-splitting organisms, will promote the formation of calculi, usually of struvite composition. Foreign bodies are a frequent cause of bladder calculi since the surface of a foreign body serves as a focus for crystal formation. Indwelling bladder catheters are often a site for crystallization and also for formation of amorphous inflammatory material. While the catheter is in the bladder, casts of its tip may be formed and, when the catheter is removed, break off and remain within the bladder, thus forming a base for further encrustation (see Fig. 5-13). The abnormal surface of bladder tumors may also permit crystal adhesion and growth of calculi (see Figs. 5-25, 5-31).

SYMPTOMS. Most bladder calculi are asymptomatic. In patients with outlet obstruction, the symptoms are predominantly those related to the obstruction. The typical presentation in those patients who become symptomatic includes pain and hematuria. The pain may be of varying quality, is usually located in the lower abdomen, and is often increased at the end of urination. The urinary stream may be interrupted intermittently by the calculus lodging within the urethral orifice at the bladder neck. Microscopic hematuria is often present, and terminal gross hematuria may develop. If a urinary infection is present, it may be very difficult to eradicate.

DIAGNOSIS. Radioopaque vesical calculi can be seen on a plain radiogram of the abdomen and pelvis (Fig. 12-1). Radiolucent calculi may appear as a filling defect in the partially filled bladder during excretory urography, while the radioopaque calculi may consequently be obscured. Urinalysis will often demonstrate microscopic hematuria and frequently pyuria as well. Many bladder calculi are associated with cystitis, and the typical findings of pyuria, hematuria, and bacteriuria may be evident on urinalysis. Crystals of the same composition as the calculi may also be detected in the voided urine.

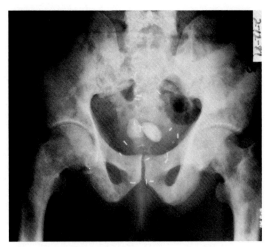

Figure 12-1. *Two radioopaque bladder calculi, composed of magnesium ammonium phosphate, are demonstrated on this plain radiogram of the abdomen in a male with a vesical neck contracture.*

The major diagnostic technique to ascertain the presence of vesical calculi is cystoscopy. Any calculi present, even within diverticula, can then be determined by direct inspection (see Figs. 5-18, 5-20). The calculi appear as crystalline structures or stones, usually moving freely within the bladder. Single or multiple calculi may be seen. The macroscopic crystalline structure typical of the chemical composition can usually be identified and is the same as that described for ureteral and renal calculi (see Chap. 6).

MANAGEMENT. Treatment of bladder stones can be divided between open surgical procedures and endoscopic procedures, which fragment the stones so that they can be removed transurethrally. Each technique has its unique advantages and complications.

Cystolithotomy. The open surgical approach, or cystolithotomy, has several advantages. If multiple calculi are present, they can all be removed at one time and even very large calculi or those adherent to the bladder can be removed. Earlier attempts at surgical removal used a perineal approach. This route had advantages that were essential before the availability of aseptic techniques and antibiotic therapy: The abdomen was not entered and dependent drainage was afforded. After aseptic techniques became accepted, the suprapubic approach was adopted as early as 1880 and remains the most frequent approach today. In many cases, the cause of obstruction can be treated and corrected at the same procedure. As an example, bladder calculi lodged in a diverticulum can be removed and the diverticulum itself can be excised. The major disadvantages of such a surgical procedure is the incision and the need for lengthy catheterization during bladder healing.

Endoscopic Treatment. The techniques available for endoscopic removal of calculi have many basic similarities in that the calculus is fragmented or crushed within the bladder into numerous, smaller pieces, which can then be removed through the urethra. These techniques have been developed and refined over more than a century. Some of the advantages of each technique and the potential complications remain basically similar, although the frequency and the techniques for avoiding and treating complications successfully have improved markedly.

Small bladder calculi (<5 mm in diameter) can be removed from the bladder with foreign body forceps or with Lowsley's forceps. Stones less than 4 mm in diameter can often be washed from the bladder through a resectoscope sheath of 26 or 28 Fr. by filling the bladder with irrigation fluid and allowing the fluid to flow from the sheath with the tip directed toward the base of the bladder where the stones rest. Small calculi can also be trapped with the resecting loop and drawn into the sheath.

LITHOTRITY. Lithotrity was the earliest endoscopic technique for treatment of bladder calculi. The calculi were detected within the bladder by passing metal sounds through the urethra and tapping on the base of the bladder until the calculus was detected or sounded. The calculus could then be crushed either with the sound or with specially designed lithotrites with opposing jaws that could be mechanically apposed to crush the calculus. The smaller fragments were then washed from the bladder through a large-eyed catheter. The patient was allowed to pass the remainder of the fragments while awaiting a future sitting for another attempt at lithotrity. This was a prolonged affair often accompanied by bladder injury and sepsis, which was frequently fatal.

Twinen[11] reviewed the early days of urology in New York City and found that the first recorded lithotrity was performed in 1846. Postoperatively, the patient passed several fragments and required a repeat operation in 9 days and was hospitalized for a total of 90 days. The hospital stay for lithotripsy varied from 25 to 180 days and required up to 6 procedures.

LITHOLAPAXY. Bigelow[3] introduced the concept of lithotrity by a single operation with irrigation of the fragments from the bladder at the same time. The procedure in which the calculus is crushed and the fragments are washed from the bladder is called *litholapaxy.* Bigelow also reported the development of a design for the lithotrite, which has as its advantage an inflow channel for irrigation fluid, opposing jaws with a wider foot plate to minimize the chance of injuring the bladder, and strong blades that could be closed with considerable mechanical advantage. In the same report he tried an evacuating apparatus with which fragments could be irrigated from the bladder. Bigelow also found that he could prolong the operation from the usual 2 to 5 minutes to the period necessary (3/4–3¾ hr) to flush and evacuate the stone entirely. The Bigelow lithotrite and procedure remained in use until the mid-twentieth century and was essentially unchanged, except for the addition of modern cystoscopic equipment for the diagnosis and irrigation of fragments. The technique continues to have its advocates but generally has been superseded by visual techniques.

Blind or tactile litholapaxy includes several steps that can be performed by a skilled urologist. (1) The bladder must be distended with irrigating fluid before the lithotrite is passed. (2) Once the jaws of the lithotrite have entered the bladder, the lower jaw is compressed against the bladder floor so that the stone or fragments of calculus can roll onto it. (3) The lithotrite is shaken gently to vibrate the fragments onto the lower jaw. (4) The jaws are totally apposed by the screw mechanism to crush any fragments between the jaws. (5) The position of the lower jaw should be changed several times and the steps for crushing repeated. (6) Fragments are evacuated through a resectoscope sheath to allow endoscopic observation for other fragments.

The potential for damage with this instrument is quite obvious. If the bladder is caught within the jaws of the instrument, with or without the calculus, it may be torn with a significant perforation. There may be rather active bleeding and extravasation of contrast outside of the bladder. In order to remove the fragments of calculus, the lithotrite must be removed and the resectoscope sheath placed through the urethra. Furthermore, if any fragments remain, the lithotrite would again have to be replaced and the procedure repeated.

Nevertheless, this procedure represented a major advance and became the standard therapy for bladder calculi for several decades. In New York City, litholapaxy with the Bigelow lithotrite was instituted as early as 1878 and reduced the average hospital stay from 70 days for a lithotripsy to 50 days for a perineal lithotomy to only 12 days for a litholapaxy[11]. More recently, Barnes, Bergman, and Worton[2] compared tactile litholapaxy with visual litholapaxy and cystolithotomy and found that litholapaxy afforded a shorter hospital stay and shorter operative procedure than cystolithotomy. Ninety-seven percent of patients required more than 5 days of hospitalization after cystolithotomy but only 50 percent of patients stayed in the hospital for more than 4 days after litholapaxy.

Visual Litholapaxy. Several disadvantages of blind litholapaxy were overcome by visual endoscopic techniques. In general, the visual lithotrite is an instrument with opposing jaws that appear within the field of vision during endoscopy. The calculus can be localized visually and grasped within the jaws of the instrument to be crushed in full endoscopic view. These lithotrites have the same propensity as blind lithotrites to damage the mucosa, and blood within the bladder may obscure the field; however, the larger fragments of stone can usually be seen and fragmented during a single procedure.

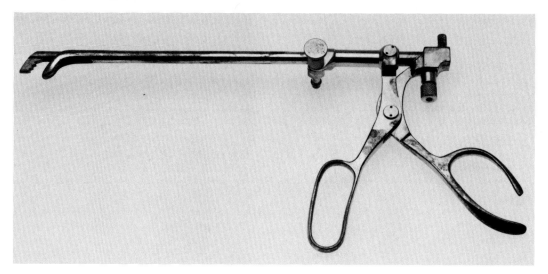

Figure 12-2. *The visual lithotrite can be used to crush calculi mechanically under endoscopic visualization.*

There are numerous designs for visual lithotrites. An instrument with laterally opposing jaws has been available but the possible disadvantage of this design is that the metal can, under rare circumstances, be twisted when force is applied to the handles and the jaws to crush the stones. This would prevent total apposition of the jaws and also prevent removal of the instrument transurethrally. Such a complication would demand surgical removal.

A second common design, known as the *Hendrickson lithotrite,* is an instrument with jaws that extend and retract to oppose in a fashion similar to the Bigelow lithotrite (Fig. 12-2). Variations of this instrument, which have different manual control mechanisms, have become available. The jaws may be closed with a handle or with rack and pinion control.

The visual lithotrite can be introduced into the bladder with a tactile technique. Although the blades of the instrument are relatively short, the angulation is more acute than that of Van Buren sounds; therefore, it may be slightly more difficult to negotiate the instrument through the urethra, over the bladder neck, and into the bladder. In order to pass it safely, the instrument should fall in the urethra to the proximal bulbous urethra and then be advanced into the bladder by lowering the end of the instrument in the operating hand. The instrument should not be lowered too soon or the tip may perforate the urethra.

Once the instrument enters the bladder, the telescope is replaced into it, and the calculus can then be visualized. The jaws of the lithotrite are opened and placed around the calculus but should be closed only after the urologist has determined that there is no bladder mucosa between the jaws. The stone is then trapped between the jaws as they are closed. The instrument is raised off the bladder floor into the lumen of the distended bladder to crush the stone completely. It may be necessary to repeat the procedure several times to crush the entire stone. The instrument is removed from the bladder after all the fragments have been reduced to a size that permits irrigation through the resectoscope sheath. The lithotrite can be replaced into the bladder as necessary to fragment the calculus further. Each passage, however, runs the risk of urethral damage with this rather large instrument.

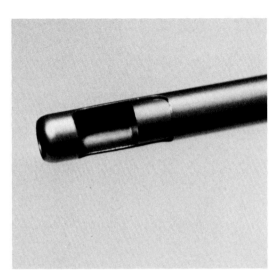

Figure 12-3. *The punch lithotrite can grasp and fragment small or irregular calculi and can be passed through an endoscopic sheath.*

Another more recent design is the punch lithotrite reported by Mauermayer (Fig. 12-3). This instrument has an inner and an outer cylinder with a slit located laterally on the distal portion of the outer cylinder into which stones can be placed endoscopically (Fig. 12-3). By sliding the cylinders together, the stone is crushed by biting pieces from the edge of the stone. It is useful for small bladder calculi but grasping the round surface of larger calculi may prove difficult with the instrument. Its major use has been for further crushing and removing calculi that have been partially fragmented with the electrohydraulic lithotriptor. This instrument affords excellent visibility of the working area and permits the operator to avoid injuring the bladder. Another major advantage is that the instrument can pass through a resectoscope sheath, thus allowing the entire procedure of stone fragmentation and irrigation through a single indwelling transurethral sheath.

Although visual lithotripsy permits safer and more accurate treatment of bladder calculi, injury to the bladder or urethra remains a potential and relatively frequent complication. There also remains a possibility of damage to the instrument itself. The instrument must be harder and stronger than the hardest stone to remain undamaged when excess force is applied to it. Although newer alloys result in much stronger instruments than the earlier versions, damage to the instrument remains a possibility. In addition, each of these instruments is limited by the size of the calculus that can be treated. Usually, the upper limit is 3 cm or less in diameter.

Ultrasonic Lithotripsy. Ultrasonic lithotripsy fragments calculi by passing ultrasonic vibrations produced in a ceramic crystal along a metal transducer in contact with the stone (see Fig. 17-2). The transducer is a hollow cylinder through which suction can be applied both to draw the stone to the transducer and to evacuate fragments with the irrigation fluid, which simultaneously cools the transducer. The transducer is rigid and straight and can be passed through a straight endoscope. The telescope, therefore, must be offset so that the head of the operator can be placed at the side of the major axis of the instrument for viewing.

To remove stones, the tip of the transducer is placed directly on the calculus, which is gradually drilled away by the ultrasonic movement of the transducer. A hole can be drilled into the calculus but, with careful change of position of the transducer, the stone can be fragmented into smaller and smaller pieces and gradually removed entirely. The transducer can be applied to the edge of the stone to prevent fragmentation into multiple small pieces and to achieve a gradual reduction in size. Although the transducer becomes quite hot after a few seconds of power application in air, the continuous circulation of irrigation solution provides cooling via the flow of water through the lumen. This is a relatively slow procedure but is also quite safe. It has achieved more popularity and success for the percutaneous removal of renal calculi (see Chap. 17). Within the bladder, more rapid procedures, which may allow escape of some of the fragments from the immediate operative area, have proved more appealing. Because of this accurate control of fragments without distention of the lumen, ultrasonic lithotripsy may also be particularly useful in a small contracted bladder containing calculi.

Electrohydraulic Lithotripsy. Electrohydraulic lithotripsy represents a major advance in the endoscopic treatment of bladder calculi. It offers the benefits of endoscopic stone removal with fewer of the disadvantages. This technique was described by Goldberg in the Latvian Urological Society in 1959. Practical therapy was established after development of the URAT-1, which was used in clinical series reported from several countries. Similar but technically advanced instruments have become available and are manufactured both in the United States and in Europe.

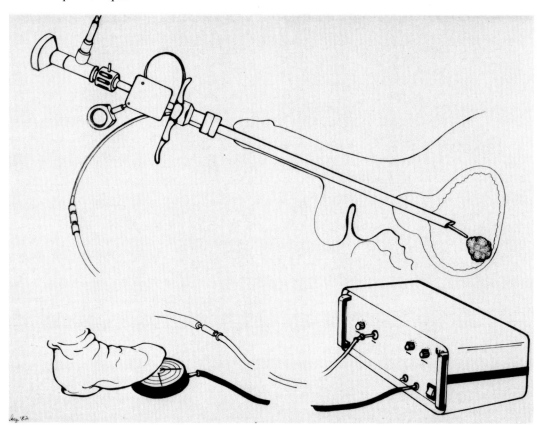

Figure 12-4. *The controls are readily accessible on both electrohydraulic lithotriptor units. The foot switch and the probe are connected to the power unit by well-insulated cables.*

The basis for this technique is spark formation within a liquid medium which, because of its incompressibility, transmits the impulses as shock waves that are destructive to rigid matter but non-injurious to pliable materials. In the electrohydraulic lithotriptor, a high voltage capacitor discharge is generated across a limited area at the tip of a coaxial cable electrode. When this occurs in a non-conductive or poorly conductive liquid medium, shock waves are established within the liquid. In a conductive medium, the current may be conducted without spark formation although saline has been used successfully in some instances. In the bladder containing a calculus, the elastic bladder walls absorb the shock waves without damage but the crystalline structure of the calculus is disrupted. By repeated application of the shock waves to the calculus, the entire stone can be fractured.

The power output can be regulated in either instrument with the higher settings required for initial fragmentation and for harder calculi (Fig. 12-4). There is a choice of single or repetitive impulses, and activation of the instrument and duration of the procedure can be controlled with a foot switch to leave both hands free for instrumentation. A well-insulated cable connects the circuitry box of the instrument to the coaxial cable transducer, which is placed into the bladder either through a standard cystoscope or a special guide element that can be passed through a resectoscope sheath (Fig. 12-5). It is most convenient to use the same sheath which will also accept the punch lithotrite for further fragmentation of the calculus.

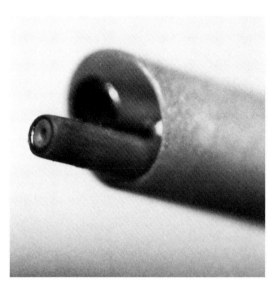

Figure 12-5. *The electrohydraulic lithotriptor probe can be used with either a standard cystoscope or a special carrier and sheath. The coaxial design of the electrode can be seen at the tip.*

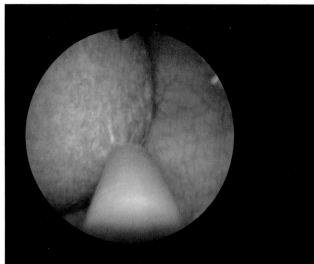

Figure 12-6. *The electrohydraulic lithotripsy (EHL) probe has been placed through the cystoscope into the bladder and the tip located near a uric acid calculus. (The same calculus appears in Figs. 12-7 to 12-11.)*

The transducer, or probe, is the working element of the lithotriptor and is subject to severe stresses in operation. It can destroy itself within 10 seconds of continuous operation but, when activated intermittently, can tolerate as long as 30 seconds of accumulated activity. The tip should be removed and inspected for damage during the procedure. Occasionally, a tear in the sheath can be seen endoscopically during the procedure (see Fig. 12-9). The probe should be replaced immediately if there is any damage to the insulation and should be limited to use in only a single procedure.

TECHNIQUE. After the bladder is inspected cystoscopically and the calculus identified, the electrohydraulic lithotriptor probe is passed through the instrument. Within the bladder, irrigation is continued with dilute saline (one-sixth or one-seventh normal) to distend the bladder sufficiently to move the bladder walls away from the calculus without overdistending the lumen. The probe of the lithotriptor is advanced under direct vision and positioned with its tip near the calculus but not in contact with it (Fig. 12-6). We prefer to place it approximately 2 to 4 mm from the surface of the calculus. A minimum distance of 1 cm should be maintained between the tip of the electrode and the lens at the tip of the telescope.

Fragmentation is then begun by activating the instrument with the foot switch to produce the spark that causes the electrohydraulic shock waves. The lower settings should be chosen and increased as necessary to produce a satisfactory shock wave to fragment the stone. The continuous, or repetitive, mode is chosen for initial fragmentation. Initial bursts of 1 to 2 seconds duration are then applied to the calculus until a fracture or break in the outer layer of the stone can be seen. As the impulse is generated across the tip of the probe, a spark develops at the tip and the calculus can be seen to be moved or fragments from the surface thrown through the irrigant (Fig. 12-7). The ideal setting for the lithotriptor is the lowest that will fragment the stone without excessive movement of the stone.

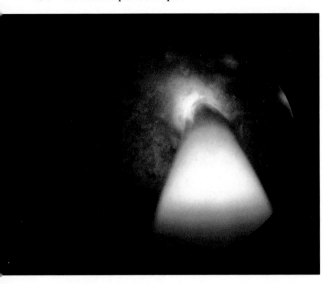

Figure 12-7. *The current is applied and a spark seen at the tip. Fragments of the stone are washed from the surface in the irrigant.*

After the outer surface has been fractured, the inner layers usually are easier to fragment. As a cavity develops in the outer surface, fragmentation of the irregular margin of the cavity is also usually easier (Fig. 12-8). If the calculus is broken into large fragments, lithotripsy should be continued and directed toward the irregular inner surface of each fragment. As smaller fragments are formed, a lower power setting of the instrument is used to minimize the scatter of fragments and the trauma to bladder mucosa. Disintegration with the electrohydraulic lithotriptor can be continued so that the fragments are no larger than gravel and can pass through the sheath (Figs. 12-9, 12-10).

Alternatively, once the calculus has been reduced to fragments no more than 0.5 to 1.0 cm, the electrohydraulic lithotriptor probe can be replaced with the punch lithotrite. The fragments are then further reduced with this instrument to particles that will pass through the sheath (Fig. 12-11). The smallest pieces can then be removed through the sheath by irrigation with the Ellik evacutor.

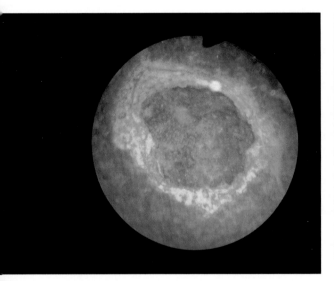

Figure 12-8. *A shallow cavity has formed with fragmentation of the surface of the stone.*

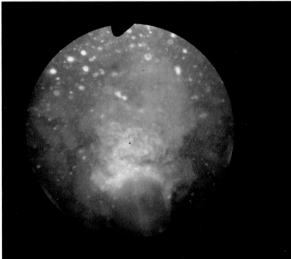

Figure 12-9. *As the stone is fragmented further, numerous particles in the irrigating fluid can be rinsed from the bladder through the sheath. The insulation of the lithotriptor probe has torn in this view (right side of probe), and the probe must be replaced.*

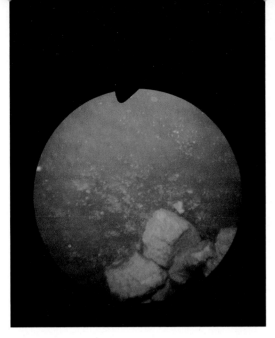

Figure 12-10. *Minute fragments, or sand, from the calculus and larger fragments requiring further breakdown are evident.*

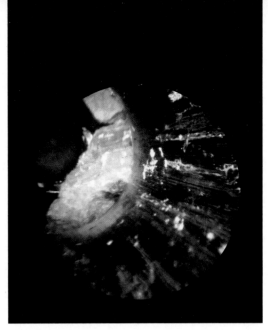

Figure 12-11. *These irregular fragments are easily broken further with the stone punch. The smaller fragments can then be irrigated through the sheath.*

Irrigation. Optimal sparking from the electrohydraulic lithotriptor probes require a very dilute electrolyte solution. The manufacturer has previously recommended using distilled water as the irrigant and relying on the residual ions in the bladder. The most reliable functioning, however, has been achieved with a dilute solution of sodium chloride (one-sixth to one-seventh normal saline). The manufacturer suggests using two methods of preparation: (1) Add 6 ml concentrated saline (23.4%) to 1 liter sterile distilled water, or (2) add 1.4 gm of NaCl to 1 liter sterile distilled water. A similar dilute solution can be made by adding 500 ml normal saline to 3 liters sterile distilled water. This final method is convenient for preparation of larger volumes of dilute saline, using readily available prepackaged solutions in standard-sized containers.

Results. Excellent results have been achieved with the use of the electrohydraulic lithotriptor for bladder calculi (Table 12-1). In collected series of several hundred patients, calculi from 0.5 to 7 cm have been fractured with a failure rate from 1 to 8 percent. In the report of 304 patients by Bulow and Frohmueller[4], electrohydraulic lithotripsy of the calculus, including removal of the fragments, required an average of 26.1 minutes with a range of 2 to 122 minutes. Uric acid, which previously had been found to be the hardest bladder stone treated, was present in 53.5 percent of the cases.

Complications have been minimal. Electrohydraulic lithotripsy causes remarkably little mucosal injury. Small fragments of calculi may become imbedded in the bladder mucosa, but this risk can be lessened by decreasing the intensity and duration of the spark applied to fragments. Excessive hematuria is only very rarely a problem but mild hematuria is expected. In one series, hematuria was noted in 9.9 percent of patients[10]. The reported incidence of postoperative fever ranged from "seldom" to 18.9%, but most series reported no major episode of sepsis[7,8,10]. Bladder perforation occurred in 6 of 304 patients studied by Bulow and Frohmueller[4], but surgical drainage was necessary in only a single patient (0.3%).

Difficult Calculi. As may be expected, soft irregular stones are fragmented much more easily than harder or smooth stones, which may reflect the shock waves more effectively. Small stones may move about as they are struck by the shock waves, but this problem can be overcome by trapping the stones between the probe and the bladder mucosa. Uric acid stones are among the hardest urinary calculi, and Raney[7] has reported the difficulty in fragmenting these stones with the electrohydraulic lithotriptor. Because uric acid stones are also soluble in an alkaline medium, however, those that will not fragment with electrohydraulic lithotripsy can often be dissolved or at least partially dissolved with irrigation or with treatment with alkalinizing agents.

Table 12-1. Bladder Calculi Treated by Electrohydraulic Lithotripsy

Series	Year	No. Patients	Size of Calculi	Failures	Complications	
					Hematuria	Fever
Reuter[8]	1970	50	1–6 cm	NS	NS	Seldom
Raney[7]	1976	34	NS	4	(No major)	(No sepsis)
Trapznikov[10]	1977	201	0.5–7.0 cm	2	9.9%	18.9%
Bapat[1]	1977	38	2.5 cm	NS	Slight	NS
Bulow[4]	1981	304	1–135 gm	24	NS	NS

NS = not studied.

We have encountered a single patient with a struvite bladder stone formed on intravesical hair that evidently had migrated into the bladder, in which an indwelling catheter had been present for years. Although the shell of the calculus fragmented easily with the electrohydraulic lithotriptor, the structure of the stone was held intact with the interwoven hairs. Some of the hair could be grasped with three-pronged grasping forceps and drawn through the sheath, leaving smaller fragments of stone within the bladder, which then could be irrigated through the sheath. We have had a similar patient in whom a stone formed on a fragment of the latex balloon of a urethral catheter. The crystalline material was fractured with the electrohydraulic lithotriptor and the piece of latex was then removed through the sheath. The fragments were subsequently removed by irrigating them through the sheath.

Calculi Within Diverticula. The calculus located within a diverticulum presents special problems in therapy. The wall of the diverticulum is considerably thinner and more delicate than the intact bladder wall. The possibility of perforating the diverticulum is much higher than the chance of injuring the bladder itself. Therefore, particular care must be taken in fragmenting these stones. The probe of the electrohydraulic lithotriptor can be placed adjacent to the mouth of the diverticulum and the calculus. Fragmentation should be initiated at the lowest possible power and increased as necessary. As soon as the fragments are sufficiently small, they should be removed from the diverticulum into the body of the bladder. Within the bladder itself, they can be fragmented further without fear of perforating the diverticulum. The entire diverticulum should be inspected at the completion of the procedure to ensure that all calculus fragments have been removed. Since it may be difficult to reach and observe the entire diverticulum with a rigid instrument, it may be advantageous to inspect the diverticulum with the flexible nephroscope used in the capacity of a cystoscope. Treatment of the diverticulum itself can then be individualized.

Simultaneous Treatment of Obstruction. As previously noted, most bladder calculi form in the presence of obstruction. The most common cause is prostatic enlargement, although urethral strictures and neurogenic bladders may also be contributing factors. It will be to the patient's benefit to treat the calculi and the obstruction at the same time if doing so will not risk an increase in mortality or morbidity. Barnes, Bergman, and Worton[2] reported the lower morbidity and mortality seen when litholapaxy was combined with prostatic resection as opposed to the combination of cystolithotomy and prostatic enucleation. The mortality was 0.6 percent after litholapaxy and resection, but the latter combination was associated with the higher mortality rate of 3.2 percent.

Electrohydraulic lithotripsy has provided a major benefit for simultaneous treatment of obstruction. In the case of a urethral stricture, visual internal urethrotomy can be combined with this procedure and, in fact, would be necessary before passing the sheath into the bladder. Transurethral resection of the prostate can also be combined with electrohydraulic lithotripsy; moreover, it can usually be performed through the same endoscopic sheath. Bulow and Frohmueller[4] found associated infravesical obstruction in 245 male patients, of whom 238 required a subsequent transurethral procedure under the same anesthesia for relief of obstruction.

Adjuvant Treatment. Since many small fragments of the stone may be adherent to the bladder mucosa following endoscopic treatment of calculi, we prefer to attempt to remove these fragments by intravesical irrigation. For uric acid stones, an irrigant of sodium bicarbonate is passed into the bladder either with a three-way Foley catheter or with a system of Munro tidal drainage[5]. This latter technique allows partial filling of the bladder before intermittent emptying and offers the advantage of contact of the irrigant with a greater surface area of the bladder.

For struvite calculi, a similar technique can be employed with an irrigant such as Urologic G solution (Suby's G), an acidic solution that contains citrate in high concentration and thus is capable of dissolving struvite stones. Hemiacidrin (Renacidin) has also been used for irrigating the bladder to dissolve struvite calculi with some success. For other calculi that are generally not specifically soluble, we have chosen to irrigate the bladder to provide a mechanical flushing of some of the remaining minute fragments. The follow-up of these few patients is limited and, therefore, the benefit of such treatment cannot be ascertained.

REFERENCES

1. Bapat, S. S. Endoscopic removal of bladder stones in adults. *Br. J. Urol.* 49:527, 1977.
2. Barnes, R. W., Bergman, R. T., and Worton, E. Litholapaxy vs. cystolithotomy. *J. Urol.* 89:680, 1963.
3. Bigelow, H. J. Lithotrity by a single operation. *Am. J. Med. Sci.* 75:117, 1878.
4. Bulow, H., and Frohmueller, H. G. W. Electrohydraulic lithotripsy with aspiration of the fragments under vision — 304 Consecutive cases. *J. Urol.* 126:454, 1981.
5. Munro, D., and Hahn, J. Tidal drainage of the urinary bladder. *N. Engl. J. Med.* 212:229, 1935.
6. Purohit, G. S., Pham, D., Raney, A. M., and Bogaev, J. H. Electrohydraulic lithotripsy: An experimental study. *Invest. Urol.* 17:462, 1980.
7. Raney, A. M. Electrohydraulic cystolithotripsy. *Urology* 7:379, 1976.
8. Reuter, H. J. Electronic lithotripsy: Transurethral treatment of bladder stones in 50 cases. *J. Urol.* 104:834, 1970.
9. Riches, E. The history of lithotomy and lithotrity. *Ann. R. Coll. Surg. Engl.* 43:185, 1968.
10. Trapeznikov, M. F., and Borodulin, G. G. Electrohydraulic impulse lithotripsy of bladder stones with URAT-1. *Endoscopy* 9:6, 1977.
11. Twinen, F. P. Early days of urology in New York City and the founding of the American Urological Association. *J. Urol.* 97:163, 1967.
12. Twinen, F. P., and Langdon, B. B. Surgical management of bladder stones. *J. Urol.* 66:201, 1951.
13. Wangensteen, O., Wangensteen, S. D., and Wiita, J. Lithotomy and lithotomists: Progress in wound management from Franco to Lister. *Surgery* 66:929, 1969.

13
URETERAL CATHETERIZATION, RETROGRADE URETEROPYELOGRAPHY, AND SELF-RETAINING URETERAL STENTS

Jeffry L. Huffman

Demetrius H. Bagley

Edward S. Lyon

URETERAL CATHETERIZATION. Ureteral catheterization, one of the basic endoscopic techniques performed by the urologist, is still used for a variety of diagnostic and therapeutic procedures. *Young's Practice of Urology* [29], published in 1928, contains a thorough description of the technique of ureteral catheterization for retrograde pyelography and for bypassing tuberculous strictures or obstructing calculi. Although the instrumentation has been improved immensely, much of Young's description of the technique for identifying the orifices and passing ureteral catheters is still applicable.

Probably the most common diagnostic use of ureteral catheterization today is for retrograde pyelography; however, the indications for this procedure have lessened since the advent of ultrasonography and tomography with an excretory urogram. Obtaining separate urine collections for culture or for split-renal function studies requires bilateral ureteral catheterization. Therapeutically, catheterization of the chronically or acutely obstructed kidney, on either a long-term or a temporary basis, is done to provide urinary drainage. Often, this procedure is performed on an emergency basis for relief of an infected hydronephrosis when open surgery is not possible or not indicated.

More recently, improvements in the variety of ureteral catheters available have led to an increase in the types of lesions that can be treated following ureteral catheterization. Gill introduced retrograde brushing of upper tract urothelial lesions for cytologic diagnosis (see Chap. 14). Brushes are available that deflect to a variety of angles to reach varied positions in the middle and lower pole of the kidney. Angioplasty balloon catheters, originally introduced for percutaneous dilation of arterial narrowings, are now also applicable for use with ureteral narrowings to facilitate stone passage or to treat ureteral strictures primarily. Finally, many other steerable or deflectable catheters that are commonly employed radiologically are directly adaptable for use in ureteral manipulations.

Modification of the same basic technique is used for performing all types of ureteral catheterizations. Locating the orifices and passing the catheters through the submucosal and intramural portions of the ureter are performed in essentially the same manner using standard ureteral catheters, stone baskets, loop extractors, or flexible tip guidewires for self-retaining stents. The following sections will review the instrumentation available to the endoscopist for ureteral catheterization and will discuss in detail the various techniques, including retrograde pyelography and the placement of self-retaining ureteral stents.

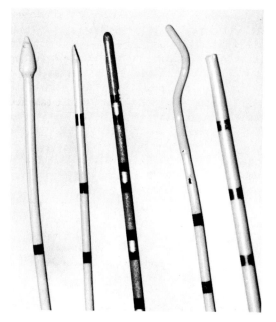

Figure 13-1. *The different types of standard ureteral catheters include (from left to right) the cone tip, whistle tip, round tip, spiral tip, and open-end catheter designs.*

Types of Ureteral Catheters. The different types of standard ureteral catheters are similar in that they are made of polyurethane and have uniform markings every 1 cm and distinguishable larger marks every 5 cm. They are characterized, however, by the configurations of their tips (Fig. 13-1). The most commonly used *whistle tip* catheter is straight and has an opening at its sharp, beveled tip as well as one on its side to provide for easier flow of urine than catheters with an opening only on the side. The *spiral tip* catheter is very useful for bypassing acutely angulating or extremely tortuous distal ureters, and the *round tip* catheter, with an opening only on the side, can be used when the ureter enters the bladder perpendicular to the mucosa. The *bulb,* or *cone tip,* catheter is used for retrograde ureteropyelography. The collar occludes the orifice and allows contrast to pass from the tip without leaking back into the bladder. The *open-end* ureteral catheter can be passed over a flexible tip guidewire, which facilitates placement in some circumstances. All of these catheters are available in a variety of sizes. A larger size is needed if occlusion of the ureter is desired; however, to help minimize traumatic injury to the ureter, it is important to select the smallest diameter that will allow a successful procedure.

Cystoscopic Instruments for Ureteral Catheterization. There are different types of cystoscopic instruments used for ureteral catheterization. The most common and probably the most useful instrument is the *Albarran bridge,* which is used in conjunction with a standard cystoscopic sheath (see Fig. 7-2). The Albarran bridge has a deflecting arm at its distal tip to deflect the catheter at an angle away from the beak of the cystoscope and toward the orifice. Endoscopes with a shorter fenestration at the tip provide greater stabilization of the catheter during passage, thus giving the endoscopist greater control in positioning the tip of the catheter and also deflecting the catheter into the field of view of the 70- to 90-degree lenses. They may have either single or double channel catheterizing ports.

The single arm and double arm bridges are also useful for catheterization when a deflecting bridge is not required. These bridges attach the telescope to the sheath and have individual catheterizing ports to guide catheters into the cystoscope sheath (see Fig. 7-1).

Various types of telescopes may be employed in combination with the catheterizing bridges. The 70-degree telescope lens in conjunction with the Albarran deflecting bridge is often useful for orifices that are difficult to catheterize, such as those in ectopic positions or located behind large prostatic median lobes. For normal orthotopic orifices, however, the standard catheterizing bridge with a forward viewing telescope is usually adequate.

Techniques of Catheterization

FINDING THE ORIFICE. Even the most expert endoscopist may have difficulty either finding the orifice or, once found, catheterizing it. There are, however, basic steps to follow in order to be successful routinely.

Initially, the catheterizing cystoscope is inserted into the bladder in a standard fashion, as discussed in Chapter 7. The most reliable method to locate the orifice is then to withdraw the cystoscope to the bladder neck in the midline. The cystoscope is then slowly advanced, proximally, along the trigone until the interureteric ridge can be identified (see Fig. 1-13). This ridge is sometimes difficult to find in the female but is usually obvious in the male unless obscured by severe trabeculation. Once the interureteric ridge has been found, the cystoscope is then rotated laterally to the right or to the left along the ridge. The right orifice is usually located at approximately the 7 o'clock position on the ridge (see Fig. 1-12) and the left at approximately the 5 o'clock position (see Fig. 1-14). The orifice should appear as a slit on the crest of the interureteric ridge or slightly inferior to the crest.

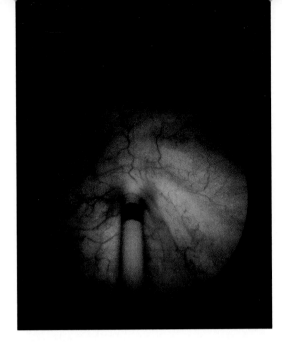

Figure 13-2. *A whistle tip catheter is placed into the right ureteral orifice using an Albarran bridge and a 70-degree lens.*

It is sometimes helpful to watch for ejection of a bolus of urine from the orifice with peristalsis of the ureter. If the orifice is difficult to locate, an ampule of indigo carmine can be given intravenously. This is excreted by a normally functioning kidney into the urine within 4 to 5 minutes and can be seen as obvious blue jets of dye from the orifices.

CATHETERIZING AN ORTHOTOPIC ORIFICE. Once the orifice has been identified, the catheter can be inserted. The catheter is initially loaded through the catheterizing port. When using the Albarran bridge, the tip of the catheter must be engaged with the deflecting arm (see Fig. 7-2). With one hand deflecting the bridge down, the other hand pushes the catheter through the cystoscope sheath until the catheter makes contact with the deflecting arm. At this point, the arm is pulled up and the catheter is slowly advanced until just the tip of the catheter is visible at the 6 o'clock position through the telescope. The catheter is then properly centered and ready to be inserted into the ureteral orifice. It is helpful to have the catheter loaded and in proper position prior to searching for the orifice so that the catheterization can be performed immediately and the position of the orifice is not lost.

The catheter is initially aligned in the same plane as the anticipated course of the intramural ureter. It is then advanced along the floor of the orifice and into the lumen of the ureter with the deflecting arm directing the tip (Fig. 13-2). Once within the orifice, it is passed proximally to the desired position in the ureter or pelvis. In passing the catheter, some tension can be applied by utilizing the deflecting bridge; however, marked buckling of the catheter is most often indicative of obstruction, tortuosity, or kinking of the ureter. It is in these instances that a spiral tip catheter may be useful to pass an obstructing region.

Difficulty may be encountered passing a catheter through the distal ureter because of an overdistended bladder. The full bladder may accentuate distal ureteral tortuosity and should not be distended during attempts at catheterization. A similar procedure is employed when performing catheterization with the single or double port bridge without the Albarran lever. Somewhat less control of the catheter tip results from this technique, however.

CATHETERIZING AN ECTOPIC ORIFICE. Catheterization of an ectopic ureter or one that has been reimplanted, either for vesicoureteral reflux or during a renal transplantation, can be difficult. Prior to beginning the procedure, it is helpful to obtain an approximate location of the orifice by examining previous excretory urograms or reviewing operative summaries. For example, it was known preoperatively that the transplanted ureter shown in Figure 13-3 had been placed on the right side of the bladder dome. Cystoscopically, the orifice was then readily identified and catheterized using an Albarran bridge and a 70-degree telescope (Fig. 13-4).

The transplanted orifice or one that has been reimplanted (Fig. 13-5) may also be surrounded by either acute or chronic inflammation secondary to the surgical procedure. The fibrous scarring that results not only makes identification difficult but can hamper catheterization due to the resulting immobility and nondistensibility of the orifice.

Catheterization in the setting where the orifice cannot be located is accomplished occasionally by gently probing the bladder mucosa with a catheter tip. Great care should be taken in this instance, however, to ensure that bleeding or mucosal swelling does not occur. It may also be helpful to watch for a bolus of urine or to inject indigo carmine to identify the orifice.

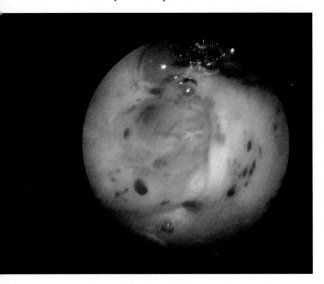

Figure 13-3. *The orifice of a ureter that has been transplanted into the dome of a bladder is viewed with a 70-degree telescope rotated 180 degrees. The orifice appears as a slit in the mucosa, which is slightly inflamed and swollen.*

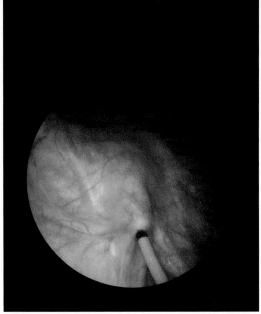

Figure 13-5. *A reimplanted orifice may be difficult to locate due to its abnormal position and distortion by scar. This orifice on the right lateral bladder has been catheterized with a 4 Fr. ureteral catheter using a 70-degree telescope.*

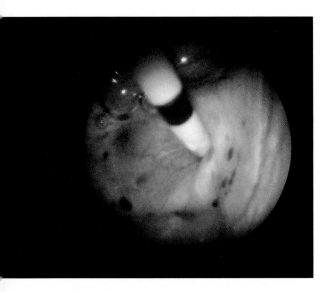

Figure 13-4. *The orifice shown in Fig. 13-3 has been catheterized using a 70-degree telescope and an Albarran bridge rotated 180 degrees.*

Complications of Ureteral Catheterization. Perforation is always a possibility during any ureteral manipulation. It is most important that a gentle touch be used for this procedure and no unnecessary force be applied during any attempt at catheterization of the ureter. If a perforation is suspected, a radiographic study, preferably injection of contrast using fluoroscopy, is mandatory. Treating a perforation generally includes leaving a ureteral catheter in place to divert urine away from the injured area and thus allow healing. Surgical exploration with ureteral repair and drainage of extravasated urine may be necessary in the presence of infected urine or large amounts of extravasation. An alternative method of treatment would be a percutaneous nephrostomy for proximal diversion followed by surgical repair or antegrade stent placement at a later setting.

RETROGRADE URETEROPYELOGRAPHY

Indications for Retrograde Ureteropyelography. The role of retrograde ureteropyelography has undergone a tremendous change during the 1970s and 1980s. Since the advent of tomography with excretory urography[12], ultrasonography[2], diuresis renography[19], and computerized tomography[17], very few indications now exist for its use as a pure diagnostic study. Localization of intrarenal and intrapelvic filling defects or calcifications, which previously required a retrograde study, can now be performed using a tomogram in conjunction with an excretory urogram. Ultrasonography can determine the presence or absence of hydronephrosis in the anuric patient, and diuresis renography can be used either to determine whether hydronephrosis is secondary to obstruction or purely on a functional basis. Computerized tomography with contrast can detect not only ureteral obstruction but can often identify the etiology of the obstruction (e.g., lymphadenopathy, aneurysm, perianeurysmal fibrosis, opaque and nonopaque calculi, and retroperitoneal metastatic disease).

Retrograde ureteropyelography continues to have definite indications, however. It is especially useful in conjunction with another transurethral procedure. For example, in the patient in whom self-retaining ureteral stents are to be placed, a retrograde pyelogram is done in order to identify the extent and level of obstruction. Also, in a patient in whom an attempt is to be made at endoscopic stone retrieval, it is useful to identify the level of the calculus by means of a retrograde pyelogram prior to an attempt at manipulation with a stone basket or ureteroscope. Conversely, however, if a supravesical diversion such as a percutaneous nephrostomy is planned, it is more convenient to do antegrade ureteropyelography in conjunction with the percutaneous procedure than retrograde ureteropyelography[22]. Antegrade ureteropyelography can also identify the extent and level of obstruction.

Another indication for retrograde ureteropyelography is a patient history of demonstrated sensitivity to parenterally administered contrast material. Witten's group[28] reported on 33,000 consecutive excretory urograms with a total incidence of 6.8 percent reactions. Only 1.7 percent of these reactions were viewed as significant and 5 percent of these (30 patients) were viewed as life-threatening reactions requiring vigorous supportive and resuscitative maneuvers. Although not an absolute contraindication to reexamination by excretory urography[11], previously demonstrated reactions usually dictate the use of retrograde pyelography or radionuclide scanning techniques if reexamination of the urinary tract is indicated. Absorption of contrast media following retrograde ureteropyelography, however, has also been shown to occur experimentally in the pelvicalyceal systems of dogs and may be a risk to the sensitive patient[15,21].

Because of these facts we suggest that when performing a retrograde ureteropyelogram on a patient who has demonstrated a previous sensitivity reaction to the parenterally administered contrast material to take great care not to overdistend the collecting system and possibly produce pyelorenal backflow. Using smaller amounts of contrast for the injection and performing the procedure under fluoroscopy are also indicated in these settings.

Techniques of Retrograde Ureteropyelography

SELECTING THE CONTRAST MATERIAL. To perform retrograde ureteropyelography, contrast media similar to that for excretory urography is used. Usually a 20 to 30% solution of the nonabsorbable water-soluble salts — sodium diatrizoate, methylglutamine diatrizoate, or methylglutamine iothalamate — is used. Many urologists routinely mix antibiotics such as neomycin with the contrast media to help lessen the chance of upper tract infection. The solution is then aspirated into a Luer-Lok syringe, which can be attached to the ureteral catheter by means of a blunt tip adaptor, a beveled needle, or a Luer-Lok adaptor that fits over the ureteral catheter (Fig. 13-6).

SELECTING A URETERAL CATHETER. The types of ureteral catheters have been described in detail previously. For retrograde ureteropyelography most urologists prefer to use a catheter with an occluding tip, such as a bulb or cone tip, because the tip fills the entire ureter and passage of the catheter beyond the lesion in question is not required. The size of the catheter depends on the caliber of the ureteral orifice. Usually, however, an 8 or 10 Fr. catheter will adequately occlude the orifice and prevent leakage of contrast during injection.

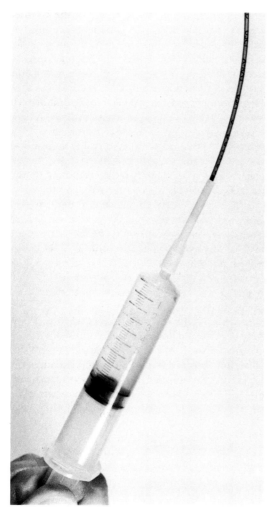

Figure 13-6. *An inexpensive, disposable ureteral catheter adaptor. The adaptor screws tightly into a Luer-Lok syringe and fits snugly over a ureteral catheter to prevent leakage during injection.*

SELECTING THE INSTRUMENT. In performing retrograde ureteropyelography, several different types of cystoscopes can be used, depending on the preference of the urologist. Generally, a forward viewing telescope in conjunction with a standard catheterizing bridge is adequate; if the orifice is difficult to identify, however, such as one located behind a prostatic median lobe, it may be necessary to use an Albarran bridge with a 70-degree telescope.

IRRIGATING THE BLADDER AND TAKING A PRELIMINARY RADIOGRAPH. There are several other steps that should be taken prior to injection of contrast material to the collecting system. First, and probably most important, it is necessary once the cystoscope is inserted into the bladder, that all debris be thoroughly irrigated from the bladder. This step lessens the risk of promoting an infection with the retrograde injection. The procedure is contraindicated in the presence of an acute cystitis, and many urologists routinely mix antibiotics with the contrast media, especially when the examination site is an obstructed collecting system. Secondly, it is very important that a plain film of the abdomen be taken prior to injection of contrast material. Any calcifications can then be identified and compared with the postinjection films. Lastly, all air remaining in the catheter should be removed prior to injection of contrast. Air bubbles in the urinary tract are often indistinguishable from filling defects such as tumors or radiolucent stones, and great care should be taken to ensure that no air remains in the system prior to injection.

PERFORMING RETROGRADE URETEROPYELOGRAPHY. The retrograde pyelogram can be performed after the above steps have been taken. The catheter is secured in the viewing field as described previously and the orifice is identified. Once the orifice is identified, the catheter is advanced while the orifice is viewed through the telescope. The tip of the catheter is inserted into the orifice to a point where the collar of the cone tip fits snugly inside the ureteral orifice (Fig. 13-7). A small amount of contrast media (5–7 ml) can then be injected, preferably under fluoroscopic control. Fluoroscopy is of great value in that much less time is needed to make the diagnosis. Filling can be evaluated and extravasation appreciated immediately. If fluoroscopy is unavailable, a film is taken following injection of 3 to 5 ml of contrast. More contrast can then be injected to obtain more distention of the collecting system and to determine the level of obstruction or the identity of any filling defects in the collecting system. It is preferable in most cases for the person performing the procedure to inject the contrast material. This enables the endoscopist to have control over the pressure that is applied while watching either fluoroscopically or endoscopically for leakage of contrast around the catheter back into the bladder. After removing the catheter, a postinjection radiograph is performed to visualize the degree of drainage of the collecting system. Because of the dependent position of the renal pelvis, it may be necessary to position the patient in an upright fashion to allow the contrast to drain.

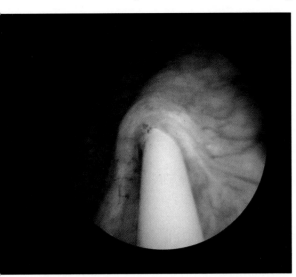

Figure 13-7. *An 8 Fr. cone tip catheter is placed into the left ureteral orifice using a 5-degree telescope. The collar occludes the orifice and helps prevent backflow of contrast into the bladder during injection.*

Complications of Retrograde Ureteropyelography. Complications of ureteropyelography include those associated with both ureteral catheterization and injection of the contrast material. The procedure should be performed with the awareness of the possible need for subsequent surgical intervention for correction of the problems.

Whenever an orifice is catheterized, a chance of perforation exists[6]. Following diagnosis of extravasation, an attempt should be made to pass a ureteral catheter into the renal pelvis to bypass the perforation and provide urinary drainage. Alternatively, percutaneous nephrostomy or open surgical exploration may be required.

A rare complication of catheterization is a submucosal injection of the contrast material. This occurs following penetration of the submucosal surface of the ureter by the catheter tip and subsequent injection of a bolus of contrast material. Although this complication does not require treatment, it usually prevents further retrograde studies until the distortion and edema that are produced subside.

In association with the injection of the contrast material and overdistention of the collecting system, the main complication encountered is pyelorenal backflow (Fig. 13-8)[27]. This may lead to bacteremia or systemic exposure to contrast media in the allergic patient. These problems must then be treated appropriately. Pyelorenal backflow can be subclassified into pyelotubular, pyelosinus, pyelolymphatic, pyelovenous, and pyelointerstitial forms. *Pyelotubular backflow* is reflux of urine into the papillary ducts due to increased pelvic hydrostatic pressure. Rupture of a calyceal fornix due to increased hydrostatic pressure will lead to *pyelosinus backflow*; once in the sinus, urine may leak into the lymphatics *(pyelolymphatic backflow)* or arcuate veins *(pyelovenous backflow)* if these structures have also been ruptured. *Pyelointerstitial backflow* results from a direct laceration involving the calyx and the corresponding renal pyramid, most commonly due to perforation by a ureteral catheter.

Inherent in the retrograde injection is the possible contamination of a previously sterile upper urinary system from urine pushed proximally with the injection from the bladder. This complication can be especially important clinically if a significant obstruction exists that is infected by the retrograde injection. The condition of these patients rapidly progresses to sepsis, and urgent drainage is necessary. The spread of malignant cells into the upper urinary tract is a theoretic possibility if a retrograde pyelogram is performed in a patient with a known bladder neoplasm[1].

SELF-RETAINING URETERAL STENTS. The use of ureteral catheters passed transurethrally has been a highly effective method of bypassing ureteral obstructions or stenting ureteral fistulas. Numerous problems arise, however, when using standard ureteral catheters for this purpose. Since a catheter must be long for cystoscopic insertion, a portion of it remains outside of the urinary system and external to the patient. As a result, the patient's mobility is markedly limited and the risk of intrarenal infection is increased. The major problem of distal migration of these catheters was obviated slightly by insertion of a Foley catheter into the bladder, to which the ureteral catheter was then secured. This system still is not suitable for long-term use. Most patients treated initially for chronic ureteral obstruction by this method subsequently do require supravesical urinary diversion by means of ureterostomy or tube nephrostomy.

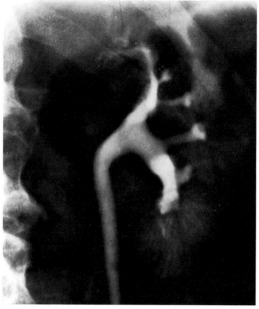

A

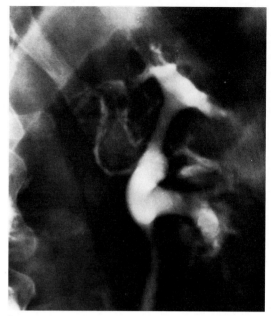

B

Figure 13-8. *A. Increased hydrostatic pressure in the renal pelvis results in reflux of contrast into the papillary ducts or pyelotubular backflow. B. Pyelolymphatic backflow (upper pole) results from absorption of contrast into lymphatics after contrast has entered the renal sinus through a ruptured calyceal fornix. An area of pyelosinus backflow is shown in the lower pole.*

Zimskind and co-workers[30], in early 1967, first reported the use of an indwelling ureteral stent in patients with ureteral obstruction. They applied silicone tubing to a 4 Fr. whistle tip catheter, which was inserted into the renal pelvis. The tubing was then held in that position with grasping forceps while the ureteral catheter was removed. The silicone was found to be less reactive and more flexible, and the authors reported good results in 13 patients treated with this method with follow-up ranging from 6 to 19 months. The major advantage of this method was that the patients were without external catheters and thus able to ambulate normally; in addition, there was less chance for retrograde infection than with the externally draining systems. The method did not ensure, however, that the catheters retained their positions.

Marmar[15], in 1970, subsequently modified the silicone catheter somewhat to facilitate insertion by sealing the proximal end of the catheter. This design enabled the catheter to be placed through more severely obstructed ureters without displacement of the silicone tubing. In 1973, Orikasa's group[21] modified the insertion technique slightly by first inserting a ureteral catheter and then passing a silicone tube over it with the help of a hard polymer tube to act as a "pusher." The silicone tube was then held in position by the pusher while the initially placed ureteral catheter was removed.

Maintaining proper position after insertion continued to be a problem with the use of the indwelling catheters. Gibbons and co-workers[5] first tried to solve the problem of upward migration by adding a distal flange to the silicone catheter. Of 12 patients, however, proximal migration occurred in 2 and expulsion of the stent in 4. Gibbons[4] subsequently added barbs that projected from the side walls of a radioopaque stent to prevent expulsion. Unfortunately, the addition of the barbs increased the stent's diameter, making passage of the stent through tight obstructions more difficult. The technique for insertion was also more complex, requiring initial ureteral dilation with successively larger ureteral catheters prior to passing the 4 Fr. ureteral catheter used as a guide for the stent. This catheter was subsequently found difficult to insert by many authors[25], including the urologists at our institution.

More recently, two types of self-retaining indwelling ureteral stents have come into widespread use. Both the double pigtail stent as described by Mardis's group[13] and the double J stent as described by Finney[3] have coils at each end of the catheter to prevent proximal or distal migration. Each catheter has its advantages and disadvantages, and each has a different insertion technique.

Double Pigtail, Self-Retaining Ureteral Stent.

The double pigtail stent was an adaptation of the "Shepherd's Crook," self-retaining ureteral catheter, which was originally described by McCullough[19]. The catheter, composed of polyethylene, had a pigtail "memory" at its proximal end, which enabled it to curl in the renal pelvis following insertion. Hepperlen and associates[8] described in 1978 a similar single pigtail ureteral stent with a distal flange, which they had used in 25 patients with excellent results. The same group developed the double pigtail catheter a year later[7].

A similar multipurpose ureteral stent is constructed of a new, less reactive elastomer, C-Flex, which resists crystal encrustation and depolymerization[14].* It is radioopaque, noncompressible, and has multiple apertures to provide internal drainage. The catheter comes with a closed proximal end to facilitate placement intraoperatively through a urethrotomy incision. This end must be cut off for transurethral passage over a guidewire. It is available in a wide range of sizes with diameters of 6 to 8 Fr. and lengths of 20 to 30 cm. A 5 Fr. catheter is also available in lengths from 10 to 30 cm. The lengths listed above include only the straight portion of the stent of each catheter and do not include the portions that coil following placement.

TECHNIQUE FOR PLACEMENT OF DOUBLE PIGTAIL URETERAL STENT

Selecting the Appropriate Catheter. An important requirement for a properly functioning double pigtail catheter is that it be of appropriate length. A catheter that is too short will not coil properly in the pelvis and bladder. A catheter that is too long may cause significant irritative voiding symptoms with excess catheter-causing mucosal irritation in the bladder.

To choose the correct length, a previous excretory urogram or retrograde study should be reviewed. The distance along the course of the ureter from the desired position in the intrarenal collecting system to the ureterovesical junction should be measured. This distance in centimeters is the length of the double pigtail stent that should be used.

Passing the Flexible Tip Guidewire. The essential feature of the technique for placement of the stent (Fig. 13-9) is passage of a guidewire with a spring tip beyond the ureteral obstruction and into the renal pelvis (Fig. 13-10). This technique, as originally described, involves passing the 6 Fr. open-end catheter beyond the obstruction and then passing the guidewire through the ureteral catheter. The 6 Fr. catheter is subsequently withdrawn, leaving the guidewire in place. Often, the 6 Fr. catheter will not pass; in these instances, we have found that using the flexible tip guidewire alone is quite satisfactory. In addition to the straight flexible tip guidewire, the flexible J-tip guidewire is occasionally useful and often, unlike the straight guidewire, will pass in a tortuous ureter.

Inserting the Double Pigtail Stent. Once the guidewire is in place, the stent is passed over it. The pigtails are straightened for passage and the stent is advanced into position by using a pusher that is supplied with the kit (Fig. 13-11). Care must be taken in passing the stent to make certain that the guidewire does not become dislodged from its initial position, either proximally or distally. When the stent has been passed proximally into position, the guidewire is removed, which allows the proximal and distal ends of the stent to coil in the renal pelvis and bladder. Radiographic control, preferably fluoroscopic control, is used to ensure proper positioning of the guidewire and to document proper placement of the stent (Fig. 13-12). The entire process is observed endoscopically to make certain that passage of the catheter into the ureteral orifice is smooth and that the distal pigtail is coiled properly in the bladder following removal of the guidewire and pusher (Fig. 13-13).

Removing or Replacing the Double Pigtail Stent. Once a double pigtail stent is no longer required, it can be removed cystoscopically, using standard techniques for foreign body removal. The distal, coiled end of the stent is located in the bladder and the end is grasped with either a rigid or flexible grasping forceps (Fig. 13-14). Since the double pigtail catheter is relatively inflexible, it can usually be removed more easily by withdrawing the entire cystoscope from the bladder while holding the stent with the forceps rather than by attempting to withdraw the stent through the sheath of the cystoscope.

Replacing or changing a double pigtail stent can be accomplished using one of three techniques. One method is first to remove the catheter completely and then repeat the placement procedure as described above. This method is subject to failure since it is often difficult to recatheterize the orifice after an indwelling stent has been removed.

---

*C-Flex thermoplastic elastomer, trademark of Concept, Inc., Clearwater, FL 33515.

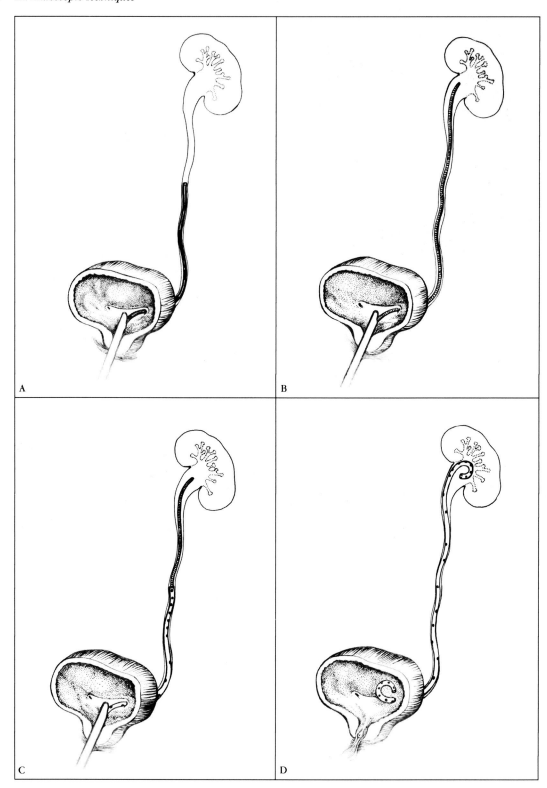

Figure 13-9. *The steps in placement of a double pigtail ureteral stent include (A) passage of a 6 Fr. open-end ureteral catheter beyond the ureteral obstruction, (B) insertion of a flexible tip guidewire through the catheter followed by removal of the catheter, leaving the guidewire in place, (C) placement of the double pigtail stent over the guidewire, using the "pusher" for advancement, and (D) removal of the guidewire, thus allowing the proximal and distal ends of the stent to coil in the renal pelvis and bladder respectively.*

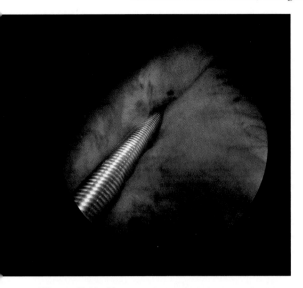

Figure 13-10. *The essential step in placing a double pigtail ureteral stent is passage of a flexible tip guidewire beyond the obstructing lesion. This guidewire has been placed into the right ureteral orifice and is advanced toward the renal pelvis. (Figs. 13-10 to 13-14 demonstrate placement of the same stent.)*

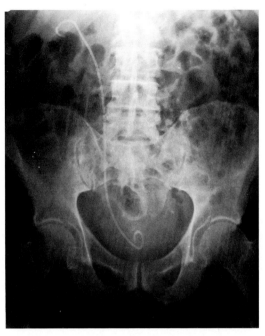

Figure 13-12. *Radiograph of the abdomen following placement of the double pigtail ureteral stent. The proximal end is coiled in the renal pelvis and the distal end in the bladder.*

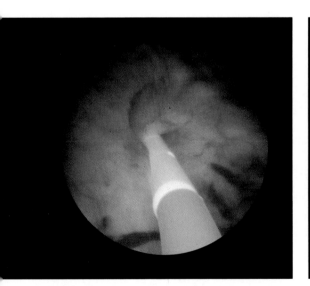

Figure 13-11. *Once proper position of the flexible tip guidewire is ensured, a pusher (green) is used to advance the double pigtail ureteral stent (white) over the guidewire.*

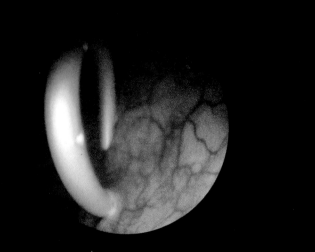

Figure 13-13. *Following removal of the guidewire, the distal end of the double pigtail stent (blue) coils smoothly in the bladder.*

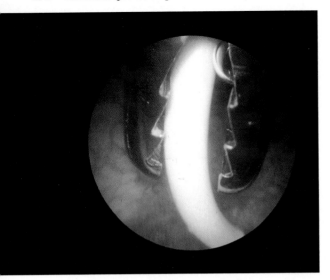

Figure 13-14. *To remove the indwelling ureteral stent, the end of the stent* (white) *is grasped with rigid grasping forceps and then withdrawn from the bladder.*

A second method of replacement involves passing the flexible tip guidewire alongside the existing catheter. Once the position of the guidewire has been documented radiographically, the old stent is removed and a new catheter is inserted over the guidewire, just as in initial placement. It may be difficult to pass the guidewire alongside the stent, particularly at the level of the obstruction. It may also be difficult to maintain the position of the guidewire while withdrawing the old stent.

The third technique allows removal of the stent over a wire with replacement of a new stent over the same guidewire. The tip of the stent is grasped cystoscopically and then withdrawn from the bladder and through the urethra only until the tip of the stent appears at the urethral meatus. The tip of the stent is then grasped manually and a flexible tip guidewire is passed through the stent and into the renal pelvis. After the proper position of the guidewire has been determined radiographically, a new double pigtail catheter can be inserted over the guidewire using the standard technique. This method cannot be used if the lumen of the stent is obstructed. It also carries the risk of forcing particulate matter from the stent back into the ureter or renal pelvis.

Double J Self-Retaining Ureteral Stent. Although the double J ureteral stent as described by Finney[3] is very similar to the double pigtail stent, it does have certain significant differences. It is made of silicone, which makes it softer and less reactive. Furthermore, because there is no proximal opening in the stent, it must be passed initially with the stylet in its lumen. It is available in diameters of 6 Fr. (length 12–30 cm), 7 Fr. (length 16–30 cm), and 8.5 Fr. (length 16–30 cm).

TECHNIQUE FOR PLACEMENT OF DOUBLE J URETERAL STENT

Selecting the Appropriate Catheter. The same guidelines apply for choosing the correct catheter size for the double J stent as were described for the double pigtail design. Initially, the ureteral length from the pelvis to the ureterovesical junction is measured on a radiograph. This distance in centimeters correlates to the length of the double J catheter required.

Inserting the Double J Stent. Compared to the double pigtail catheter, the increased flexibility and larger size of the double J catheter sometimes makes its passage difficult or impossible in cases of significant obstructions. If the catheter is not positioned correctly, the entire stylet and catheter must be removed and the procedure started over. This drawback is not shared by the double pigtail catheter, in which the guidewire can be left in place and only the stent changed.

The double J ureteral stent comes without a proximal or distal opening; therefore, prior to endoscopic insertion, the very distal end of the catheter must be cut off to expose the lumen. The inner stylet is then inserted into the lumen and pushed to the proximal enclosed end. Next, the catheter and stylet are loaded into the catheterizing cystoscope. The orifice is identified and the catheter advanced into the ureter. It is important throughout the insertion that the stylet is not withdrawn. This maneuver would allow the proximal end of the catheter to become disengaged from the stylet and make further catheter advancement impossible.

Once the stent is in proper position in the collecting system (documented by radiographic means), the pusher is inserted through the cystoscope over the stylet. When this catheter makes contact with the indwelling stent, the stylet can be safely removed. The pusher catheter holds the stent in position and allows the proximal and distal ends to coil in the renal pelvis and bladder. Cystoscopically, the proper coiling of the stent in the bladder can be observed and a radiographic film should be taken to ensure proper positioning in the renal pelvis.

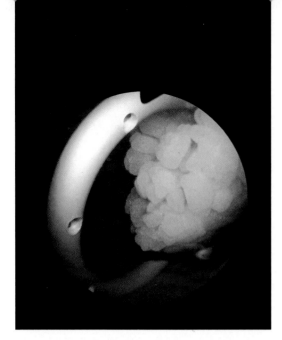

Figure 13-15. *This double pigtail ureteral stent became obstructed after being left in place for 9 months. A large calculus is seen surrounding the coil of the stent in the bladder and plugging the drainage holes with encrustation.*

Removing and Replacing the Double J Ureteral Stent. The technique for removing the double J stent is identical to that described for the double pigtail design. The distal coiled end of the catheter in the bladder is grasped cystoscopically using rigid or flexible forceps. The instrument and catheter are then removed together.

Replacing double J stents may often be more difficult. For this catheter design, the original stent must be removed entirely and a new stent inserted using exactly the same steps as outlined above.

Complications Associated with Self-Retaining Stents.

There are several problems that may be encountered with the self-retaining ureteral stents. These include obstruction due to the crystal encrustation[9], infection, reflux, irritative voiding symptoms from the catheter tip, and perforation. These complications will be discussed in more detail in the following sections. Other authors have also reported more serious complications including perforation of the ureter and renal vein, which requires open surgical correction[10].

OBSTRUCTION. The major problem encountered with the double pigtail stents has been obstruction of the stents by crystal encrustation (Fig. 13-15). Because of the high rate of obstruction, the catheters should be changed at least every 3 months.

INFECTION. Infections in the presence of a foreign body may present a significant problem for treatment. The potential for infection, however, is certainly minimized by the presence of a closed, internally draining system as opposed to an externally draining ureteral catheter. Prophylactic antibiotics are routinely used to cover initial stent placement and the changing of the stents in our patients and those of other groups[9].

REFLUX. Vesicoureteral reflux may occur with internal ureteral stents. If, however, intravesical chemotherapy is considered in patients with stents in place (e.g., those undergoing formalin therapy for hemorrhagic cystitis), the urologist should be aware of the possibility of supravesical reflux. If a cystogram does show reflux in these patients, temporary removal may be required.

IRRITATIVE VOIDING SYMPTOMS. Irritative voiding symptoms may be caused by the catheter tip overriding the trigone. This risk, however, is minimized when the proper catheter is used. Prior to insertion, the catheter of appropriate length is chosen so that the distal tips do not protrude into the bladder mucosa.

PERFORATION. Perforation remains a potential problem whenever the ureter is catheterized. If a perforation is suspected, a contrast study should be done to identify the site and extent of extravasation.

Treatment of a perforation is directed toward ensuring upper tract drainage. An attempt should be made at passing a ureteral catheter beyond or above the affected area. If catheterization is unsuccessful, diversion can be accomplished by percutaneous nephrostomy or, alternatively, open surgical exploration with repair of the perforation, drainage of the upper tract, and drainage of any extravasated urine.

Antegrade Placement of Indwelling Ureteral Stents. Refinements in the technique of percutaneous nephrostomy placement have allowed it to become a routine procedure for most hospitals. This antegrade access to the collecting system allows placement of flexible tip guidewires past obstructing lesions from above in a manner similar to that previously described for transurethral passage [17,24]. The double pigtail stent adapts readily to this technique, as does the Universal ureteral stent described by Smith [26]. The catheter is an 8 Fr. silicone rubber tube that is 90 cm in length and must be cut for appropriate length. Its drainage holes are placed in the bladder and pelvis. The distal end coils in the bladder while the proximal end is secured at the level of the skin and plugged. It may then be unplugged for irrigation or, if obstruction occurs, changing.

REFERENCES

1. Boreham, P. The surgical spread of cancer in Urology. *Br. J. Urol.* 28 : 163, 1957.
2. Ellenbogen, P. H., Scheible, F. W., Talner, L. B., and Leopold, G. R. Sensitivity of gray scale ultrasound in detecting urinary tract obstruction. *Am. J. Roentgenol.* 130 : 731, 1978.
3. Finney, R. P. Experience with the new double J ureteral catheter stent. *J. Urol.* 120 : 678, 1978.
4. Gibbons, R. P., Correa, R. J., Jr., Cummings, K. B., and Mason, J. T. Experience with indwelling ureteral stent catheters. *J. Urol.* 115 : 22, 1976.
5. Gibbons, R. P., Mason, J. T., and Correa, R. J., Jr. Experience with indwelling silicone rubber ureteral catheters. *J. Urol.* 111 : 594, 1974.
6. Goldstein, A. G., and Conger, K. B. Perforation of the ureter during retrograde pyelography. *J. Urol.* 94 : 658, 1965.
7. Hepperlen, T. W., Mardis, H. K., and Kammandel, H. The pigtail ureteral stent in the cancer patient. *J. Urol.* 121 : 17, 1979.
8. Hepperlen, T. W., Mardis, H. K., and Kammandel, H. Self-retained internal ureteral stents: A new approach. *J. Urol.* 119 : 731, 1978.
9. Kearney, G. P., Mahoney, E. M., and Brown, H. P. Useful technique for long-term urinary drainage by inlying ureteral stent. *Urology* 14 : 126, 1979.
10. Kidd, R. V., Confer, D. J., and Ball, T. P., Jr. Ureteral and renal vein perforation with placement into the renal vein as a complication of the pigtail ureteral stent. *J. Urol.* 124 : 424, 1980.
11. Lalli, A. F. Urography, shock reaction and repeated urography. *Am. J. Roentgenol.* 125 : 264, 1975.
12. Lloyd, L. K., Witten, D. M., Bueschen, A. J., and Daniel, W. W. Enhanced detection of asymptomatic renal masses with routine tomography during excretory urography. *Urology* 11 : 523, 1978.
13. Mardis, H. K., Hepperlen, T. W., and Kammandel, H. Double pigtail ureteral stent. *Urology* 14 : 23, 1979.
14. Mardis, H. K., Kroeger, R. M., Hepperlen, T. W., Mazer, M. J., and Kammendel, H. Polyethylene double-pigtail ureteral stents. *Urol. Clin. North Am.* 9 : 95, 1982.
15. Marmar, J. L. The management of ureteral obstruction with silicone rubber splint catheters. *J. Urol.* 104 : 386, 1970.
16. Marshall, W. H., Jr., and Castellino, R. A. The urinary mucosal barrier in retrograde pyelography. *Radiology* 97 : 5, 1970.
17. Mazur, M. J., LeVeen, R. F., Call, J. E., Wolf, G., and Baltaxe, H. A. Permanent percutaneous antegrade ureteral stent placement without transurethral assistance. *Urology* 14 : 413, 1979.
18. McClennan, B. L., and Fair, W. R. CT scanning in urology. *Urol. Clin. North Am.* 6 : 343, 1979.
19. McCullough, D. L. "Shepherd's Crook" self-retaining ureteral catheter. Urologists' Letter Club, May 24, 1974.
20. O'Reilly, P. H., Testa, H. J., Lawson, R. S., Farrar, D. J., and Edwards, E. C. Diuresis renography in equivocal urinary tract obstruction. *Br. J. Urol.* 50 : 76, 1978.
21. Orikasa, S., Tsuji, I., Siba, T., and Ohashi, N. A new technique for transurethral insertion of a silicone rubber tube into an obstructed ureter. *J. Urol.* 110 : 184, 1973.
22. Payne, W. W., Morse, W. H., and Raines, S. L. A fatal reaction following injection of urographic medium. A case report. *J. Urol.* 76 : 661, 1956.
23. Pfister, R. C., and Newhouse, J. H. Interventional percutaneous pyeloureteral techniques. *Rad. Clin. North Am.* 17 : 341, 1979.
24. Pingoud, E., Bagley, D. H., Zeman, R. K., Glancy, K. E., and Pais, O. S. Percutaneous antegrade bilateral ureteral dilatation and stent placement for internal drainage. *Radiology* 134 : 780, 1980.
25. Schneider, R. E., DePauw, A. P., Montie, J. E., and Thompson, I. M. Problems associated with Gibbons ureteral catheter. *Urology* 8 : 243, 1976.
26. Smith, A. D. The Universal ureteral stent. *Urol. Clin. North Am.* 9 : 103, 1982.
27. Thomsen, H. S., and Dorph, S. Pyelorenal backflow during retrograde pyelography in adult patients. *Scand. J. Urol. Nephrol.* 15 : 65, 1981.
28. Witten, D. M., Hirsch, F. D., and Hartman, G. W. Acute reactions to urographic contrast medium. *Am. J. Roentgenol.* 119 : 832, 1973.
29. Young, H. H., and Davis, D. M. *Young's Practice of Urology.* Philadelphia: Saunders, 1928.
30. Zimskind, P. D., Fetter, T. R., and Wilkerson, J. L. Clinical use of long-term indwelling silicone rubber ureteral splints inserted cystoscopically. *J. Urol.* 97 : 840, 1967.

14
BRUSH BIOPSY OF THE UPPER URINARY TRACT

W. B. Gill

Retrograde brushing of the kidney and ureter was developed in response to the need for accurate determinations of the etiologies of radiolucent filling defects found by urography of the upper urinary tract[13]. The diagnostic dilemma with urinary collecting system tumors is the differentiation between benign and malignant lesions, which produce similar radiographic, radiolucent filling defects on intravenous and retrograde pyelograms. The differential diagnosis of radiolucent filling defects in the renal collecting system is outlined in Table 14-1[10]. From this table it is apparent that some of these lesions should be treated by radical nephrectomy or nephroureterectomy without exposing the lesion while others should be treated medically. Therefore, it is of paramount importance to establish accurately the etiology of the radiolucent filling defect in question. The diagnostic aids in the evaluation of radiolucent filling defects in the renal collecting system are outlined in Table 14-2. These methods will be briefly discussed before retrograde brush biopsy is more extensively reviewed.

DIAGNOSTIC AIDS IN EVALUATION OF RENAL COLLECTING SYSTEM RADIOLUCENT FILLING DEFECTS

History and Physical Examination. The signs and symptoms of renal transitional cell carcinomas are highly variable, ranging from silent growth to metastases to early bleeding. Schapira and Mitty[26] reviewed the literature on tumors of the renal pelvis and concluded that the main manifestation was total gross hematuria occurring in about 80 percent of patients. Because of the nonspecificity of the signs and symptoms and the usual absence of endocrinic-metabolic effects, the history and physical examination at best are usually only suggestive.

Anatomic-Radiographic Studies. The anatomic-radiograpic studies are very helpful in revealing the presence of a lesion (a radiolucent filling defect) but usually do not contribute significantly to establishing the etiology. The intravenous and retrograde urograms may at best suggest a tumor versus a benign lesion by the smoothness (suggestive of a stone) or irregularity (suggestive of a tumor) of the filling defect. Since most transitional cell tumors exhibit definite vascular changes (see Chap. 11) that are not demonstrable radiographically[30], angiography is usually nondiagnostic unless the lesion is a renal parenchymal tumor invading the collecting system.

Table 14-1. Differential Diagnosis of Radiolucent Filling Defects in the Renal Collecting System

1. Tumors
   a. Transitional cell carcinomas arising from urothelial lining
   b. Renal cell adenocarcinomas invading the collecting system
   c. Benign tumors (e.g., angiomas, fibromas, lipomas)
   d. Cysts (pyelitis cystica)
2. Stones
   a. Uric acid stones (also other purine analogs, e.g., xanthine, hypoxanthine, allopurinol, and metabolites)
   b. Matrix (mucoprotein) stones
3. Blood clots (from any cause of renal bleeding)
4. Sloughed tissue
   a. Sloughed renal papillae
   b. Necrotic tissue (often characterized by inspissated pus associated with infections, e.g., nonspecific bacteria, tuberculosis, fungi)
5. Extrinsic compression
   a. Normal variations in anatomy of crossing blood vessels indenting infundibulae
   b. Extrinsic tumors (directly extending and/or metastatic to periaortic-pericaval lymph nodes)

Table 14-2. Diagnostic Aids in the Evaluation of Radiolucent Filling Defects in the Renal Collecting System

1. History and physical examination
   a. Usually nonspecific hematuria, flank pain, and/or mass
   b. Usually no endocrinic-metabolic manifestations of tumors
2. Anatomic-radiographic studies (urography)
   a. Intravenous pyelography
   b. Retrograde pyelography
   c. Angiography
   d. Ultrasound
   e. Computed tomography scan
3. Biochemical-immunologic studies
   a. Urinalysis (cells, casts, crystals, protein, sugar, microorganisms)
   b. Urinary enzymes
   c. Urinary biochemicals
   d. Urinary and serum immunologic biochemicals
4. Pathology studies
   a. Urinary cytology
   b. Retrograde renal brushing (histology and cytology)
   c. Transurethral ureteroscopy and pyeloscopy
5. General screening studies
   a. Hematologic profile
   b. Metabolic screening
   c. Metastatic evaluation (e.g., liver, lung, bone)

Ultrasonic differentiation of larger uric acid calculi from noncalculous (nonacoustic shadowing) lesions in the renal pelvis has been reported by Mulholland's group [21]. Computerized tomography has recently been employed to demonstrate a nonopaque calculis in the ureter [1]. The ability to differentiate noncalculous lesions with ultrasound or tomography, or both, remains uncertain. Transurethral ureteroscopy and pyeloscopy are becoming more generally available and will enhance our diagnostic capabilities in identifying the nature of filling defects (see Chap. 15).

Biochemical-Immunologic Evaluations. The theoretic relationship between urinary carcinogenic metabolites and the development of transitional cell carcinomas in the urinary tract has long been studied in experimental as well as clinical situations. Several tryptophan metabolites (3-hydroxykynurenine, 3-hydroxyanthranilic acid, xanthurenic acid), which are normally excreted in the urine [5] (and are increased in cigarette smokers' urines [18]), can produce bladder cancer under experimental conditions in animals [7]. Benassi and co-workers [2] have demonstrated that 10 of 20 patients with bladder tumors excreted increased amounts of 3-hydroxykynurenine and 9 of 32 patients with renal carcinomas excreted abnormally large amounts of 3-hydroxyanthranilic acid. Large quantities of 3-hydroxyanthranilic acid have been reported [28] in the urine of a patient with asynchronous bilateral papillary tumors of the renal pelvis. Although these relationships are very intriguing, they have not yielded a practical diagnostic test of urinary chemical excretion pattern(s) for the presence of a transitional cell carcinoma.

Urinary enzyme excretion patterns (lactate dehydrogenase, alkaline phosphatase) have been considered as a possible diagnostic test for urinary tract tumors. Wacker[27] has demonstrated an elevated urinary alkaline phosphatase and lactate dehydrogenase in 3 of 4 patients with transitional cell carcinoma of the renal pelvis, but these 3 also had hydronephrosis, which would produce a leak of enzymes from the cytoplasm. Although these enzymes are frequently elevated with both renal parenchymal and renal collecting system tumors, they are also frequently elevated with benign conditions (urinary tract infections, prostatitis, benign prostate hypertrophy). Because of the nonspecificity of the elevation in urinary enzymes plus the difficulty in assays, which required dialysis to remove naturally occurring enzyme inhibitors, the determination of urinary enzymes has not gained wide acceptance[29].

The identification of tumor-specific or at least tumor-associated antigens and/or antibodies in the serum or urine of patients with transitional cell carcinomas appears to be a promising area for investigation. Carcinoembryonic antigen (CEA) levels are detectable in human urines, with increased levels being found proportional to the mass and surface area of transitional cell bladder carcinomas[16]; infected urines also give increased levels, however, so CEA urinary levels may merely reflect tissue breakdown. Sera from patients with transitional cell carcinomas have been shown to have complement-dependent cytotoxicity (presumably cytotoxic antibodies) against transitional cell carcinoma target cells in tissue culture[17]. Cutaneous antigen testing in patients with transitional cell bladder carcinoma has shown varying degrees of defective cell-mediated immunity, with more severely diminished immunologic competence found to be associated with active, progressive, extensive disease[22]. The various immunologic techniques seem to be primarily of value in immunologic staging of patients with known tumors diagnosed by other means, and are neither specific enough nor sufficiently sensitive to serve as a practical primary diagnostic tool at this time.

Angiogenesis factor has been detected at elevated levels in the urine of patients bearing uroepithelial carcinomas. Chodak, Scheiner, and Zetter[8] reported good correlation between levels of angiogenesis factor, as assayed by endothelial cell migration in urine of bladder cancer patients, and the presence of recurrent tumors.

Pathology Studies. Urinary cytology has been applied to the diagnosis of urinary tract tumors since its early application by Papanicolaou and Marshall[23] in 1945. Unfortunately, urinary tract cytology has been found to give a high rate of false negatives with upper tract tumors. Winter's group[15] found a false-negative rate of 67 percent with urinary cytology in 15 patients with renal pelvis transitional cell carcinomas. Sarnacki and co-workers[25], despite examining retrograde collections of urine for cytology, reported a false-negative rate of 41 percent in 22 cases of renal pelvis transitional cell carcinoma. Because of this limitation of urinary cytology, our group developed retrograde brushing to provide histologic specimens as well as improved cytologic materials from tumors in the upper urinary tract[3,13].

RETROGRADE RENAL AND URETERAL BRUSHING (TRANSCATHETER BIOPSY TECHNIQUES). We believed that the application of Fennessy's[9] bronchial brushing to the upper urinary tract could be a natural solution to the problem of obtaining specimens for making a histopathologic and/or cytopathologic diagnosis of radiolucent filling defects in the renal collecting system.

Retrograde ureteral or renal collecting system brushing, as developed by our group, consists of the following steps:

1. Retrograde brushing is readily performed with analgesic and sedative premedications such as Demerol and Vistaril plus topical intraluminal urethral anesthesia (1% Metycaine or 5% Xylocaine) in male patients.
2. An angiographic spring guidewire is passed up the ureter via a cystoscope to approximately the level of the lesion.
3. An open-end ureteral catheter (8.4, 6.5, or 5.5 Fr., depending on the anatomy of the orifice) is passed over the guidewire. Intraluminal ureteral injection of a few milliliters of 1% Carbocaine or Xylocaine may be used to facilitate passage of the open-end ureteral catheter.
4. The catheter is then positioned adjacent to the lesion with radiographic contrast media (Renografin-60 undiluted or diluted 1:1 with 0.5 gm neosporin in 0.9% NaCl) injected through the catheter during fluoroscopy (preferably television-monitored and image-intensified), which enables the urologist to see the brush directly passing back and forth over the lesion.

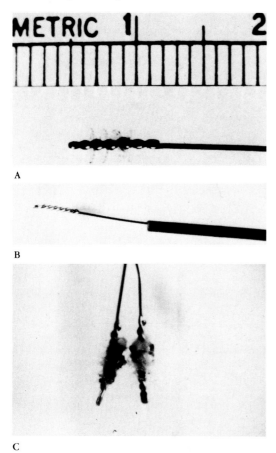

A

B

C

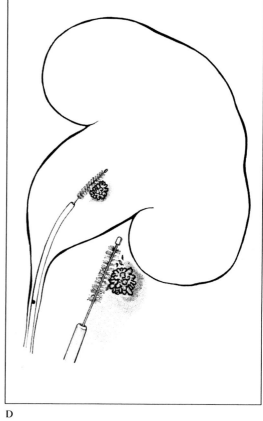

D

Figure 14-1. *A. Brush with nylon bristles 2.5 mm in diameter. B. Brush protruding from open-end ureteral catheter. C. Brushes with entrapped tissue immersed in tube containing formalin. D. Brush sampling renal pelvic tumor.*

5. After removing the contrast medium by washing with normal saline, which helps to prevent cytologic distortion by the hypertonic contrast medium, nylon or steel bristle brushes (Fig. 14-1A) on long wires are passed up the ureteral catheter (Fig. 14-1B) and the lesion is brushed vigorously back and forth six times (Fig. 14-1D). The center wire of the spring guidewire may be removed by cutting off a few millimeters of the end and withdrawing the inner straight wire. The hollow coiled guidewire may then be passed over the straight brush wire to give more rigidity to the brushing.

6. The brush is removed and a touch smear preparation is made on a slide, which is immediately placed in a solution of 95% ethanol for subsequent Papanicolaou staining.

7. The brush tip is then cut off the long wire handle and immediately immersed in 10% phosphate-buffered formalin (Fig. 14-1C) for at least 1 hour before the urologist gently teases the fixed material from the brushes and wraps the fragments in tissue paper for further fixation and processing.

8. After approximately six brushings, using the wire brushes if insufficient tissue is obtained with the softer nylon bristle brushes, the catheter is irrigated with saline to remove other fragments and cells loosened by the brushing for cytologic, histologic, and microbiologic evaluations.

9. Postbrushing voided urines are also sent for cytology.

A variety of open-end catheters and brushes on long wires are available commercially.* They can also be readily fashioned from Kifa angiographic catheter tubing and brushes, which are stocked in radiology departments. Although the 8.4 Fr. gray Kifa catheter is preferred because both the nylon and wire bristle brushes can be readily passed, the smaller, thin-walled 6.5 Fr. red Kifa catheter, which will accept only nylon brushes, may be used if difficulty in passing the larger catheter is encountered.

Modifications to Facilitate Specific Renal Calyceal Brushings. Several techniques have been found useful for placement of the open-end catheter in the middle or inferior renal calyces. After passing the open-end catheter to the renal pelvis, the stiffer end of an angiographic guidewire, bent to the approximate angle between the pelvis and the desired calyx, is passed up the previously passed open-end catheter into the calyx. Following placement of the bent guidewire, the open-end catheter is advanced over the guidewire into the calyx and the guidewire is removed before brushing is commenced. Unless the infundibulum is quite large, the catheter will usually stay in the lower or middle calyx being brushed. A second technique of positioning the open-end catheter in the middle or inferior calyces is to use an angiographic catheter with a preshaped curve that is straightened out over the guidewire until it arrives at the end of the guidewire in the renal pelvis. With this technique it is sometimes hard to negotiate the lower ureter. A third technique for lower calyceal placement is to use the "joy stick" manipulator developed by Medi-Tech for angiographic maneuvers, whereby the distal 2 or 3 cm of the catheter tip can be manipulated by a set of control wires built into the catheter wall, as originally reported by Brown, Hawtrey, and Pixley[6]. Alternately, a much cheaper manipulable brush is the controlled bronchial brush as reported by Cole's group[24] and Gittes[14]. These manipulable catheters and brushes, however, can be used only with smaller brushes.

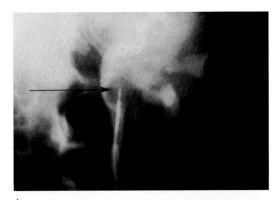

A

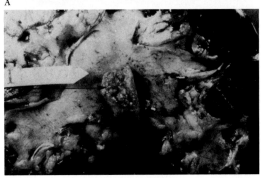

B

Figure 14-2. *A. Retrograde brushing x-ray showing brush protruding from an open-end ureteral catheter over a radiolucent filling defect in the left renal pelvis. B. Surgical specimen (nephroureterectomy) showing papillary transitional cell carcinoma that accounts for the radiographic defect in A.*

Results. The entire spectrum of lesions producing radiolucent filling defects in the ureter, renal pelvis, and renal calyces has been diagnosed preoperatively by retrograde brushing. No false-positive or known false-negative results have been encountered to date in our series of over 75 cases. The following lesions have been correctly diagnosed by retrograde brushing: transitional cell carcinomas of the ureter, renal pelvis, and renal calyces; uric acid stones in the ureter and renal collecting system; mucoprotein matrix stones; ureteral polyps; sloughed renal papillae; ureteritis cystica; extrinsic ureteral compression by iliac artery aneurysm; extrinsic calyceal compression by renal vessels; renal cell carcinomas (hypernephromas); and multiple myelomas involving the kidney. Illustrative cases are presented in Figures 14-2 through 14-4.

---

*Sage Products, Elk Grove, IL 60007; Vantec Products, Spencer, IN 47460; Mill Rose Brush Co., Mentor, OH 44060.

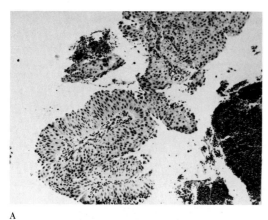

A

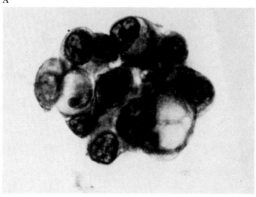

B

Figure 14-3. *A. Brushing histology (same case as Fig. 14-2). Hematoxylin-eosin stain reveals fragments of moderately differentiated papillary transitional cell carcinoma (150×). B. Brushing cytology (same case as Fig. 14-2). Papanicolaou stain shows moderately differentiated malignant transitional cells; note coarse chromatin pattern (800×).*

Postbrushing morbidity has been limited in about one-third of patients to transient colic, which has cleared spontaneously in a matter of hours. Antibiotic coverage is routinely used and morbidity from instrumentation infection has not been encountered. Perforations of the ureteral wall have not occurred. The main technical problem experienced has been difficulty in negotiating the ureteral orifice or lower ureter in men with significant trigonal elevation from prostatic enlargement.

The foregoing is a description of our personal results. Like most developers and proponents of new techniques, we have probably exercised unusual perseverance and compulsiveness, which would favor unusually good results.

GITTES STUDY. Ruben Gittes and colleagues[14] have recently both reported their own experiences with 21 patients over a 6-year period and conducted an extensive survey of other urologists concerning their experiences with this new technique during the year 1978. Of the urologists surveyed, 70 reported a total 177 retrograde brush biopsies, 47 of which were described in detailed reports, giving Gittes a total of 68 cases on which to report.

Major complications occurred in 5 of the 68 patients, an incidence rate of 7 percent. Of these 5 patients with major complications, 3 had hemorrhage necessitating exploration, 1 had gram-negative sepsis, and 1 had ureteral perforation; no deaths occurred. Tumor complications of clot colic or flank pain occurred in 15 percent of these 68 patients.

The overall diagnostic accuracy was reported as 78% in these 68 cases, with 31 cases of transitional cell carcinoma (all but 5 were low grade) and 1 case of renal cell carcinoma that had invaded the renal pelvis. Incorrect diagnoses were reported in 22 percent of the 68 patients. An incorrect diagnosis of malignancy was made in 2 patients with chronic inflammation of the urothelium and 1 patient with a stone, leading to 3 false-positive results. Inaccurate placement of the brush may have caused 8 other false-negative results since some cases were performed without fluoroscopic and/or urographic localization of the lesion. Gittes concluded that "our results support the conclusion that this procedure is of value in the management of selected patients with problem radiolucent filling defects of the renal pelvis and ureter."

LANG STUDY. Lang's group has reported renal brush biopsy with a percutaneous translumbar approach to the renal pelvis. This technique seems to be most useful when the ureter is obstructed or a ureterovesical structure precludes retrograde catheter passage, such as an enlarged median lobe with benign prostatic hyperplasia. This percutaneous technique runs the risk of tumor spillage, however, and some workers consider this procedure to be contraindicated.

CONCLUSIONS. It needs to be emphasized that retrograde brush biopsy includes both brushing histology and brushing cytology of saline washes postbrushing. Also included is all material filtered or centrifuged from the saline washes (i.e., bacteria and crystals as well as cells).

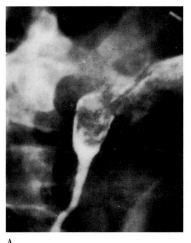 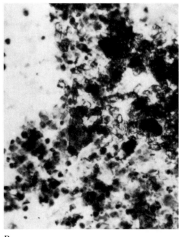 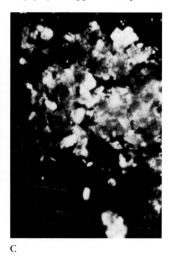

A   B   C

Figure 14-4. *Uric acid stone in renal pelvis. A. This retrograde urogram shows a somewhat irregular radiolucent filling defect, which partially obstructs the left ureteropelvic junction. B. Retrograde brushing histology. Transmitted ordinary light shows nonmalignant urothelial cells plus crystalline material (Pap stain, 128×). C. Retrograde brushing histology. Transmitted polarized light (same field as B) shows high birefringence and habit of uric acid.*

After 6 weeks of urinary alkalization and use of an internal double pigtail ureteral catheter to relieve the obstruction, the filling defect disappeared. The patient has done well following removal of the ureteral catheter.

The importance of crystals found in the cytologic preparations should be stressed because in our experience cytopathologists tend to overlook or ignore crystals while they concentrate on cellular morphology. We routinely review the cytologic brushing specimens with both transmitted and reflected polarized light so as not to miss uric acid, struvite, or calcium oxalate crystals, which may be somewhat obscured by clumps of cells (Fig. 14-4).

Aids to facilitate passage and manipulation of the brushing catheter have previously been discussed. An additional option to consider is the technique of transurethral ureteroscopy (see Chap. 15), which has been used on several occasions to dilate the ureteral orifice and negotiate the lower ureter with the brushing catheter[20]. Additionally, ureteropyeloscopy has been used to brush lesions in minor calyces that could not be approached for forceps biopsies.

Tailoring the catheter size to the anatomy of the ureteral orifice and using image-intensified, television-monitored fluoroscopy markedly enhanced the success rate of performance of this procedure and the accuracy of obtaining specimens from the lesion being evaluated[11,12].

The final arbitrator of the accuracy of all diagnostic procedures remains the direct microscopic identification of tissues on histology, cells on cytology, and crystals under the polarizing microscope.

REFERENCES

1. Alter, A.J., Peterson, D.T., and Plautz, A.C., Jr. Non-opaque calculus demonstrated by computerized tomography. *J. Urol.* 122:699, 1979.
2. Benassi, C.A., Perissinotto, B., and Allegri, C. The metabolism of tryptophan in patients with bladder cancer and other urological diseases. *Clin. Chim. Acta* 8:822, 1963.
3. Bibbo, M., et al. Retrograde brushing as a diagnostic procedure on ureteral, renal pelvic, and renal calyceal lesions. A preliminary report. *Acta Cytol.* 18:137, 1974.
4. Blute, R.D., Jr., Gittes, R.R., and Gittes, R.F. Renal brush biopsy: Survey of indications, techniques and results. *J. Urol.* 126:146, 1981.
5. Boyland, E., and Williams, D.C. The metabolism of tryptophan. 2. The metabolism of tryptophan in patients suffering from cancer of the bladder. *Biochem. J.* 64:578, 1956.
6. Brown, R.C., Hawtrey, C.E., and Pixley, E.E. Brush biopsy of the renal pelvis: A preliminary report. *Am. J. Roentgenol. Radium Ther. Nucl. Med.* 119:779, 1973.
7. Bryan, G.T., Brown, R.R., and Price, J.M. Mouse bladder carcinogenicity of certain tryptophan metabolites and other aromatic nitrogen compounds suspended in cholesterol. *Cancer Res.* 24:596, 1964.
8. Chodak, G.W., Scheiner, C.J., and Zetter, B.R. Urine from patients with transitional cell carcinoma stimulates migration of capillary endothelial cells. *N. Engl. J. Med.* 305:869, 1981.
9. Fennessy, J.J. Bronchial brushing in the diagnosis of peripheral lung lesions. A preliminary report. *Am. J. Roentgenol.* 98:474, 1966.

10. Gill, W. B., et al. Evaluation of renal masses: Including retrograde renal brushing. *Surg. Clin. North Am.* 56:149, 1976.

11. Gill, W. B., Lu, C. T., and Bibbo, M. Retrograde ureteral brushing. *Urology* 12(3):279, 1978.

12. Gill, W. B., Lu, C. T., and Bibbo, M. Retrograde brush biopsy of the ureter and renal pelvis. *Urol. Clin. North Am.* 6(3):573, 1979.

13. Gill, W. B., Lu, C. T., and Thomsen S. Retrograde brushing: A new technique for obtaining histologic and cytologic material from ureteral, renal pelvic, and renal calyceal lesions. *J. Urol.* 109:573, 1973.

14. Gittes, R. R. S. Retrograde renal and ureteral brush biopsy. *Am. J. Nurs.* 78:410, 1978.

15. Grace, D. A., Taylor, W. N., Taylor, J. N., and Winter, C. C. Carcinoma of the renal pelvis: A 15-year review. *J. Urol.* 98:566, 1968.

16. Guinan, P., et al. Urinary carcinoembryonic-like antigen levels in patients with bladder carcinoma. *J. Urol.* 111:350, 1974.

17. Hakala, T. R., Castro, A. E., Elliott, A. Y., and Fraley, E. E. Humoral cytotoxicity in human transitional cell carcinoma. *J. Urol.* 111:382, 1974.

18. Kerr, W. K., et al. The effect of cigarette smoking on bladder carcinogenesis in man. *Can. Med. Assoc. J.* 93:1, 1965.

19. Lang, E. K., Alexander, R., Barnett, T., Palomar, J., and Hamway, S. Brush biopsy of pyelocalyceal lesions via a percutaneous translumbar approach. *Radiology* 129:623, 1978.

20. Lyon, E. S., Banno, J. J., and Schoenberg, H. W. Transurethral ureteroscopy in men utilizing juvenile cystoscopy equipment. *J. Urol.* 123:17, 1980.

21. Mulholland, S. G., Arger, P. H., Goldberg, B. B., and Pollack, H. M. Ultrasonic differentiation of renal pelvic filling defects. *J. Urol.* 122:14, 1979.

22. Olsson, C. A., Rao, C. M., Menzoian, J. O., and Byrd, W. E. Immunologic unreactivity in bladder cancer patients. *J. Urol.* 107:607, 1972.

23. Papanicolaou, G. N., and Marshall, V. F. Urine sediment smears as a diagnostic procedure in cancers of urinary tract. *Science* 101:519, 1945.

24. Parra, G., Seery, W., Khashu, B., and Cole, A. T. Retrograde brushing: Improved technique using a catheter-tip deflector system. *J. Urol.* 117:693, 1977.

25. Sarnacki, C. T., et al. Urinary cytology and the clinical diagnosis of urinary tract malignancy: A clinicopathologic study of 1,400 patients. *J. Urol.* 106:761, 1971.

26. Schapira, H. E., and Mitty, H. A. Tumors of the renal pelvis: Clinical review with emphasis on selective angiography. *J. Urol.* 106:642, 1971.

27. Wacker, W. E. C. Lactic Dehydrogenase and Alkaline Phosphatase Activities in the Diagnosis of Renal Cancer. In J. S. King, (Ed.), *Renal Neoplasia.* Boston: Little, Brown, 1967. P. 87.

28. Wallace, D. M. Clinico-pathological Behavior of Bladder Tumors. In D. M. Wallace (Ed.), *Tumours of the Bladder.* Edinburgh: Churchill Livingstone, 1959.

29. Wilkinson, J. H. Enzyme Tests in Renal Diseases. In F. W. Sunderman and R. W. Sunderman, Jr. (Eds.), *Laboratory Diagnosis of Kidney Diseases.* St. Louis: Warren H. Green, 1970. P. 243.

30. Young, J. M., and Morrow, J. W. Problems in interpretation of angiograms in renal mass lesions. *J. Urol.* 107:925, 1972.

15
TRANSURETHRAL URETEROPYELOSCOPY

Jeffry L. Huffman

Edward S. Lyon

Demetrius H. Bagley

Lesions within the ureter had been accessible only by open surgical approaches until the 1970s, when the extension of standard endoscopic procedures and the availability of rigid and flexible fiberoptic ureteroscopes made it possible to diagnose and treat many ureteral and renal pelvic lesions endoscopically. Hugh Hampton Young[13], in 1912 unexpectably was able to pass a pediatric cystoscope into a massively dilated ureter and renal pelvis in a child with posterior urethral valves (Fig. 15-1). In 1971, Aso's group[11] described a flexible pyeloureteroscope that could be passed in a retrograde fashion to visualize the entire ureter and kidney. In 1977, Lyon, Kyker, and Schoenberg[9] described the use of rigid pediatric instruments in the distal ureter.

Several rigid instruments have subsequently become available specifically for endoscopy of the ureter and renal pelvis. In collaboration with Lyon's group[8] in 1978, Richard Wolf Instruments developed special instrumentation to facilitate ureteroscopy for observation, diagnosis, and surgery in the distal ureter. Perez-Castro Ellendt and Martinez-Pineiro subsequently described in 1980 the use of a rigid ureterorenoscope that could reach the level of the renal pelvis when passed transurethrally. We have called this same instrument the *ureteropyeloscope*, a more accurate descriptive term since the instrument visualizes only the ureter and renal pelvis. Combination of these instruments with standard technology used intravesically has resulted in a new, expanded role for endoscopic diagnosis and treatment of lesions of the upper urinary tract.

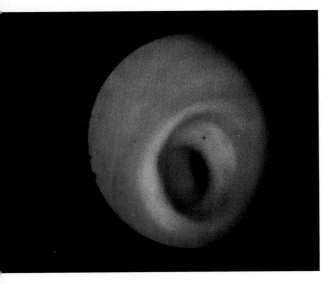

Figure 15-1. *The distal ureter of a newborn is visualized after insertion of a pediatric cystoscope through a dilated ectopic ureteral orifice.*

RIGID INSTRUMENTATION FOR URETEROPYELOSCOPY

Rigid Ureteroscope. The rigid ureteroscope, with a 23-cm working length, was the first instrument designed specifically for observation and surgical manipulation within the distal ureter[8]. The instrumentation included separate ureteroscope sheaths, telescopes and a resectoscope working element. Ureteroscope sheaths come in 3 sizes — 13, 14.5, and 16 Fr. The telescopes are smaller in diameter (2.7 mm) than the standard cystoscopic telescope and have a 5- or 70-degree viewing angle. The resectoscope is 14.5 Fr. and is designed with a short excursion of the working element; both the 14.5 and 16 Fr. instruments, however, permit passage of additional catheters or instruments sized up to 5 Fr.

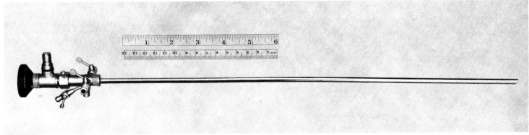

A

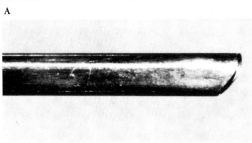

B

Figure 15-2. *A. The rigid ureteropyeloscope has a working length of 41 cm. The 11.5 Fr. instrument has a 5 Fr. working channel and interchangeable telescopes. B. The tip of the ureteropyeloscope is smoothly beveled to facilitate insertion and passage in the ureter.*

Rigid Ureteropyeloscope. The longer rigid ureteropyeloscope, with a working length of 41 cm, can reach transurethrally to the level of the renal pelvis in both male and females.* With the original design, the Wolf observation sheath was 11 Fr. and the operating sheath was 12 Fr. The newer model has a 10 Fr. sheath for observation and an 11.5 Fr. sheath for procedures (Fig. 15-2). The telescope is only 2.7 mm in diameter and has viewing angles of 5 degrees and 70 degrees for the renal pelvis; no deflecting bridge is available for use with the 70-degree telescope, however. Although the 10 Fr. instrument is for observation only and does not have a working channel, the 11.5 Fr. sheath will accept forceps, electrodes, or other instruments sized up to 5 Fr. There is also an integral 9.5 Fr. sheath with a 5 Fr. working channel; the telescope, however, cannot be removed.

*Richard Wolf Instruments, Inc., Rosemont, IL 60018.

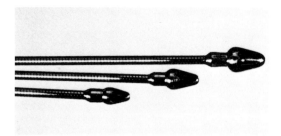

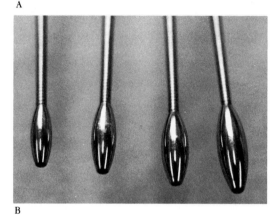

A

B

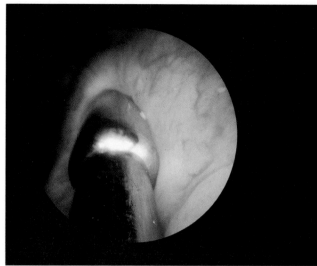

Figure 15-4. *The tip of a 12 Fr. ureteral dilator is passed into the left ureteral orifice.*

Figure 15-3. *A. Attached to a flexible carrier are 10, 12, and 15 Fr. conical metal ureteral dilators. B. The olive-shaped metal dilators are sized 10.5, 12.0, and 15.0 Fr. They are attached to a flexible carrier and fit over a 0.038-inch guidewire.*

The Karl Storz ureteropyeloscope has an 11.0 Fr. sheath with interchangeable bridges for using either the 0-degree or the 70-degree telescope.† The sheath will accept catheters, baskets, or forceps sized up to 5 Fr. There is also an integral 9.0 Fr. sheath with a 5 Fr. working channel and a 0-degree telescope that cannot be removed.

Both manufacturers have also introduced ureteropyeloscopes with an offset 0-degree telescope. These are designed specifically for use with ultrasonic lithotripsy transducers to enable ultrasonic stone fragmentation under direct vision.

TECHNIQUE OF RIGID TRANSURETHRAL URETEROSCOPY

Dilation of the Ureteral Orifice and Intramural Ureter. As discussed in Chapter 2, the narrowest portion of the ureter encountered during passage of the ureteroscope is the distal intramural ureter. Some authors recommend placing a ureteral catheter for several days prior to the procedure in order to dilate this segment while other authors blindly pass the ureteroscope sheath over a catheter.

We recommend dilation of the orifice and intramural ureter under direct vision. This type of ureteral dilation is well established and was used initially by early urologists to facilitate stone passage. It can be done with either conical metal dilators, olive-shaped metal dilators, or angioplastic balloon catheters.

The conical metal dilators come in sizes 10, 12, and 15 Fr. (Fig. 15-3A). The dilating tip fixed to the flexible carrier can be passed through the 25 Fr. cystoscope sheath under direct vision into the ureteral orifice (Fig. 15-4). Once inside the orifice the dilator must be aimed along the projected course of the ureter and slowly advanced through the intramural ureter (Fig. 15-5). This ensures that the dilating tip will pass smoothly within the ureteral lumen, without applying force to the ureteral wall.

Occasionally, the ureteral catheter or flexible tip guidewire may be passed to define the course of the distal ureter. The dilator may then be passed alongside the catheter or after its removal. The orifice and intramural ureter are initially snug, even to passage of the 10 Fr. dilator, but gradually accommodate the larger dilating tips. It is necessary to dilate sequentially only the intramural portion of the ureter to 15 Fr. since the more proximal extravesical ureter will usually distend easily with irrigation and the passage of the instrument itself. The orifice and intramural ureter may show submucosal hemorrhage or ecchymosis after dilation (Figs. 15-6, 15-7), but mucosal tears are rare.

†Karl Storz Endoscopy—America, Inc., Culver City, CA 90230.

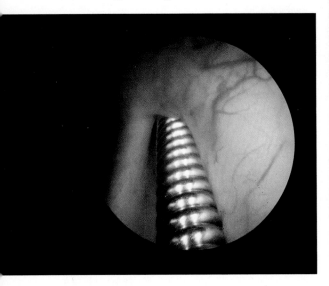

Figure 15-5. *The 12 Fr. ureteral dilator has been passed through the entire intramural ureter. Only the flexible carrier outside the orifice remains visible.*

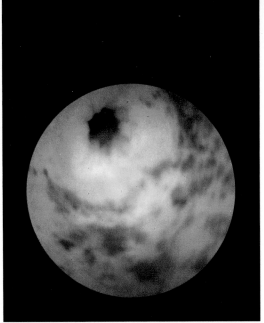

Figure 15-7. *The same portion of the ureter shown in Fig. 15-6 is seen here during peristaltic constriction of the proximal lumen.*

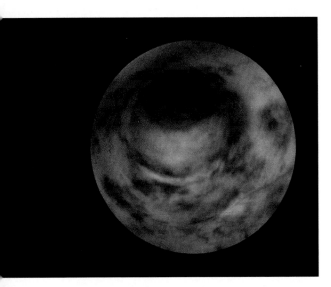

Figure 15-6. *Submucosal hemorrhage and ecchymosis are seen in the intramural ureter following dilation to 15 Fr. The more capacious extravesical ureter is visible in the background.*

A false passage may be produced when excessive force is applied during the dilation or when the ureteral lumen is not well defined and the dilator is misdirected. It is mandatory that only gentle force be applied to the flexible carrier and dilator during the dilation to allow the orifice and intramural ureter to accommodate slowly to the successive increases in the size of the dilating tip.

If the conical metal dilator does not pass smoothly through the entire intramural ureter, a different method must be used to dilate prior to passage of the ureteroscope. The olive-shaped metal dilators come in sizes 10.5, 12.0, 13.5, and 15.0 Fr. (see Fig. 15-3B). These dilators are passed over a 0.038-inch guidewire that has been initially passed to negotiate tortuosity withing the intramural ureter. In a sequential fashion under cystoscopic observation, the dilators slide over the guidewire through the intramural ureter and detrusor hiatus. The preplaced guidewire ensures that the dilator follows the course of the intramural ureter and helps prevent false passages at this level. Alternatively, an angioplastic balloon catheter may be used. The catheter is passed through the intramural ureter, usually over a previously inserted flexible tip guidewire. Once in position, the balloon is inflated under endoscopic observation. After approximately 15 to 30 seconds, the balloon is completely deflated and removed so that the ureteroscope can be inserted. Various types and sizes of balloon-dilating catheters are available; we have found the 5 or 6 Fr. catheter with a 6 × 30-mm balloon to be the most effective variety.

Lower ureteral injury from prior basketing of stones or operative procedures at the uretero-vesical junction, either reimplantation of the orifice or ureterolithotomy, often renders the terminal ureter inelastic from the resulting fibrosis. Consequently the dilating process becomes both difficult and more hazardous. Under these circumstances it is advisable to dilate along a ureteral catheter or over a guidewire, which can be positioned in the ureter with great safety. The guidewire not only gives direction to the dilating instrument but also, by the feel of the dilator slipping over the guidewire, indicates that the dilator is advancing intraluminally rather than causing a perforation. Small dilators will pass through the working channel of large cystoscopes to permit direct observation of the initial stages of the dilating process. Larger dilators that do not fit through the cystoscope port should be passed over the guide through an empty endoscopic sheath and monitored fluoroscopically. The variety of instruments for dilating the ureteral orifice and intramural ureter with this technique permits selection of the dilator most appropriate for the individual circumstance encountered.

Insertion of the Rigid Ureteroscope. After ureteral dilation, the 13 Fr. ureteroscope with a forward viewing (5-degree) lens is placed transurethrally into the bladder. The inflow irrigation pressure is lowered to 30 cm so that the ureter will not become overdistended. The ureteral orifice is identified and approached by the instrument, which is directed toward the center and inferior margin of the orifice (a position similar to that used when passing a ureteral catheter). The tip of the ureteroscope is then placed on the floor of the bladder to allow the upper lip of the orifice to pass over the telescope and sheath. As the instrument enters the orifice, vision is obscured only for several millimeters. The lumen becomes visible as the tip of the ureteroscope is advanced into the intramural portion of the ureter.

Difficulty may be encountered in entering the ureteral orifice. The instrument may pass over the orifice or may tear the mucosa. These problems can be avoided by adequately depressing the tip of the instrument at the ureteral orifice and by directing the ureteroscope along the path of the ureter. Once again, excessive force must be avoided throughout the procedure.

Insertion of the Rigid Ureteropyeloscope. In the original description of the technique, the ureteropyeloscope sheath was inserted blindly over an 8 Fr. ureteral catheter. We have found, however, that the technique for insertion under direct vision, as described for the rigid ureteroscope, is easy and reliable. After ureteral dilation, the ureteropyeloscope with a forward viewing lens is placed transurethrally into the bladder. The ureteral orifice is approached in the same fashion as described for the ureteroscope but, at a point just outside the orifice, the instrument is gently rotated 180 degrees and advanced slightly into the orifice (Fig. 15-8). This maneuver allows the beveled tip of the instrument to slip underneath the superior margin of the orifice. The instrument is then returned to its upright position and the ureteral lumen can be visualized. The slight angulation of the tip of the ureteropyeloscope facilitates this insertion (see Fig. 15-2B).

As discussed in Chapter 2, the ureter courses laterally and slightly posteriorly away from the bladder (Fig. 15-9). The instrument is advanced proximally along this course so as to keep the lumen in the center of the viewing field. The lumen then courses anteriorly and medially over the pelvic brim and iliac vessels. It is occasionally necessary to rotate the instrument 180 degrees in order to cross the iliac vessels. The ureter achieves its most anterior position over the psoas muscle (Fig. 15-10). At this point, the lumen is followed posteriorly and laterally toward the ureteropelvic junction and then into the renal pelvis. As the ureteropelvic junction is approached, the movements of the kidney with respiration are immediately noticeable. The ureteropelvic junction is identified as a slightly narrowed portion in the ureter with the large renal pelvis visible in the distance. As the instrument enters the renal pelvis, the infundibula are usually evident, and the lateral collecting system may be seen with the 70-degree lens (Fig. 15-11). The instrument can often be advanced into the upper pole infundibula. The corresponding endoscopic views are shown in Figures 2-1 through 2-8.

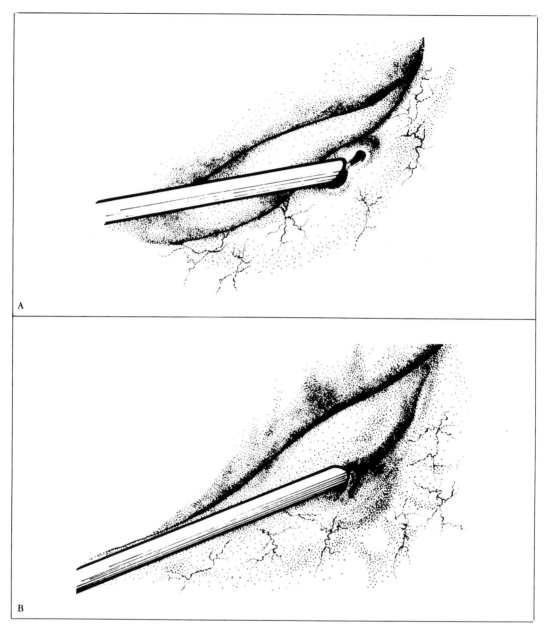

Figure 15-8. *As the ureteral orifice is approached (A), the ureteropyeloscope is gently rotated 180 degrees to allow its beveled tip to slide under the lip of the orifice (B). It is advanced slightly within the orifice (C) and then returned to its upright position inside the ureteral lumen (D).*

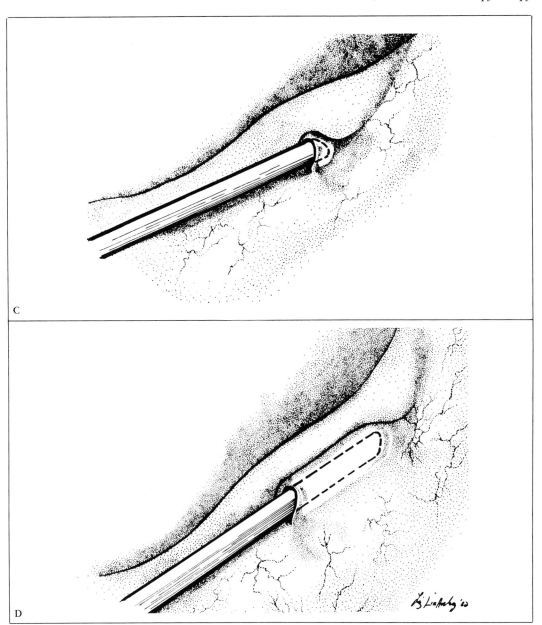

C

D

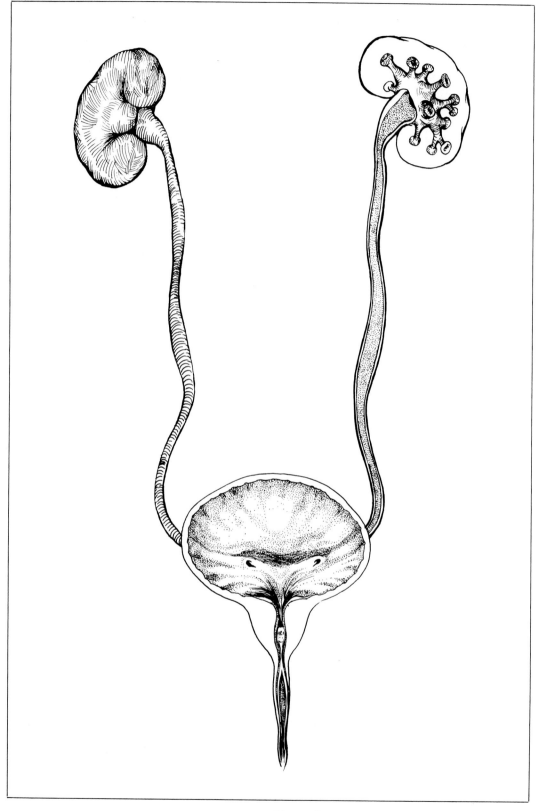

Figure 15-9. *The course of the ureter is represented from the kidney to the bladder in an anterior view.*

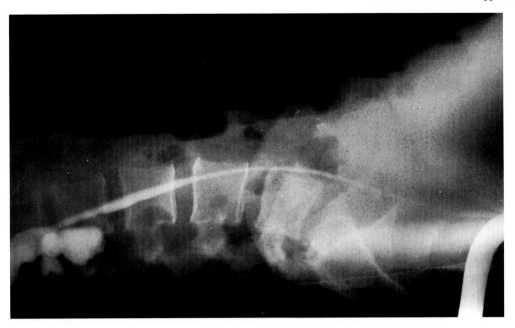

Figure 15-10. *A lateral retrograde pyelogram outlines the gentle curvature of the ureter from the bladder to the renal collecting system.*

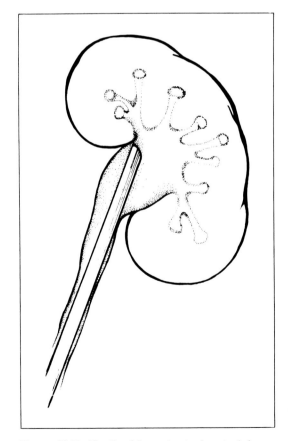

Figure 15-11. *The tip of the ureteropyeloscope is located in the renal pelvis. By interchanging the 5- and 70-degree telescopes, a large portion of the pelvis can be seen.*

PROBLEMS ENCOUNTERED DURING INSERTION OF THE URETEROPYELOSCOPE. As discussed in Chapter 6, narrowed portions of the supravesical ureter are occasionally encountered during ureteropyeloscopy. Although these narrowings are not strictures in the sense of causing significant obstruction to the flow of urine and increased proximal hydrostatic pressure, they are significant in that they may prevent passage of the ureteropyeloscope. As the instrument is advanced, the ureter will be telescoped ahead of the viewing field, where one of these narrowings or "subclinical" strictures will be encountered. The lumen is not of sufficient caliber to accept the instrument and, unlike that of the normal ureter, will not distend with irrigating fluid. It is critical in these instances that the instrument *not* be forcefully advanced. These subclinical strictures must be dilated before ureteropyeloscopy can proceed; otherwise, perforation of the ureter is likely to occur.

After identifying the narrow region through the ureteropyeloscope, two methods may be employed for dilation (Fig. 15-12). The preferred method is to use a small coronary angioplastic balloon catheter, which can be inserted through the working channel of the ureteropyeloscope to permit dilation under direct vision. The 4.2 Fr. catheter with a 3.7 × 30-mm balloon is utilized and, while watched through the telescope, the balloon is inflated exactly at the point of ureteral narrowing. It is held inflated for 15 to 30 seconds and then deflated completely. Usually the instrument can then be advanced either partially or completely past the narrowed region. Occasionally, repetition of the dilation is required.

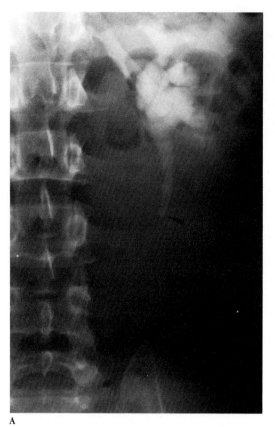

A

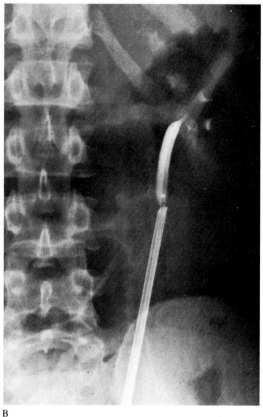

B

Figure 15-12. *Ureteroscopic dilation of a ureteral stricture using an angioplasty balloon catheter. A. Narrow segment of the left ureter opposite the third lumbar vertebral body. B. Dilation of the stricture. The balloon is inflated across the stricture just distal to the tip of the instrument.*

The alternative method is to use a larger balloon catheter (e.g.,5 Fr. with 5 × 30-mm balloon). After the narrow region has been identified endoscopically, the telescope is removed and the ureteropyeloscope sheath is left in place so that its tip is immediately distal to the narrowed region. The balloon catheter is then inserted through the sheath and aligned in proper position with the aid of fluoroscopy. Using a dilute mixture of contrast media and normal saline, the balloon is inflated once again under fluoroscopic observation. After 15 to 30 seconds of dilation, the balloon is deflated completely and the catheter removed so that the telescope can be replaced for continuation of the procedure.

Another commonly encountered problem is poor visualization during the procedure, due to debris or blood. For instance, should an impacted ureteral stone be present, the irrigation does not flow well through the instrument because of the obstructing stone and often chronic inflammatory debris and blood result. In these instances, it is helpful to pass a 4 Fr. ureteral catheter through the instrument. Hand irrigation can then be performed through the catheter to remove the debris and provide better ureteral distention and clearer visualization.

INDICATIONS FOR URETEROPYELOSCOPY. Initially, the availability of the ureteroscope allowed endoscopic procedures to be performed only in the lower ureter. Many techniques performed cystoscopically in the urethra and bladder could similarly be used ureteroscopically in the lower ureter. With the added length of the ureteropyeloscope, indications for urologic endoscopy were again expanded to include lesions located in the proximal ureter or renal pelvis (Table 15-1)[5].

Table 15-1. Indications for Ureteropyeloscopy

1. Filling defects
2. Hematuria
3. Positive cytology
4. Obstruction
5. Lithiasis
6. Foreign bodies

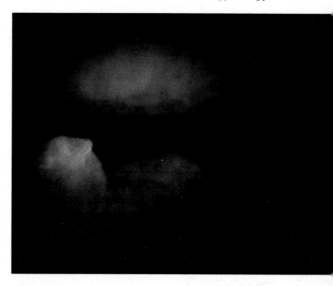

Figure 15-13. *These struvite calculi were located in the renal pelvis and successfully removed ureteroscopically. Areas of chronic pyelitis cystica (see Chap. 6) with mucosal edema and inflammation are present.*

Suspicion of Urothelial Tumor. An important indication for the use of ureteropyeloscopy is suspicion of a urothelial malignancy of the ureter or renal pelvis. Previously, these lesions could be identified by indirect radiographic studies or cytologic techniques and the diagnosis confirmed by open surgical exploration. The ureteropyeloscopic technique gives the urologist an alternative approach to establish the diagnosis. A variety of circumstances may lead to the suspicion of a malignancy of the upper urinary tract.

The surveillance of the patient who has undergone a partial ureterectomy for tumor can readily be accomplished. Ureteropyeloscopy can be performed and the site of resection inspected for tumor recurrence in the same fashion as cystoscopic surveillance of bladder tumors.

Filling Defects. If a filling defect is identified on excretory urography or retrograde ureteropyelography, this suspicious area can then be visualized directly and usually identified. If the diagnosis is not obvious, then the lesion can be biopsied. By obtaining tissue transurethrally for histologic examination, the possibility of tumor spillage and local recurrence following open surgical or nephroscopic biopsy (see Chap. 8)[12] can be avoided.

Obstruction. Ureteral obstruction not readily identified by standard radiographic techniques lends itself to the ureteropyeloscopic approach. Examination of the site of obstruction allows identification of the obstruction and, if necessary, biopsy. With either intrinsic or extrinsic obstruction, ureteropyeloscopy is often essential to pass a ureteral catheter.

Hematuria. In the presence of documented unilateral hematuria and radiographically normal structure, ureteropyeloscopy allows direct examination of the urothelium. The site of bleeding may be identified and suspicious lesions visualized or biopsied. In the case of intrarenal bleeding, the source may be localized to a particular major calyx. Arteriography can then be performed with particular attention to that portion of the kidney. Gittes and Varady[2] have reported similar findings using operative nephroscopic techniques.

Suspicious Cytology. As in the patient with unilateral hematuria, the recovery of malignant cells from one collecting system, with or without radiographic changes, presents a clinical situation in which ureteropyeloscopy is indicated. Any suspicious lesions can then be biopsied. If there are no suspicious lesions, random biopsies can be taken within the pelvis and ureter to identify carcinoma in situ.

Lithiasis. Initially, the ureteroscopic technique was used for diagnosis and extraction only of distal ureteral calculi[6]. The longer ureteropyeloscope and the longer ultrasonic transducer, however, extended this technique to larger stones located in the midureter and proximal ureter and occasionally in the renal pelvis (Fig. 15-13)[7]. Many factors, including size and location of the stone and anatomy of the collecting system, determine the success of stone extraction.

Foreign Bodies. A less common indication is a retained foreign body in the ureter or renal pelvis. Occasionally, a ureteral stent will migrate proximally[4] or, rarely, a stone basket will fragment[1], or its filiform tip separate. Such foreign bodies justify an attempt at ureteroscopic removal before performance of an open operation. Long-term presence of a foreign body produces inflammatory reaction with edema and granulation, which hampers ureteroscopic visualization.

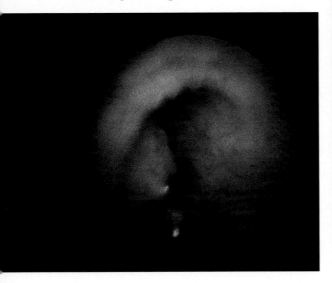

Figure 15-14. *Biopsy of a lower ureteral tumor with 5 Fr. flexible cup-biopsy forceps.*

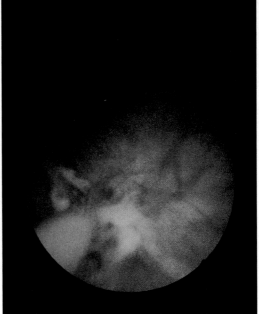

Figure 15-15. *Fulguration of the base of the ureteral tumor shown in Fig. 15-14 with a 5 Fr. Bugbee electrode.*

INTRAURETERAL PROCEDURES. As a suspicious region is approached within the ureter or renal pelvis, it is often difficult to identify the lesion visually because of overlying debris or blood clot. In these instances, it is necessary to wash off the object with irrigation fluid. Following this maneuver, a stone can be identified by the presence of crystals (see Figs. 6-3 to 6-7), a transitional cell tumor by the fine papillary fronds (see Figs. 6-10 to 6-14), or an inflammatory cyst by its smooth spheroid surface (see Fig. 6-8).

After the diagnosis has been established with the 10 Fr. ureteropyeloscope or the ureteroscope, the larger operating sheaths must be inserted for any procedure. All procedures that can be performed through a 5 Fr. working channel cystoscopically within the bladder can be performed ureteroscopically within the ureter. These include biopsy, fulguration, and resection of tumors, as well as extraction of stones and passage of catheters. Throughout the procedure it is necessary to keep the inflow irrigation pressure at less than 30 cm of water and to empty the upper tract intermittently to prevent overdistention of the proximal collecting system and fluid absorption.

Tumors. When a suspicious lesion or an obvious ureteral or renal pelvic tumor is encountered, several options are available. A biopsy can be obtained with the 5 Fr. flexible cup biopsy forceps (Fig. 15-14) or a flexible ureteral brush (see Chap. 9). The lesion can be fulgurated with a Bugbee electrode (Fig. 15-15). If fulguration is performed, we recommend that a very low current be used and that consideration be given to leaving a ureteral catheter in place for several days following the procedure.

A feature of the ureteroscope and ureteropyeloscope is a resectoscope sheath and working element that can be used to resect and fulgurate lesions in the ureter, once again using a very low setting on the fulgurating current. The resecting is done by starting at the top of a tumor and working toward its base. Irrigation must be maintained and the upper tract emptied intermittently. Even though the ureter and pelvis are very thin, the small size of the resectoscope loop and the fine control afforded by the working element allow transurethral tumor resection and fulguration to be performed without perforation.

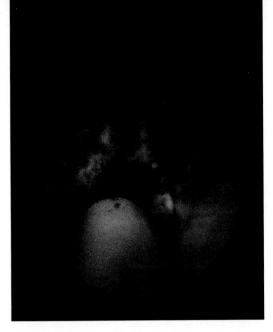

Figure 15-16. *This patient had a staghorn calculus in addition to this completely obstructing proximal ureteral calculus. It was not possible to pass a catheter cystoscopically. Ureteroscopically, however, a catheter could be passed between the stone and the ureteral wall.*

Obstruction. Occasionally, it is impossible to pass a ureteral catheter using standard cystoscopic approaches. In these cases, it is often helpful to insert the ureteroscope to the level of the obstructing lesion or past the tortuous section of an otherwise impassable ureter. At this level, there can often be seen one small opening in the ureteral lumen through which a catheter may pass under direct vision (Fig. 15-16). Once this opening is found, a 5 Fr. ureteral catheter or guidewire can be passed under direct vision, bypassing the obstruction.

Calculi. Advances in ureteroscopic instrumentation have led to great improvements in the endoscopic treatment of upper tract calculi. As noted earlier, the short ureteroscope initially permitted removal of only small distal ureteral calculi. The longer ureteropyeloscope enabled small calculi to be removed from the entire ureter and renal pelvis. The greatest improvement, however, was the development of ultrasonic and electrohydraulic lithotripsy instrumentation for the rigid ureteropyeloscope, an advance that allowed much larger calculi to be removed.

DIRECT BASKET EXTRACTION. Ureteroscopic extraction of calculi should be preceded by a retrograde ureteropyelogram to define the ureter distal to the obstruction site. Often, an excretory urogram does not show ureteral anatomy distal to the obstructing stone and the retrograde study must verify ureteral course and caliber. This study helps in the planning of ureteroscopic passage by identifying narrowed or tortuous portions of the ureter that may require dilation prior to encountering the calculus. The ureteropyeloscope is then inserted under direct vision in the fashion described previously. It is mandatory that the inflow irrigation pressure be lowered to an absolute minimum (<30 cm of water) so that the stone will not be washed proximally into the kidney.

The patient with a ureteral calculus should be in a reverse Trendelenburg's position to maintain the lower ureter in a dependent position. Any free-floating calculus or fragment would then be carried distally in the ureter by the force of gravity. In the supine position, calculi proximal to the most anterior point of the ureter (over the psoas muscle) tend to move proximally into the renal pelvis and possibly into the posterior and lateral calyces (see Fig. 15-10). Renal pelvic calculi may be approached ureteropyeloscopically with the patient in the lateral position, which causes the renal pelvis to become the most dependent portion of the renal collecting system (Fig. 15-17). The instrument is then advanced to the level of the calculus. Once the calculus is identified, the stone basket is inserted through the instrument to the level of the stone. We prefer to use a six-wire basket with a Teflon-coated sheath that holds the stone securely and slides easily through the instrument. Occasionally, the stone is adherent to the ureter and the basket will pass at only one area between the stone and the ureteral mucosa. The basket is opened under direct vision and closed to engage the stone tightly within the wires of the basket (Figs. 15-18, 15-19). The entire instrument, stone basket, and stone are then gently extracted. It can be observed during the extraction that the stone is being removed freely and the ureteral mucosa is not trapped in the basket. Following successful removal of the calculus, the instrument is reinserted into the ureter to ensure that no stone fragments remain and that no damage has been inflicted on the ureteral mucosa. We prefer to leave a ureteral catheter in place for 48 hours following successful removal.

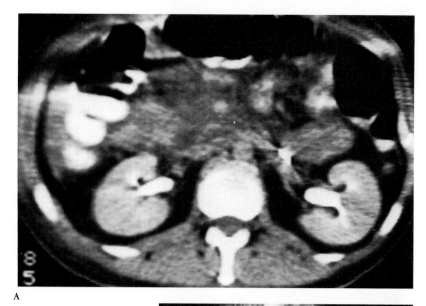

A

B

Figure 15-17. *A. CT scan shows the posterior and lateral position of the renal pelvis. (Note the left ureter and renal pelvis.) B. In the lateral position the renal pelvis becomes the most dependent portion of the renal collecting system.*

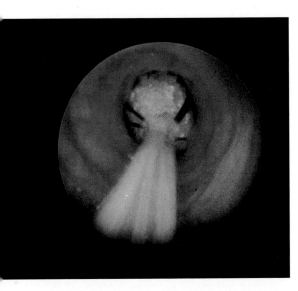

Figure 15-18. *Cystine calculus engaged within a stone basket. The basket holds the stone securely and there is no ureteral mucosa trapped between the wires.*

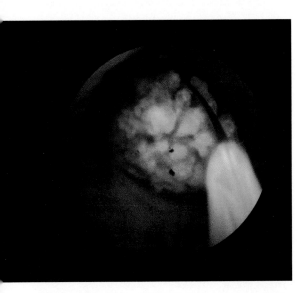

Figure 15-19. *This calcium oxalate calculus is firmly trapped within the wires of a stone basket and is being withdrawn through the ureter.*

ULTRASONIC LITHOTRIPSY. Stones too large to be pulled down the ureter safely can be disintegrated ultrasonically once they are visualized and engaged in a stone basket (Fig. 15-20)[7]. A long ultrasonic transducer similar to that used in percutaneous nephrostolithotomy (see Fig. 17-2) can be inserted through the ureteropyeloscope sheath after the telescope is removed. Prior to removing the telescope, however, the stone, secure within the wires of the basket, is positioned directly at the tip of the ureteropyeloscope sheath and held in position. Consequently, the ultrasonic transducer, when inserted, will make contact with the stone held at the end of the instrument.

There is also a rubber diaphragm on the ultrasonic transducer that locks into the ureteropyeloscope sheath to form a water-tight seal. This maintains a closed system for irrigation, which is vital in order to dissipate the heat and remove the fragments produced by the disintegration process.

Once the transducer has been partially inserted and the rubber diaphragm locked in position, the tip of the transducer is slowly advanced until it makes contact with the stone. This maneuver is observed fluoroscopically (Fig. 15-20). The irrigation fluid should be flowing and the suction through the transducer should be started; the disintegration can then proceed. Usually only a short burst (<10 sec) is required to cause partial disintegration of the stone, and often the wires of the stone basket can be felt to close as the stone's size diminishes. Following partial disintegration, the transducer is replaced by the telescope. Often, a groove is visible where the transducer has passed (Figs. 15-21, 15-22). Occasionally, the stone is small enough following partial disintegration to be pulled down the ureter safely; if it still is too large and continues to adhere to the ureteral wall, further disintegration is required.

Following stone removal, the ureteropyeloscope is reinserted and the site of stone impaction inspected. Smaller stone fragments are occasionally identified, and these can be removed with a three-prong grasping forceps or a stone basket. If there is any mucosal damage, dye extravasation, or edema, a ureteral catheter is left in place for 48 hours.

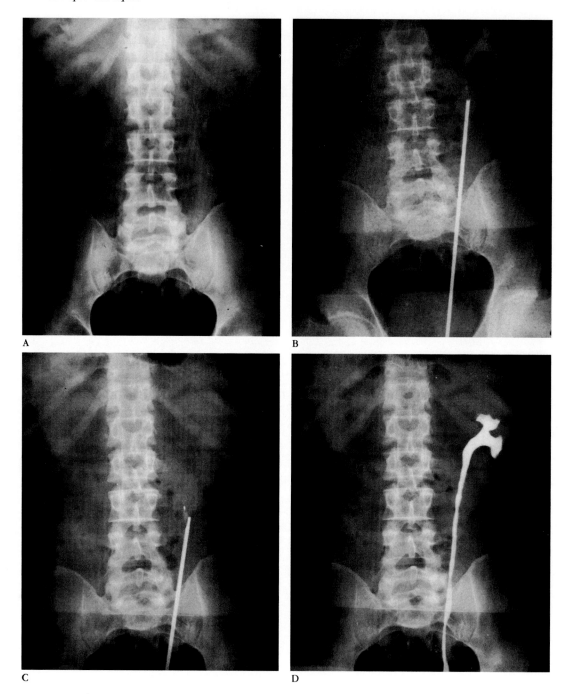

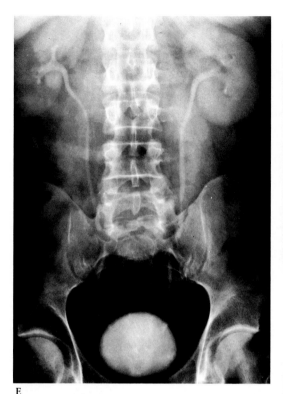

E

Figure 15-20. *The technique of ureteroscopic ultrasonic lithotripsy. A. Proximal left ureteral calculus lodged between the second and third lumbar vertebral bodies. B. Following a retrograde pyelogram, the ureteropyeloscope is inserted and the stone visualized. C. The stone is engaged in a basket and positioned at the tip of the instrument. The telescope is removed and the ultrasonic transducer is inserted to make contact with the stone. D. A contrast study is done immediately following successful stone removal. There is no extravasation of contrast or edematous obstruction. E. Excretory urogram performed 1 month following the procedure. There is no ureteral narrowing at the site of stone impaction and there is good renal function. (From J. L. Huffman, D. H. Bagley, H. W. Schoenberg, and E. S. Lyon, Transurethral removal of large ureteral and renal pelvic calculi using ureteroscopic ultrasonic lithotripsy. J. Urol. 130 : 31, 1983.)*

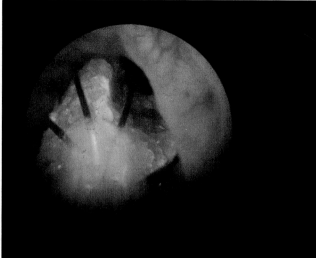

Figure 15-21. *Following one application of the ultrasonic transducer, a groove is seen in the stone corresponding to the path of disintegration.*

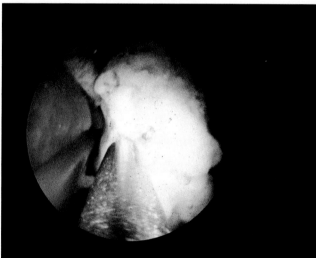

Figure 15-22. *Using the offset telescope, ultrasonic lithotripsy is performed under direct vision. This calculus is trapped by a Fogarty balloon (catheter at 8 o'clock), and the ultrasonic transducer (6 o'clock) is applied while viewing endoscopically. A guidewire is also visible at the 10 o'clock position.*

Several points regarding the use of ultrasonic disintegration through the ureteropyeloscope should be emphasized. First, this is a relatively blind procedure. Even though the stone has been positioned at the tip of the instrument, the procedure should be watched fluoroscopically to make sure that the tip of the transducer does not pass too far and damage the ureter proximal to the stone. The disintegration should be done only in short bursts and the telescope should be replaced frequently to assess progress. Secondly, Howards and co-workers[3] have shown experimentally that urothelial damage may occur with ultrasound if heat is allowed to accumulate. This can result in a thermal injury to the ureteral mucosa. To prevent heat buildup, irrigation must be kept flowing through the instrument during the disintegration process to dissipate the heat. It flows in through the ureteropyeloscope sheath and out through the lumen of the transducer with the small stone particles that are produced. Also, only short bursts (<10 sec) of ultrasound are required; thus heat buildup is offset by short periods of disintegration.

ELECTROHYDRAULIC LITHOTRIPSY. Destruction of upper tract calculi can also be accomplished ureteroscopically using electrohydraulic lithotripsy. There is a 5 Fr. coaxial probe that can pass through the working channel of the instrument. A shock wave is generated from the tip of the probe and directed toward the calculus.

The advantage of this technique is that the entire process can be watched endoscopically, unlike ultrasonic lithotripsy. The probe is placed directly adjacent to the stone under endoscopic observation, and the magnitude of the shock wave produced is slowly increased to a level sufficient to fracture the calculus.

The disadvantage of the technique is that no provision is made for recovery of the fragments that are produced. Suction is not provided, as it is with the ultrasonic transducer, and the shock wave often causes an "uncontrolled" fragmentation, resulting in loss of fragments proximally in the kidney.

Experience thus far with this technique is highly limited. We have used it only once in the renal pelvis and never in the ureter. At this time, its use cannot be recommended for primary treatment.

Table 15-2. Ureteroscopic Procedures

Procedure	Ureteroscope (no. procedures)	Ureteropyeloscope (no. procedures)	Total (no. procedures)
Calculi	20	107	127
Tumor	29	21	50
Hematuria	10	14	24
Catheterization	2	10	12
Filling defects	0	8	8
Positive cytology	0	1	1
Foreign bodies	1	3	4
Total	62	164	226

RESULTS OF URETEROPYELOSCOPY. At the University of Chicago, 226 ureteroscopic procedures were performed from 1976 through 1983 (Table 15-2). These 226 procedures were performed on 161 patients, 73 of whom were female and 88 of whom were male. The ages of the patients ranged from 20 to 83 years. In some instances, the procedures were performed on multiple occasions with the same patients or on both ureters. Of these 226 procedures, 164 were performed with the ureteropyeloscope, which became available in 1981, and 62 with the ureteroscope.

The majority of the procedures were performed for extraction of ureteral stones and diagnosis or follow-up of ureteral tumors. The remainder of the procedures were done for diagnosis of unexplained hematuria, ureteral obstruction, and filling defects, and for passage of ureteral catheters and removal of foreign bodies.

Table 15-3. Success Rate in Performing Procedure

Technique	Successful Cases		Unsuccessful Cases	
	No.	Percent	No.	Percent
Ureteroscope	57	92%	5	8%
Ureteropyeloscope	157	96%	7	4%
Total	214	94%	12	6%

Table 15-4. Reasons for Failures

Cause	Ureteroscope (no. patients)	Ureteropyeloscope (no. patients)	Patients (total)	
			No.	Percent
Unable to dilate orifice	1	7	8	3%
Unable to insert scope	4	0	4	2%
Total	5	7	12	5%

Table 15-5. Treatment of Calculi

Result	Ureteroscope (no. patients)	Ureteropyeloscope (no. patients)	Ureteropyeloscope Plus Ultrasonic Disintegration (no. patients)	Patients (total) No.	Percent
Successful removal of stones	13	28	38	79	72%
Unsuccessful, surgery required	4	4	1	9	8%
Unsuccessful, no further procedure required	0	12	0	12	11%
Unsuccessful, percutaneous nephrostolithotomy done	0	6	4	10	9%
Total	17	50	43	110	100%

The success rate for performing the procedure (i.e., dilating the intramural ureter and then passing the ureteroscope into the ureteral lumen), has been 94 percent (Table 15-3). The reasons for failure have been either that the ureteral orifice is inaccessible or could not be dilated or that the instrument could not be passed into the ureter (Table 15-4). Factors that prevent the passage of a ureteral catheter may also prevent the performance of ureteroscopy. Some of these factors include a tortuous distal ureter, one made immobile by previous pelvic surgery or radiation, or a nondistensible ureter secondary to stricture or fibrosis. A patient with a high posterior bladder neck or large prostatic median lobe may also have a relatively inaccessible ureteral orifice. Also, intramural ureters with a direct lateral course away from the orifice may be extremely hard to dilate.

Calculi. Our initial experience has shown ureteropyeloscopic treatment of calculi to be successful without significant complications. In our total series of 110 patients who otherwise would have been treated by open lithotomy, 79 (72%) of the patients had successful results (Table 15-5). This finding includes 7 patients in whom a calculus lodged in the renal pelvis was successfully removed (Table 15-6).

In analyzing the results of this series, it is helpful to examine the success rate according to the type of instrument used (see Table 15-5). Initially, the ureteroscope, capable of extracting only those calculi located in the distal ureter, was used[6]. With the development of the longer ureteropyeloscope, smaller calculi located anywhere within the ureter or renal pelvis could be approached. With the addition of the long ultrasonic transducer, larger calculi in the upper tract could be extracted endoscopically[7].

Table 15-6. Location of Stones

Location	No. Stones (total)	Stones Removed No.	Percent
Lower ureter	54	48	89%
Upper ureter	39	24	62%
Renal pelvis	17	7	41%
Total	110	79	72%

Of the 43 patients treated with the ureteropyeloscope plus the ultrasonic transducer, only 1 patient required open pyelolithotomy and 4 patients percutaneous nephrostolithotomies following incomplete stone removal ureteroscopically. Ureteroscopic ultrasonic lithotripsy proved successful and no further procedures were required in 38 patients (see Table 15-5). The average size of the stones removed in this fashion was 1.1 × 0.7 cm (Table 15-7).

The reasons for failures were mainly related to position of the calculi. Prior to the availability of the ureteropyeloscope, four of the calculi could not be reached by the shorter ureteroscope. Eight other calculi could not be visualized by the ureteropyeloscope because of their location in a lower pole calyx. At the start of these procedures, the calculi were lodged at the ureteropelvic junction; on insertion of the instrument, however, they were dislodged and subsequently migrated to the dependent lower pole calyx. In these locations, they were not amenable to retrieval by the rigid ureteropyeloscope. Another calculus was visualized in the ureter, and engaged in the stone basket, but a constricted portion of the distal ureter prevented its withdrawal. At that time, ultrasonic lithotripsy was unavailable and there had been no experience with dilation of ureteral strictures by angioplastic catheters. Since this study, however, 3 cases of ureteral strictures have been successfully dilated with angioplastic balloon catheters.

Table 15-7. Size of Stones Removed

Technique	Stones Removed (no.)	Average Size (cm)
All techniques	79	0.8×0.7
Ultrasonic lithotripsy	38	1.1×0.7

Urothelial Tumors. A total of 50 ureteropyeloscopic procedures involving 8 patients have been performed for diagnosis, treatment, and follow-up of ureteral or renal pelvic tumors. Of these patients, 1 underwent 16 procedures and another 13 procedures following diagnosis of a low-grade transitional cell tumor of the lower ureter. Each was evaluated at 3-month intervals over 5 years and each had occasional recurrences, which were biopsied and fulgurated. Neither required surgical intervention.

A recurrence in the renal pelvis was diagnosed pyeloscopically in 1 of these 2 patients. She had a history of recurrent bladder cancer and vesicoureteral reflux and had originally been diagnosed with the ureteroscope as having a grade I lower ureteral transitional cell carcinoma. With the longer ureteropyeloscope it was possible to examine the upper ureter and renal pelvis. In the renal pelvis, a cluster of low-grade papillary fronds was identified and biopsied (see Fig. 6-11). Prior to the procedure, an excretory urogram and retrograde pyelogram failed to identify the lesion. The patient will continue to be followed at 3-month intervals with repeat ureteropyeloscopies.

A third patient had agreed to only partial ureterectomy as treatment of an invasive grade II transitional cell carinoma diagnosed ureteroscopically. Nine subsequent ureteropyeloscopic procedures have been performed on this patient, including three fulgurations of low-grade recurrences near the region of the ureteral anastamosis.

A fourth patient underwent two ureteroscopic procedures for biopsy and fulguration of tumors in the intramural ureter. After refusing appropriate therapy of a preexisting advanced bladder cancer, she died of the disease.

A fifth patient presented with gross hematuria and positive cytology from a solitary kidney. Despite a normal-appearing excretory urogram, ureteropyeloscopy revealed a solid mass extending into the renal pelvis. The mass was biopsied and confirmed to be a grade IV transitional cell carcinoma. She refused nephroureterectomy and hemodialysis; therefore, she was treated with intrapelvic chemotherapy. The patient had no further hematuria and repeat pyeloscopy 6 weeks later showed a substantial decrease in tumor size. The patient has had 4 more follow-up procedures over a 12-month period and thus far metastatic disease has not developed and the primary tumor has steadily decreased in size.

A sixth patient who was 83 years old had a history of recurrent transitional cell bladder carcinoma. He developed a filling defect in the lower ureter on his excretory urogram. Ureteroscopic biopsy showed this 1-cm papillary lesion to be a grade II transitional cell carcinoma. Transurethral resection of the tumor using the ureteroscopic resectoscope was subsequently performed on this patient without complication. Final pathology sections showed no tumor penetration into the muscularis. He was also treated with intraureteral chemotherapy and will be followed initially at 6-week intervals with repeat ureteroscopy.

The remaining 2 patients each underwent nephroureterectomy following ureteropyeloscopic diagnosis of extensive renal pelvic tumors. In each patient the final pathologic mapping of the tumors correlated well with the preoperative ureteropyeloscopic mapping.

Hematuria. Ureteroscopic evaluation for unilateral gross hematuria was performed in 24 patients. The procedure in 5 of these patients could not be performed because of an inaccessible ureteral orifice. In 13 patients, the procedure was completed but no source of bleeding was identified.

The remaining 5 patients all had positive findings at endoscopy. Of these, 1 patient with a known squamous cell carcinoma of the lung was found to have a metastatic lesion in the renal pelvis. Small uric acid calculi in the kidneys were diagnosed in 2 other patients. In a fourth patient, bleeding was shown to be localized to the lower pole infundibulum; no cause for the bleeding was identified, however. The fifth patient had gross hematuria with excretory urography showing a renal mass impinging on the renal pelvis. Ureteropyeloscopy revealed distortion of the renal pelvis by the mass but no urothelial lesion. He later was diagnosed as having a renal cell carcinoma and underwent radical nephrectomy.

Table 15-8. Complications of Successful Ureteroscopy Procedure

Complication	Ureteroscope (no. procedures)	Ureteropyeloscope (no. procedures)	Procedures (total)	
			No.	Percent
None	51	150	201	94
Minor mucosal injury not requiring surgery	6	5	11	5
Ureteral disruption requiring surgery	0	1	1	0.5
Pyelonephritis	0	1	1	0.5
Total	57	157	214	100

COMPLICATIONS OF URETEROPYELOSCOPY.
The possible complications of the ureteropyeloscopic technique are very similar to those encountered during cystoscopy and ureteral catheterization (Table 15-8). Perforation of the ureter has not been a major problem in our initial experience. Although several false passages of the submucosal ureter resulted, there have been no cases of severe extravasation outside the collecting system. Several patients underwent radiographic evaluation following the procedure and were found to have no abnormalities resulting directly from the procedure.

Most patients experience lower quadrant discomfort in the side in which the procedure was performed. This pain is thought to be secondary to dilation of the ureter or possibly postoperative edema of the intramural ureter. These patients seldom require analgesics and the pain usually disappears after 24 to 48 hours.

There have been no cases of ureteral stenosis or stricture in all of the patients in our series. One patient underwent 13 ureteroscopic procedures over a 5-year period. She had a recurrent, low-grade distal ureteral tumor and showed no radiographic abnormalities of the ureter or intrarenal collecting system. She subsequently died following a myocardial infarction. A second patient has undergone eight ureteroscopic and several pyeloscopic procedures for follow-up on a urothelial tumor in the submucosal ureter. She has shown no renal deterioration in a 5-year follow-up period and her ureteral orifice has remained cystoscopically normal. Initially, voiding cystourethrograms were done following the procedures. These were performed on approximately the first 15 patients and there was no vesicoureteral reflux.

One patient developed pyelonephritis following ureteropyeloscopy. She had a left renal pelvic filling defect with gross hematuria and negative cytology. Although pyeloscopy showed the defect to be a uric acid calculus, 24 hours following the procedure, the patient developed left flank pain and fever to 39.5°C. Urine culture following the procedure grew more than 100,000 colonies of *Proteus mirabilis,* and blood cultures were all negative. The patient subsequently responded well to intravenous antibiotics and an excretory urogram following the procedure showed no obstruction or extravasation.

Routinely, the patients are placed on preoperative prophylactic antibiotics. These are continued postoperatively for 24 hours unless the urine is infected, in which case they are continued for a longer course.

We have encountered no significant complications after using the ultrasonic transducer in the ureter or renal pelvis. Howard's group[3], in 1974, reported their experimental work with the effects of ultrasound on the mucosa of dog bladders. They found that severe changes in the microscopic appearance of bladder mucosa occurred only when the ultrasonic tip was placed in direct contact with the tissue. By engaging the calculus in a basket, positioning it directly at the tip of the instrument, and watching fluoroscopically while the transducer is functioning, there is little chance of direct contact between the urothelium and the tip of the transducer. As noted earlier (see Ultrasonic Lithotripsy), thermal energy produced by the ultrasonic disintegration is also potentially injurious to tissues; short bursts (<10 sec) of ultrasound with constant fluid irrigation through the ureteroscope, however, prevents a significant increase in temperature.

REFERENCES

1. Beall, M., and Kidd, R. Stone basket rescue. *Urology* 17:590, 1981.

2. Gittes, R.F., and Varady, S. Nephroscopy in chronic unilateral hematuria. *J. Urol.* 126:297, 1981.

3. Howards, S.S., Merrill, E., Harris, S., and Cohn, J. Ultrasonic lithotripsy—Laboratory evaluation. *Invest. Urol.* 11(4):273, 1974.

4. Huffman, J.L. Ureteroscopic stone basket retrieval. *Urology* 180:325, 1981.

5. Huffman, J.L., Bagley, D.H., and Lyon, E.S. Extending cystoscopic techniques into the ureter and renal pelvis—Experience with ureteroscopy and pyeloscopy. *J.A.M.A.* 250:2002, 1983.

6. Huffman, J.L., Bagley, D.H., and Lyon, E.S. Treatment of distal ureteral calculi using a rigid ureteroscope. *Urology* 20:574, 1982.

7. Huffman, J.L., Bagley, D.H., Schoenberg, H.W., and Lyon, E.S. Transurethral removal of large ureteral and renal pelvic calculi using ureteroscopic ultrasonic lithotripsy. *J. Urol.* 130:31, 1983.

8. Lyon, E.S., Banno, J.J., and Schoenberg, H.W. Transurethral ureteroscopy in men using juvenile cystoscopy equipment. *J. Urol.* 122:152, 1979.

9. Lyon, E.S., Kyker, J.S., and Schoenberg, H.W. Transurethral ureteroscopy in women: A ready addition to urologic armamentarium. *J. Urol.* 119:35, 1978.

10. Perez-Castro Ellendt, E., and Martinez-Pineiro, J.A. Transurethral ureteroscopy—A current urological procedure. *Arch. Esp. Urol.* 33:445, 1980.

11. Takagi, T., Go, T., Takayasu, H., and Aso, Y. Fiberoptic pyeloureteroscope. *Surgery* 70:661, 1971.

12. Tomera, K.M., Leary, F.J., and Zincke, H. Pyeloscopy in urothelial tumors. *J. Urol.* 127:1088, 1982.

13. Young, H.H., and McKay, R.W. Congenital valvular obstruction of the prostatic urethra. *Surg. Gynecol. Obstet.* 48:509, 1929.

16
FLEXIBLE FIBEROPTIC URETEROPYELOSCOPY

Demetrius H. Bagley

Jeffry L. Huffman

Edward S. Lyon

The development of fiberoptic instruments for medical use was a major advance for diagnostic and therapeutic endoscopy. Although the phenomenon of transmission of light through glass fibers had been known since the late 1920s [3,8], it was not until Curtiss, Hirschowitz, and Peters [4] introduced in 1956 a practical fiberscope for transmitting images that the real advantages of fiberoptics in medicine became evident. The clinical use of the gastroscope by Hirschowitz's group [9] in 1958 allowed direct visualization of a duodenal ulcer through a completely flexible instrument composed of a light-conducting bundle and an image-transmitting bundle of glass fibers. For image transmission, the fibers were arranged identically at the proximal and distal ends of the bundle to allow coherent transmission of the image.

Since their introduction, fiberoptic bundles have been widely used both for illumination in the lighting systems for rigid endoscopes and for image transmission in instruments such as the uretero-scope [10], choledochoscope [11], arterioscope [7], cardioscope [6], bronchoscope [5], and nasopharyngoscope [12]. Marshall [10], in 1964, reported using a 9 Fr. fiberscope or ureteroscope developed by American Cystoscope Makers, Inc., which was passed through a 26 Fr. cystoscope into the distal ureter where a ureteral stone was visualized at 9 cm. Although transmission of light and images proved excellent, there was no method for changing the direction of the tip of the instrument and no channel for working instruments or for irrigation to provide a clear field and adequate distention of the ureter.

Takagi and co-workers [13] began in 1966 to work with a flexible fiberoptic endoscope, 2.7 mm in diameter and 70 cm in length. They reported its use in a patient undergoing an open operation during which the instrument was passed through a ureterotomy to visualize and photograph the renal pelvis and papillae. Once again, problems caused by the lack of an irrigation channel and the inability to change the direction of the tip of the instrument were encountered. It became evident, however, that it was possible to visualize portions of the urinary tract previously undetectable through rigid endoscopes.

Takagi's group [14] in 1971 reported the successful use of a "pyeloureteroscope," which had been passed transurethrally in 23 patients. The instrument was an Olympus model KF, 2 mm in diameter and 75 cm in length. The addition of a 2.5-cm angulating section at its distal end enabled the urologist to pass the instrument into the ureteral orifice and through the intramural ureter with the help of fluoroscopy in the same fashion as a ureteral catheter. It also enabled passage through the ureter and into the major calyces within the renal pelvis. Despite its advantage of a flexible distal tip, this instrument still did not have an irrigating system and was difficult to pass through the intramural ureter. This difficulty resulted in breakage of the glass fibers.

To circumvent the problem of ureteral insertion, Takayasu and Aso[15] introduced a Teflon guide tube, which initially was passed through a special cystoscope with an ocular lens system that protruded at a 45-degree angle from the shaft. The angulation of the lens helped to prevent fracture of the glass fibers of the instrument during passage through the cystoscope, and a special deflecting bridge limited sharp angulation of the instrument following passage from the end of the cystoscope. The guide tube was passed into the bladder and engaged by the deflecting bridge. A ureteral catheter was then passed through the guide tube into the ureteral orifice. Once the ureteral catheter was passed proximally, approximately 10 cm into the ureter, the guide tube was pushed over the ureteral catheter to a position proximal to the junction of the intramural ureter. The ureteral catheter could be removed and replaced with the flexible pyeloureteroscope, which consequently was in a position for observation. The authors reported a success rate of 100 percent in 19 patients using this guide tube method compared to an 80-percent success rate in 50 patients prior to its use. Irrigation was obtained only through the guide tube or by inducing a mannitol diuresis. Observation of the upper urinary tract, therefore, was difficult or impossible in the presence of debris or hematuria.

FEATURES OF FLEXIBLE URETEROPYELOSCOPY. This early experience demonstrated the value of the flexible ureteropyeloscope as well as the importance of the instrument's many different features. Flexibility is a major advantage of the ureteropyeloscope, which, as a result, can pass tortuosities within the lumen of the urinary tract. A flexible instrument has the potential advantage of passing angularly within the urinary tract, specifically of passing posteriorly and laterally into the renal collecting system. This same flexibility also may be a source of difficulty in handling since the shaft may be too flexible to pass into the ureter but rather coils within the bladder. It may also be too flexible to pass throughout the length of the ureter but merely buckles within the distal ureter.

A directable, maneuverable tip is a decided advantage for any flexible instrument. Maneuverability is essential for accurate placement within the bladder and the tortuous ureter or for exploration of the intrarenal collecting system. The mechanism within the instrument that deflects the tip uses space that would otherwise be available for the working channel, but this loss is more than offset by the gain in maneuverability.

Another essential feature of a ureteroscope is a channel for irrigation and for passing working instruments. Irrigation is used, as for other urologic instruments, to clear the field of debris and blood and also to distend the lumen. The working channel must be adequate for passing useful working instruments and should allow a reasonable flow of irrigant even when an instrument is in place.

When compared with rigid urologic instruments, flexible fiberoptic instruments are inferior in two major respects. First, the grid pattern of the fiberoptic viewing channel provides less accurate visual resolution than the solid lens system of the rigid instrument. The flexible instrument can be focused, however, and is quite adequate for identification of abnormalities within the ureter or kidney. Second, the flexible instrument has a much smaller working channel relative to that of a rigid instrument of the same outside diameter. Nevertheless, the advantage of maneuverability in some specific cases may outweigh these disadvantages.

INSTRUMENTATION. Several flexible instruments are now available that have been used as pyeloureteroscopes. These either have been designed primarily for use in the urinary tract or were used initially as pediatric bronchoscopes and have been adapted for use in the upper urinary tract only by constructing them with a longer flexible shaft. These instruments range in diameter from 1.8 to 3.6 mm, and each individual instrument has its own advantages and disadvantages (Table 16-1). The smallest, a 1.8-mm instrument, has the major advantage of its size but is limited by its nondeflectable tip and lack of a working channel. The next size, 2.7 mm in diameter, gains maneuverability with a directable, maneuverable tip. Although the instrument still has no irrigating or working channel, when used in conjunction with the rigid instrument, irrigation can be provided through the outer sheath[1].

Table 16-1. Flexible Ureteropyeloscopes*

Feature	Diameter at Tip (mm)			
	1.8	2.7	3.2	3.6
Deflection (degrees)	None	160 and 90	160 and 90	160 and 90
Working length (mm)	300, 500, or 800	300, 500, or 800	300, 500, or 800	600
Irrigation and working channel (mm)	None	None	0.5	1.2

*Olympus Corp., New Hyde Park, NY   11040.

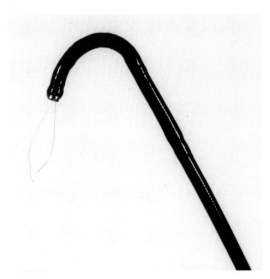

Figure 16-1. *A flat wire snare is protruding from the working channel at the tip of this 3.6-mm ureteropyeloscope, which has been flexed fully at 160 degrees. The snare is closed as it is withdrawn into the channel.*

The larger 3.2- and 3.6-mm instruments are both deflectable and have small working channels, 0.5 mm in diameter in the former and 1.2 mm in the latter. The 1.2-mm channel is adequate for the standard (0.038 in.) guidewire (Fig. 16-1). Neither graspers nor baskets are available in diameters small enough to allow them to fit through this channel. A brush will fit and a sheathless snare can be used through the working channel; in order to close the snare, however, it must be drawn against the tip of the ureteropyeloscope, thereby presenting the risk of damage to the objective lens if a stone is encountered (Figs. 16-1, 16-5).

TECHNIQUES

Retrograde Pyelography. The anatomy of the upper urinary tract should be delineated prior to ureteropyeloscopy. Although an intravenous pyelogram will demonstrate the calyces and ureter in most patients, we prefer a retrograde pyelogram for more accurate definition of the calyces and demonstration of the distensibility and tortuosity of the ureter. The retrograde pyelogram often indicates areas of the ureter that will not distend adequately with irrigation alone. The pyelogram must be available in the operating room to serve as a road map for placement of the ureteropyeloscope. This precaution is even more important with the flexible instrument since the urologist will be attempting to place the tip of the instrument into specific calyces.

Dilation of Orifice. Dilation of the ureteral orifice and intramural ureter is essential for passing the flexible ureteropyeloscope just as it is for the rigid instrument. The same technique for dilation as described in Chapter 15 is employed. After the orifice has been adequately dilated, the technique for passage varies with the instrument used.

Passage Over a Guidewire. The larger (3.6 mm in diameter) ureteropyeloscope can be passed most easily over a guidewire[2]. After the ureteral orifice has been dilated with a cone tip dilator or through one of the other techniques discussed in Chapter 15, a floppy tip guidewire (0.038 in.) is passed through the lumen of the ureter to the renal pelvis. The cystoscope used for placing the guidewire is then removed, leaving the wire in place within the renal pelvis. The flexible ureteropyeloscope is then passed onto the guidewire by placing the wire into the working channel at the tip of the instrument and bringing it out the sidearm near the eyepiece. As the channel is filled with the wire an even higher irrigation pressure is needed. It is helpful to use a pressure bag, as for blood administration, to ensure an adequate flow.

The instrument is then advanced along the guidewire, which is kept taut to prevent coiling of the instrument within the bladder. The landmarks, already inspected with the cystoscope, can be seen and the orifice recognized as the instrument approaches them along the guidewire. Just as the tip enters the ureter, mucosal pressure against the objective lens may cause loss of visibility until the lumen can be distended with irrigating fluid. The field of view, including the lumen and walls of the ureter, as well as the guidewire, can then be appreciated (Fig. 16-2).

The position of the tip of the guidewire lying within the renal pelvis should be rechecked fluoroscopically during passage to ascertain that the wire has not withdrawn into the ureter. The position and progression of the endoscope should also be confirmed fluoroscopically during the procedure to ensure that the instrument does not coil in the bladder despite the presence of the guidewire. Fluoroscopic exposure should be as brief as possible to minimize the radiation dosage to the urologist, patient, and instrument. Radiation adversely affects the fiberglass bundles as well by causing them to discolor.

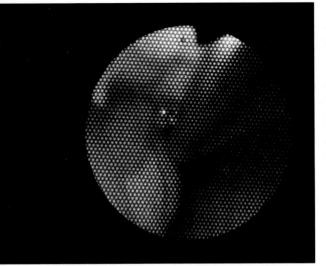

Figure 16-2. *As the flexible ureteropyeloscope is advanced through the ureter, the guidewire and an inflammatory lesion, typical of ureteritis glandularis, are seen.*

If narrowings within the ureter are encountered, it may not be possible to pass them with the instrument. In order to dilate the upper ureter, the flexible instrument must be removed. It can be replaced with the rigid instrument, through which an angioplastic dilating balloon catheter can be passed to the level of the obstruction. Dilation is then accomplished as described in Chapter 15. In order to avoid this exchange of instruments, it may be best to pass the rigid instrument before attempting to pass the flexible endoscope so that any strictures within the ureter can be adequately dilated primarily. Alternatively, after removal of the flexible endoscope, the dilating catheter can be passed over the guidewire and the dilation performed under fluoroscopic control.

As the tip of the instrument advances proximally within the ureter, it is usually not necessary to move the kidney manually to render the ureter accessible since the tip can be deflected as necessary to follow the curvature of the ureter. The maneuverability of the instrument will usually permit the ureteropyeloscope to course posteriorly in the ureter as it lies proximal to the psoas muscle and to course laterally within the kidney (Fig. 16-3).

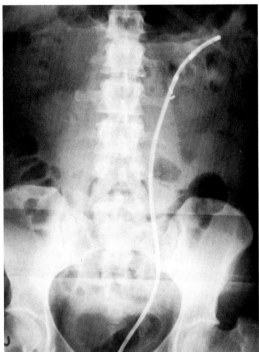

A

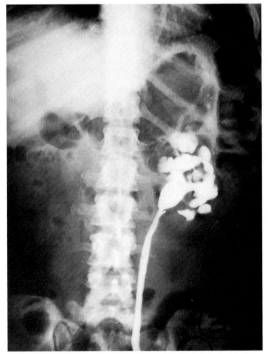

B

Figure 16-3. *A. The flexible ureteropyeloscope (3.6 mm) has been passed to the level of the renal pelvis and is shown with the tip in an anterior upper pole calyx. B. A retrograde pyelogram demonstrates the intrarenal anatomy in the same patient, who had undergone anatrophic nephrolithotomy for staghorn calculi 3 years earlier.*

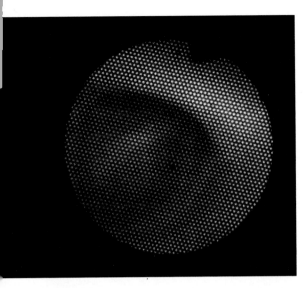

Figure 16-4. *This flattened papilla within a dilated calyx, typical of hydronephrosis and infection from calculi, was found in the patient shown in Fig. 16-3.*

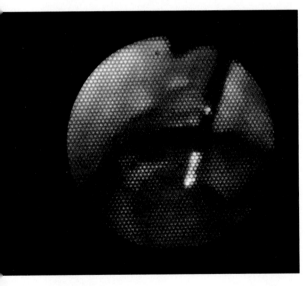

Figure 16-5. *A wire snare appears in the right and midlower field of view in a calyx viewed through the flexible ureteropyeloscope (3.6 mm).*

When the instrument reaches the desired location within the upper urinary tract, the guidewire can be removed and irrigation maintained or a brush or a snare passed through the working channel to sample or grasp objects within the field of view (Figs. 16-4, 16-5). Selective cytologic specimens can also be obtained by irrigating and aspirating through this channel once the suspicious lesion is visualized.

Passage Through a Rigid Endoscope. The smaller instruments can be passed through a rigid endoscope used as a guide tube. The 3.2-mm flexible ureteropyeloscope will pass through a 16 Fr. cystoscope or short ureteroscope (Figs. 16-6, 16-7), and the even smaller 2.7- or 1.8-mm instrument can be combined with the sheath of the rigid ureteropyeloscope, which is used as a guide tube and irrigation sheath. In the latter instance, the flexible ureteropyeloscope functions as a flexible telescope for the rigid instrument and, in addition, can be passed beyond the tip of the rigid sheath and maneuvered through the urinary tract to pass through narrower portions of the ureter and to reach laterally and inferiorly into the renal calyces (Fig. 16-8)[1].

For the guide tube technique, after dilation of the ureteral orifice, the selected rigid instrument is passed through the bladder into the distal ureter to the desired level[2]. The rigid telescope is then removed and the flexible instrument passed through a rubber diaphragm in the rigid sheath to the proximal ureter. Irrigation is maintained through the rigid sheath and drained through it as necessary. The flexible instrument is then passed under direct vision proximally within the ureter and renal pelvis. The tips of the maneuverable (2.7- or 3.2-mm) instruments can be directed into the intrarenal collecting system.

The rigid sheath thus serves as a (1) conduit for entrance of the flexible instrument into the ureteral orifice, (2) sheath for irrigation, and (3) guide to prevent coiling of the flexible instrument in the bladder. The working channel of the rigid instrument remains available for passage of working instruments, and deflectable instruments, which can be passed into the calyces laterally, can be moved into the field of vision of the flexible ureteropyeloscope (Fig. 6-9).

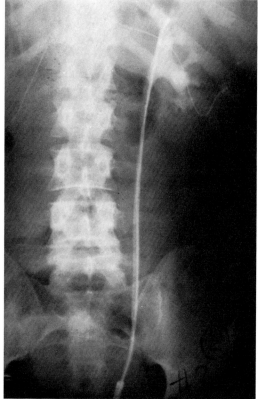

A

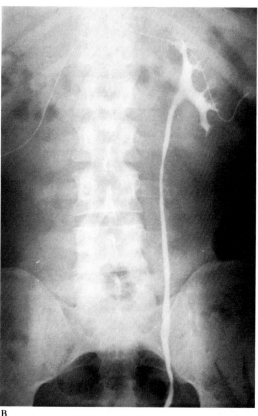

B

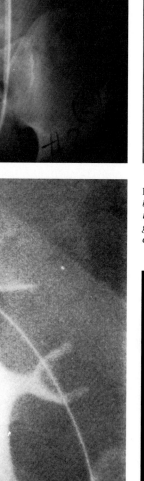

C

Figure 16-6. *A. The ureteropyeloscope (3.2 mm) has been passed through the 16 Fr. ureteroscope and the ureter to a calyx in the upper pole. B, C. A retrograde pyelogram demonstrates irregularity of the papilla within the calyx shown in A, which corresponds to a hemangioma.*

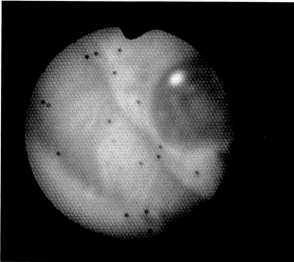

Figure 16-7. *A hemangioma is located at the tip of this papilla in the upper pole of the kidney in the patient shown in Fig. 16-6, who was evaluated for recurrent gross hematuria. The black spots indicate individual broken glass fibers.*

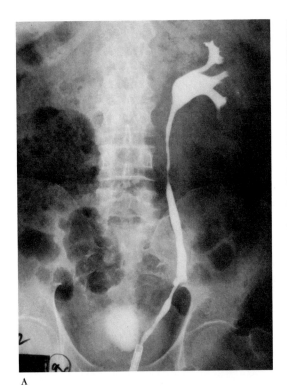

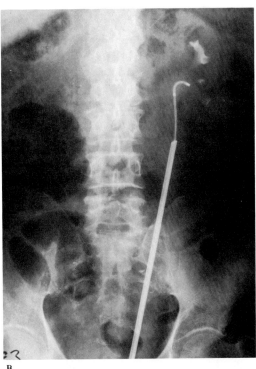

A

B

Figure 16-8. *A. A retrograde pyelogram indicates the anatomy of the upper urinary tract in a patient with narrowing of the proximal ureter. B. The rigid uretero-pyeloscope (12 Fr.) has been passed to the level of narrowing in the ureter, and the flexible ureteropyeloscope (2.7 mm) has been passed through the sheath into the renal pelvis and is within the lower infundibulum. (From D. H. Bagley, J. Huffman, and E. S. Lyon, Combined rigid and flexible ureteropyeloscopy. J. Urol. 130: 243, 1983.)*

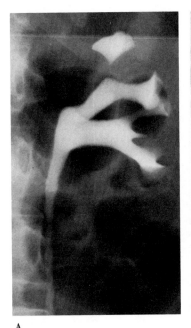

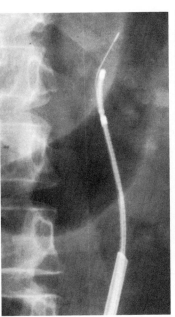

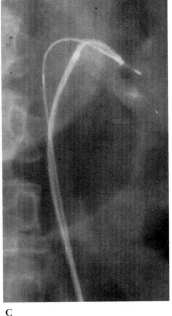

A   B   C

Figure 16-9. *A. A retrograde pyelogram outlines the intrarenal collecting system, demonstrating narrow infundibula. Urinary cytology from this patient had been suspicious for malignancy. B. The lumen of the narrow infundibulum in the upper pole was localized with the 2.7-mm flexible ureteropyeloscope and under direct vision a brush was placed into the infundibulum. C. The narrow infundibulum in the lower pole was similarly localized and brushed. Flexible endoscopes and working instruments can be used in conjunction.*

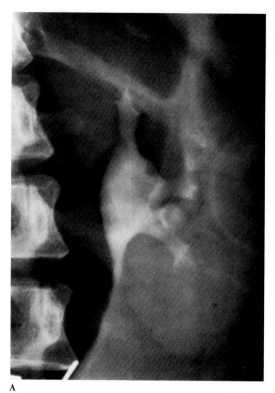

A

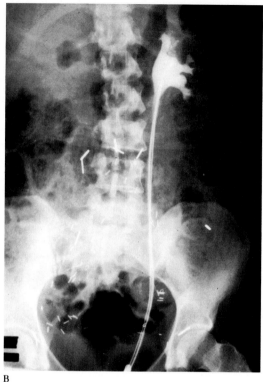

B

Figure 16-10. *A. A filling defect consistent with an aberrant papilla is confirmed by direct endoscopic visualization. B. The 3.2-mm flexible ureteropyeloscope has been passed through a 23 Fr. cystoscope into the ureteral orifice and proximally into the renal pelvis.*

A larger cystoscope that will not pass into the ureter, such as a 23 Fr. instrument, can be placed transurethrally and serve as a guide tube for the 3.2-mm flexible ureteropyeloscope. The flexible instrument can then be passed through this sheath, which is held in position near the dilated orifice so that the flexible instrument can advance directly into the orifice without risk of coiling within the bladder (Fig. 16-10). This is a very cumbersome technique and should be employed only when other more efficient instruments are not available.

Passage Through a Flexible Guide Tube. Flexible guide tubes can also be employed. The technique of Takayasu and Aso[15] was described earlier. More recently, we have employed a flexible Teflon guide tube that is passed over the 12 Fr. flexible ureteral dilator. To introduce this sheath, the ureter is dilated by any of the techniques described above to 14 Fr. and the guidewire left in place. A 12 Fr. flexible dilator with the Teflon guide tube as an outer sheath is then introduced into the ureter to carry the sheath through the intramural portion. The 12 Fr. flexible dilator is then removed, leaving the guide tube or sheath in place passing from the urethra through the bladder into the ureter, thus providing a direct conduit into the ureteral lumen. The 3.2-mm ureteropyeloscope can be passed through this sheath directly into the ureter and advanced directly under vision and fluoroscopic control (Fig. 16-11). The lumen of this guide tube is sufficiently large to allow egress of irrigant and simultaneous passage of a small working instrument alongside the flexible ureteropyeloscope.

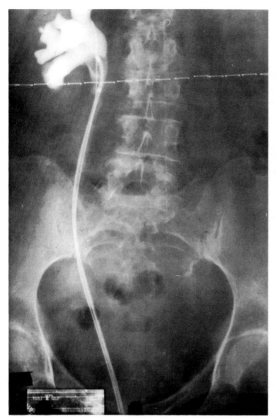

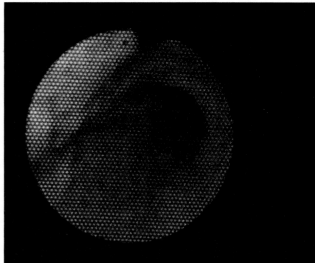

Figure 16-12. *The midureteral lumen is only partially distended with irrigant, and the normal mucosa appears redundant.*

Figure 16-11. *The 3.2-mm ureteropyeloscope has been passed through a flexible guide tube into the renal pelvis in a patient with a papillary renal pelvic tumor. The lesion was biopsied under direct vision. A guidewire is in place through the guide tube alongside the ureteropyeloscope. The metallic densities are staples on the otherwise radiolucent operating table.*

Passage Through a Ureterostomy. In patients with an established cutaneous ureterostomy, a flexible ureteropyeloscope can be passed directly into the ureter if the lumen is adequate to accept the instrument (Fig. 16-12). Since the instrument enters the confined ureteral lumen immediately, it can be advanced manually without concern for its coiling, as may occur during passage through the bladder. The deflectable tip is used as described above to maneuver the instrument through the ureter and to inspect the intrarenal collecting system.

Alternatively, the larger (3.6-mm) ureteropyeloscope can be passed over a guidewire as described above. This technique ensures accurate placement if bleeding obscures the distal lumen as the ureter passes through the abdominal wall, if inflammation of the ureter results from an indwelling stent or catheter, or if the ureter bifurcates (Fig. 16-13). After instrumentation, the guidewire can be used for placement of a stent or catheter to maintain intubation of the ureterostomy.

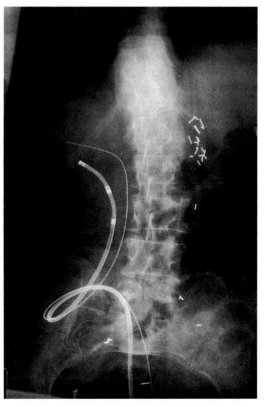

Figure 16-13. *The flexible ureteropyeloscope (3.6 mm) has been placed through a cutaneous ureterostomy into the renal pelvis. A guidewire is located within the other ureteral lumen in the double collecting system (same patient as shown in Fig. 16-12).*

Similar techniques can be used for ureteroscopy through a surgical ureterotomy. Since some bleeding is almost always present in this case, irrigation must be provided. The most efficient and satisfactory technique is to use the larger (3.6-mm) instrument with the irrigation channel. Satisfactory results are often obtained, however, by using one of the smaller instruments while irrigating through a ureteral catheter passed through the same ureterotomy.

Maneuverability Within the Kidney. The flexible ureteropyeloscopes can often be placed into even laterally located calyces and the collecting system of the lower pole. Although their flexibility allows much greater maneuverability than is possible with the rigid instruments, there are many limitations to the placement of the flexible ureteropyeloscopes within the kidney. The instrument cannot pass an infundibulum narrower than the diameter of the instrument itself and, because of the limited irrigation through these instruments, any bleeding will seriously impair the visibility. The same difficulty may occur when using the rigid endoscope sheath as a guide tube since the flow of the irrigant from the tip of the sheath may be at some distance from the tip of the flexible endoscope.

It may be very difficult or even impossible to pass the instrument into an infundibulum in the lower pole. The tip of the instrument can be deflected into the infundibulum to inspect the area, yet it may be impossible to pass the instrument farther into the calyces (see Fig. 16-8). Rather, as the instrument is advanced farther through the ureter, the tip only is withdrawn from the infundibulum. Occasionally, it is possible to pass the angled portion of the tip against the collecting system in the upper pole and deflect the tip farther into the infundibulum of the lower pole. This maneuver is often not possible, in which case inspection is limited to the lower portion of the infundibulum.

It is very helpful to opacify the collecting system by irrigating with a dilute ($\leq 30\%$) solution of radiographic contrast material and to observe the position of the flexible ureteropyeloscope fluoroscopically within the kidney. Orientation, which may be lost by endoscopic vision alone with the flexible instrument, can be confirmed radiographically, and it becomes quite easy to determine the exact location of the instrument within the collecting system.

CARE AFTER URETEROPYELOSCOPY. The same guidelines noted in Chapter 15 are used for urinary diversion after ureteropyeloscopy with the flexible instruments. If there is a threat of ureteral edema because of dilation or mucosal injury, then a ureteral catheter can be placed. If the 3.6-mm instrument has been used and a guidewire is in place, the wire is left after removal of the endoscope and a diversionary ureteral catheter is passed into the renal pelvis and, following removal of the guidewire, left for drainage. If a rigid sheath has been used for passage of the flexible instrument, then a catheter can be placed through the same sheath into the upper collecting system. If the procedure in the ureter has been simple and atraumatic, no ureteral stent is employed.

ROLE OF FLEXIBLE URETEROPYELOSCOPY. In their present state of refinement, flexible ureteropyeloscopes can be used mainly for diagnostic purposes [2]. A greater portion of the intrarenal collecting system can be visualized with these instruments than with the rigid instruments, but working maneuvers are extremely limited because of the size of the working channel. Presently available instruments have considerable limitations, yet in specific circumstances may have particular advantages, unshared by other techniques, that will provide a diagnosis.

Improving technology will undoubtedly result in more useful, flexible ureteropyeloscopes, which should become widely available and useful to the practicing urologist. The development of lasers or flexible ultrasound transducers that can be adapted to the flexible fiberoptic instruments will open new areas in the endoscopic treatment of upper urinary lesions.

REFERENCES

1. Bagley, D. H., Huffman, J., and Lyon, E. S. Combined rigid and flexible ureteropyeloscopy. *J. Urol.* 130:243, 1983.

2. Bagley, D. H., Huffman, J., and Lyon, E. S. Flexible ureteropyeloscopy. In press, 1984.

3. Baird, J. L. British Patent 285,738, February 15, 1928.

4. Curtiss, L. E., Hirschowitz, B. I., and Peters, C. W. A long fiberscope for internal medical examination. *J. Opt. Soc. Am.* 46:1030, 1956.

5. Faber, L. P., Monson, D. D., Amato, J. J., and Jenski, R. J. Flexible fiberoptic bronchoscopy. *Ann. Thorac. Surg.* 16:163, 1973.

6. Gamble, W. J., and Innis, R. F. Experimental intracardiac visualization. *N. Engl. J. Med.* 276:1397, 1967.

7. Greenstone, S. M., Shore, J. M., Heringman, E. C., and Massell, T. B. Arterial endoscopy (arterioscopy). *Arch. Surg.* 93:811, 1966.

8. Hansell, C. W. U.S. Patent 1,751,584, 1930.

9. Hirschowitz, B. I., Curtiss, L. E., Peters, C. W., and Pollard, H. M. Demonstration of a new gastroscope, the "fiberscope." *Gastroenterology* 35:50, 1958.

10. Marshall, V. F. Fiberoptics in urology. *J. Urol.* 91:110, 1964.

11. Shore, J. M., and Lippman, H. N. A flexible choledochoscope. *Lancet* 1:1200, 1965.

12. Silberman, H. D., Wilf, H., and Tucker, J. A. Flexible fiberoptic nasopharyngolaryngoscope. *Ann. Otol. Rhinol. Laryngol.* 85:640, 1976.

13. Takagi, T., Go, T., Takayasu, H., and Aso, Y. A small caliber fiberscope for visualization of the urinary tract, biliary tract and spinal canal. *Surgery* 64:1033, 1968.

14. Takagi, T., Go, T., Takayasu, H., and Aso, Y. Fiberoptic pyeloureteroscope. *Surgery* 70:661, 1971.

15. Takayasu, H., and Aso, Y. Recent development for pyeloureteroscopy: Guide tube method for its introduction into the ureter. *J. Urol.* 112:176, 1974.

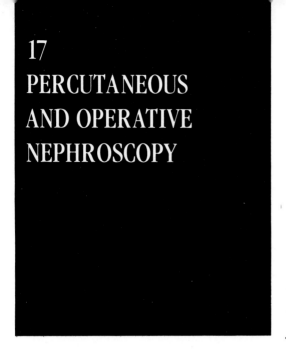

17
PERCUTANEOUS AND OPERATIVE NEPHROSCOPY

Demetrius H. Bagley

Edward S. Lyon

Jeffry L. Huffman

Nephroscopy is a procedure for visualization of the interior of the collecting system of the kidney. Through the advent of techniques of percutaneous nephroscopy, inspection of the intrarenal collecting system has assumed greater importance and wider application. It is a technique that should become available to every urologic endoscopist.

Early reports described endoscopy of the kidney through a nephrostomy tract utilizing a urethroscope for removal of stones[6]. In the 1940s Trattner[9] also reported operative pyeloscopy utilizing a straight nephroscope, which was extremely difficult to maneuver to provide full visualization of the collecting system. Leadbetter[4] reported the design and use of a right-angled nephroscope similar to present-day instruments. The nephroscope was introduced into the kidney through a pyelotomy, and the angle permitted sufficient maneuverability to view most of the calyces.

Development of the Hopkins lens system and fiberoptic light transmission has made possible the manufacture of smaller, angled rigid nephroscopes calibrated less than 15 Fr. with wide viewing angles. Development of glass fiberoptic viewing as well as lighting systems has resulted in flexible fiberoptic nephroscopes, which offer many advantages in maneuverability yet have their own disadvantages[7].

Successful clinical use of any of these instruments demands familiarity with the particular instrument employed, knowledge of the basic techniques of operative nephroscopy, and familiarity with intrarenal anatomy.

INSTRUMENTATION

Rigid Operative Nephroscope. The rigid operative nephroscope is designed with an angled shaft that can be inserted into the kidney through a pyelotomy after the latter has been exposed surgically (Fig. 17-1). The angled portion then can be directed into most of the infundibula. The angulation of the instrument prevents its use percutaneously. Operative nephroscopes are available in two designs from different manufacturers.

The right-angle nephroscope is designed in a 15 Fr. caliber.* The distal portion of the instrument extends 4 cm at a 90-degree angle from the major axis of the instrument. This nephroscope has three channels: (1) a fiberoptic bundle for viewing, (2) a fiberoptic bundle for the light source, and (3) an open channel for irrigation. The working elements attach to the shaft of the instrument and include biopsy forceps, stone forceps, grasping forceps, and a channel for an electrode or flexible instrument.

A rigid operative nephroscope is also available with the distal limb at an angle of 135 degrees from the major axis of the instrument.† Because the distal portion of the tip is only 8 Fr., this nephroscope must be protected with an attached sheath when in use. An 11 Fr. examining attachment, which permits inspection and irrigation but has no working channel, is available, as is a 15 Fr. attachable working sheath, which has a working channel of 5 Fr. to accept flexible instruments. Rigid biopsy and stone forceps can also be obtained.

*Karl Storz Endoscopy-America, Inc., Culver City, CA 90230.

†Wolf Medical Instruments, Rosemont, IL 60018.

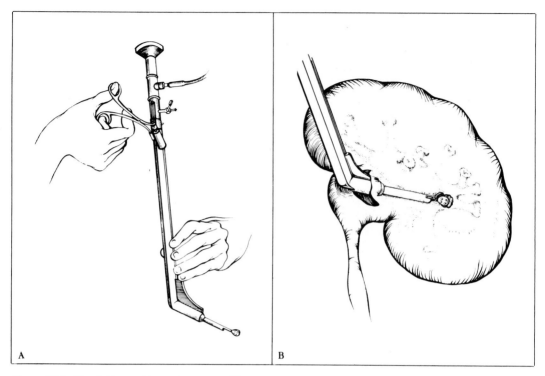

Figure 17-1. *The rigid operative nephroscope with attached stone forceps (A) has been introduced into the collecting system through a pyelotomy (B).*

Rigid Percutaneous Nephroscope. Rigid percutaneous nephroscopes possess specific features of design that make them uniquely useful for percutaneous insertion, manipulation, and stone removal (Fig. 17-2). The major axis of the instrument is straight and the working channel passes directly through the shaft of the instrument. The telescope and viewing channel, however, are offset with two 90-degree angles. Thus, the operator's viewing eye is moved away from the central axis of the instrument. The sheath of the nephroscope has a diameter of 8 mm (24 Fr.) and a removable obturator with a central channel that will accept a guidewire. The telescope has fiberoptic illumination and a rigid lens system including prisms to deflect the eyepiece from the central working channel of the instrument. The working channel passes directly through the sheath and the channel of the telescope to provide a straight lumen that will accept the rigid ultrasound probe. Irrigant can flow through the working channel into the field of view and then drain through the outer sheath of the nephroscope. Thus, continuous flow of irrigant is provided.

Each major manufacturer now makes percutaneous nephroscopes that are basically similar.

Numerous working instruments are available, both in rigid and flexible designs, which can be passed through the working channel to retrieve calculi or fragments or to be used for other intrarenal procedures. Since a relatively large lumen is available, these instruments include three-pronged grasping forceps, alligator forceps, baskets, and snares.

Ultrasonic Lithotrite. The ultrasonic lithotrite has proved to be the key to successful percutaneous removal of large renal calculi. In general, calculi are fragmented through contact with a metal probe, which is set to high-frequency vibrations with an ultrasonic transducer. Piezoceramic elements are powered by an external generator to vibrate at a frequency of 20 to 27 kHz. These ultrasonic vibrations are carried along a hollow steel tube, and thus converted into longitudinal and transverse vibrations (Fig. 17-2). The device impacts on the crystalline structure of the stone, fracturing the crystal lattice. It has been postulated that cavitation at the tip of the probe results in fragmentation of the calculus; nevertheless, immediate, firm contact between the probe and the stone is necessary for fragmentation. The ultrasound probe has also been termed a *transducer, sonotrode,* or *wand.*

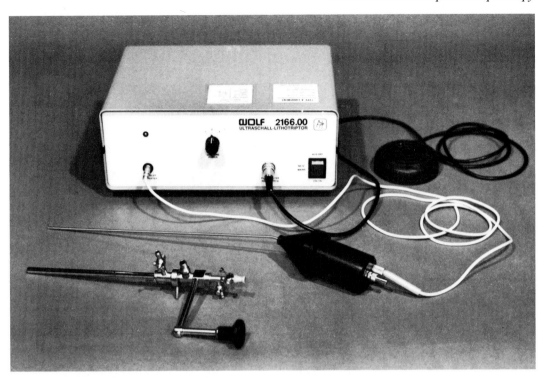

Figure 17-2. *The rigid percutaneous nephroscope in the foreground has an offset lens and a straight working channel through the instrument. The ultrasound probe, which is connected to the generator, will fit through the straight channel. The lumen of the probe can be connected to suction to remove fragments of stone. The generator can be set at three levels of intensity, and its activation is controlled by a foot switch.*

The lumen of the metal tip of the probe is hollow in order that suction can be applied through it. In this way, irrigant for cooling is drawn through the transducer and fragments are simultaneously aspirated. Marberger[17] has documented that an irrigation rate of 30 ml per minute results in a maximal temperature increase at the tip of the probe of 1.4°C.

Just as with electrohydraulic lithotripsy (see Chap. 12), different calculi may vary in their resistance to fragmentation with the ultrasonic lithotrite. Round stones with dense, smooth surfaces are usually much more difficult to fragment than irregular, spiculated calculi. Often the inner layers are easier to fragment than the outer surfaces. More time is required to fragment larger and harder stones.

Flexible Fiberoptic Nephroscope. A fiberoptic nephroscope offers the advantage of increased maneuverability. Since the instrument is flexible, it is less traumatic and can enter many portions of the intrarenal collecting system that are inaccessible to a rigid instrument. These instruments are available from several manufacturers in basically similar designs. With a caliber of approximately 15 Fr., each fiberoptic nephroscope has a long (20–30 cm) flexible segment and a tip that can be deflected by a thumb control mounted on the control unit near the eyepiece. The cylindrical shaft of this unit contains a fiberoptic viewing bundle, a fiberoptic light transmission bundle, and a single channel (5–6 Fr.), which can be used for working instruments and irrigation (Fig. 17-3). When an instrument is in the channel, the tip may not attain full deflection. It may then be necessary to increase the pressure of the irrigant to force the fluid through the channel alongside the instrument. A blood transfusion pressure pump can be placed on the bag of irrigant, but the pressure should never exceed 150 mm Hg. When pressure irrigation is used, special care should be taken to be certain that there is a low pressure outflow either alongside the instrument in the nephrostomy tract or pyelostomy or distally through the ureter.

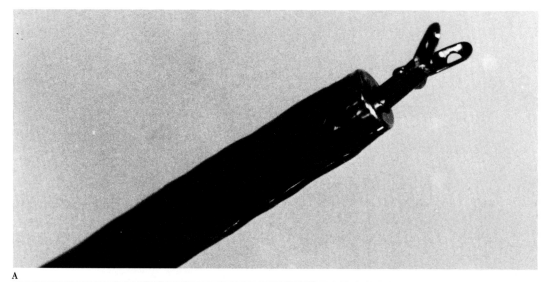

A

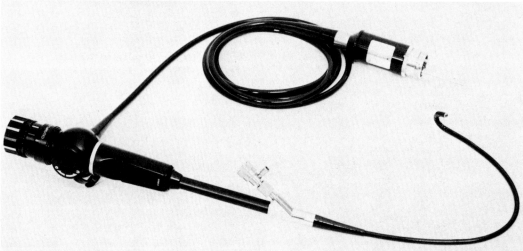

B

Figure 17-3. *A. A biopsy forceps is protruding from the working channel of the Olympus flexible nephroscope. The same channel is used for irrigation, which is partially impeded when an instrument is in place. B. The tip of the Olympus flexible nephroscope is fully angulated. The working channel and connecting light bundle are shown.*

The fiberoptic viewing bundle gives a satisfactory view in which the individual fibers are seen and resolution is thereby limited (Fig. 17-4). After extended exposure to X-ray irradiation, glass fibers become discolored wih a yellowish cast[15].

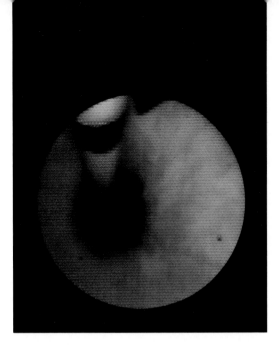

Figure 17-4. *A ureteral catheter enters the renal pelvis at the ureteropelvic junction and provides a recognizable landmark in this flexible nephroscopic view.*

It may be difficult to maintain orientation when working with the flexible instrument. It is relatively easy to know exactly where the tip of a rigid angled nephroscope is directed, but the tip of the flexible instrument can be deflected actively in two directions and, because it is flexible, can be deflected by the renal tissue in any direction. The operator should be thoroughly familiar with the instrument and able to recall readily the direction of deflection obtained with the control. A more accurate orientation can be gained by using a fluoroscopic unit to visualize the instrument within the kidney. This is particularly useful for percutaneous nephroscopy. A ureteral catheter entering the renal pelvis from the ureter can serve as a reliable landmark for orientation (Fig. 17-4).

Since the shaft of the instrument is flexible, it cannot be maneuvered by holding just the control unit. The second hand must be placed on the shaft of the instrument near its insertion into the kidney or the nephrostomy tract to provide rigidity at that point and to move the instrument. Simply maneuvering the flexible nephroscope, therefore, usually requires the operator's two hands. An assistant may be necessary to place any working instruments through the channel and to maneuver those instruments. It is helpful to have an assistant's viewing attachment so that the assistant will have the same endoscopic view as the operator and will be able to use working instruments with visual control.

LEARNING THE TECHNIQUE. Since many urologists have had either no or relatively rare experience with nephroscopy, practice in a nonpatient setting is important in order to master and perfect the techniques[10]. We prefer to instruct residents and to practice with the instruments in cadaveric kidneys. The greatest value is gained from this exercise when a pyelogram of the kidney with contrast injected into the collecting system is taken. Views should be obtained of both the anteroposterior and oblique positions to determine the number and location of the calyces. A pyelotomy is made and stay sutures placed on either side (as described in the following section, Operative Nephroscopy) to permit retraction and partial closure of the pyelostomy once the nephroscope has been placed into the collecting system. After inspecting the pelvis, the operator proceeds to place the nephroscope into a major infundibulum, preferably at one of the poles of the kidney. The operator then inspects the calyces sequentially, using the radiograms to ensure that each calyx has been inspected. The nephroscope is removed to the next infundibulum and, similarly, the calyces are inspected. In this way, the nephroscopist should progress systematically to inspect each calyx in the kidney.

As a second exercise, the first operator may place a stone into a calyx with the nephroscope and remove the instrument. The second operator is then allowed the task of finding the stone with the nephroscope. Although greater maneuverability is possible with the cadaveric kidney and there is no bleeding, the experience gained in inspecting each calyx and finding stones will be of value in the clinical setting.

The instrumentation employed in this exercise is the same as that used for clinical nephroscopy. Both the rigid and the flexible nephroscopes should be employed. The rigid instrument is first used with only the inspection sheath; after the stone has been found and the calyx identified, the stone forceps may also be attached and the calyx again localized. Although there is some risk of being unable to find the offending calyx on the second attempt, the risk of either not entering the appropriate infundibulum or damaging it with the stone forceps in place during the inspection phase may be greater.

For these exercises, irrigation is necessary but sterility is not essential. Therefore, an empty bag from the cystoscopy suite may be filled with tap water to be used for irrigation.

OPERATIVE NEPHROSCOPY. Intraoperative inspection of the intrarenal collecting system is performed with the operative nephroscope. Either the rigid angled instrument or the flexible endoscope may be employed[1,5]. The kidney must be surgically exposed and should be fully mobilized to achieve the best results with nephroscopy. In some patients who have had previous surgical procedures, it may be extremely difficult to mobilize the kidney fully; nephroscopy may then be performed after exposing only the renal pelvis. After the pelvis has been exposed, a simple pyelotomy is made. We prefer to place stay sutures prior to opening the pelvis and to make the pyelotomy in a gentle U shape extending toward the infundibula so that any tear of the pyelotomy will extend along the infundibula rather than into the ureteropelvic junction, as would occur with a linear pyelotomy (see Fig. 17-1). The stay sutures can be used both to retract the pyelotomy to permit introduction of the instrument or removal of calculi and to provide a means for partial reclosure of the pyelotomy during nephroscopy. Closure of the pyelotomy allows retention of enough irrigation fluid within the kidney to distend the collecting system slightly. Any stones clearly evident within the pelvis should be removed if possible. Immediately at this point, before any further trauma to the collecting system and before any bleeding occurs, the nephroscope should be introduced.

The nephroscope itself, the light source, and the irrigation fluid should be prepared by the nursing staff in the operating room prior to initiation of the procedure. Only sterile irrigation fluid suitable for intravenous administration can be employed. We use physiologic saline at body temperature since there is a possibility of absorption of the fluid from either the kidney or the wound.

The tip of the nephroscope is introduced through the pyelotomy with the irrigation flowing to avoid bubbles. An assistant must provide suction in the wound to remove irrigation fluid flowing from the renal pelvis and to prevent irrigant overflow from the open wound. Systematic inspection of the collecting system is then begun. The pattern of inspection should be individualized on the basis of the patient's disease. The technique in patients with a single renal or "staghorn" calculus may differ from that used in patients with a filling defect or hematuria. When nephroscopy is being performed for nephrolithotomy, it is essential to have available a radiogram indicating the expected position of the stone.

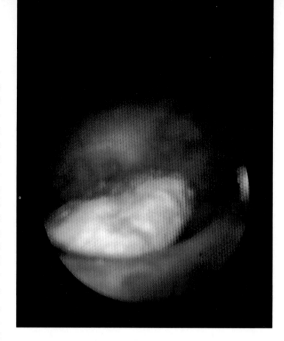

Figure 17-5. *A solitary struvite calculus is located in a dilated calyx adjacent to a papilla. There is moderate mucosal edema (flexible percutaneous nephroscopic view).*

After the ureter has been partially occluded with a retracting loop to prevent distal migration of calculi, we prefer to examine the entire renal pelvis to the level of the ureteropelvic junction nephroscopically. Attention is then turned to the infundibulum thought to contain the stone, as indicated on the preoperative studies. If the position of the stone is unknown, as may happen when the position has changed, then all the infundibula must be examined, if possible. We prefer to approach the examination systematically, proceeding from the infundibulum to either the upper or lower pole of the kidney and continuing sequentially through the remainder of the collecting system. The pyelogram must be available in the operating room as a road map to allow the nephroscopist to determine the number of calyces and the location of each infundibulum. As the instrument is introduced through the infundibulum, each calyx must be inspected to avoid missing any calculi and to provide orientation (Fig. 17-5).

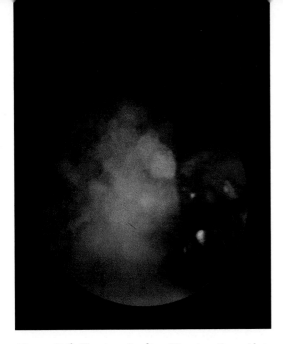

Figure 17-6. *The stone forceps of the operative nephroscope is located adjacent to a calculus, which can be grasped and removed.*

When the infundibulum containing the calculus has been located, the rigid instrument may be removed from the kidney to attach the stone forceps. The entire instrument may then be replaced into the kidney and into the infundibulum containing the stone. A working instrument may be passed through the channel of the flexible nephroscope. When the position of the calculus is known from the radiogram, the nephroscope may be introduced initially with the stone forceps in place. The combined size of the nephroscope with the attached stone forceps may be too large, however, to enter many of the infundibula and, therefore, the inspecting sheath alone is usually preferred for initial examination of the entire kidney. If the calculus is of appropriate size, it can be grasped and removed through the infundibulum and pyelotomy with the stone forceps (Fig. 17-6).[3]. If the calculus is too large to pass through the infundibulum, its location can be determined by light passing from the nephroscope through the parenchyma of the kidney. A nephrotomy is then made over the calyx localized by the nephroscope, and the calculus is removed. In some cases, this procedure can be observed through the nephroscope, which remains in place within the kidney.

An attempt should be made to inspect the entire kidney prior to performing nephrotomy since the bleeding resulting from that procedure will obscure vision and prevent completion of inspection of the collecting system. Gittes[1] has indicated that the most commonly overlooked calyx is located in the posterior midportion of the kidney, the area closest to the surgeon who is approaching the kidney through a posterior pyelotomy. The kidney should be rolled anteriorly and the nephroscope withdrawn partially to inspect the posterior wall of the intrarenal pelvis in order to find the infundibulum.

In surgery for staghorn calculi, nephroscopy may be a valuable adjunct. After the major portion of the calculus has been removed by pyelotomy or extended pyelotomy by the Gil-Vernet approach, the nephroscope can be introduced to detect any additional fragments invisible on radiogram, such as minute stone fragments and proteinaceous matrix material. This material can be removed with the stone forceps or by irrigation. Some authors have employed a pulsatile irrigation jet to improve removal of fragments from the kidney. When an anatrophic nephrotomy is performed, the infundibula are open and the calyces can be seen directly. The nephroscope is not usually necessary in these cases. In some kidneys with long upper or lower pole infundibula, however, the incision may not extend into the calyces, and the nephroscope can be used to inspect within that portion of the collecting system.

All patients treated surgically for stone disease should have intraoperative radiographs of the kidney taken prior to completion of the procedure[11]. Since portions of the collecting system may be overlooked and others may be inaccessible to the nephroscope, the operator can never be certain that residual stones or fragments have not been overlooked by nephroscopy. The radiogram is a more sensitive indicator. It can provide total visualization of the kidney and help localize residual calculi.

PERCUTANEOUS NEPHROSCOPY. Techniques of percutaneous nephrostomy and percutaneous endoscopy have radically changed the approach to urinary calculi, as well as drastically altered the morbidity of pyelolithotomy. Although a detailed treatise on the techniques of catheter placement is beyond the scope of this manual, a general description of the techniques should be known to all urologists. In addition, percutaneous instrumentation can become as familiar as transurethral endoscopy and should be available in the urologist's armamentarium.

Preparation of the Patient. The patient must be informed of the technique, the risks, and the alternative techniques. We attempt to stress to the patient that, although the plan will be to avoid open surgery by the percutaneous procedure, an open surgical procedure may become necessary. We also emphasize that long-term follow-up of patients treated by these techniques is limited. It is also valuable in the preoperative period to stress to the patient the need, when it is indicated, for full metabolic evaluation.

The anatomy of the intrarenal collecting system, particularly that portion containing the calculus, must be thoroughly defined prior to placement of a nephrostomy or even consideration for percutaneous lithotomy. The location and potential movement of the calculus should be considered. The best approach can then be planned to place the nephrostomy tract directly to the calculus. The possibility of the calculus changing location will also determine to some extent the positioning of the patient and the need for catheters to obstruct the ureter or infundibula.

The patient is positioned so that the nephrostomy site is available to the surgeon; usually the prone position is necessary. When under general anesthesia, the patient must be sufficiently padded and supported to provide room for respiratory excursion of the chest. If local anesthesia is used, there must be sufficient padding for the patient's comfort. A drainage catheter should be passed into the bladder prior to the procedure to allow drainage of urine and irrigant passing to the bladder during the procedure.

We have routinely treated patients with antibiotics preoperatively. If the urine culture is positive or the stone is of infectious origin, the antibiotic should be continued for at least 24 hours prior to manipulation. In other patients we start an antibiotic parenterally immediately before manipulation and continue it for 24 hours or less.

Anesthesia. Percutaneous nephrolithotomy has been performed under local, epidural, and general anesthesia (see Chap. 20). All forms provide adequate anesthesia and the choice must be guided by both the surgeon's experience and the preference of the individual patient. Since many of these procedures require several steps, there is some advantage in avoiding general anesthesia. The patient is in the prone position for the procedure, so there is also some risk of dislodging the endotracheal tube when moving the patient; in addition, it may be difficult to ventilate the patient. On the other hand, general anesthesia provides the best muscular relaxation and will allow greater manipulation of the rigid nephroscope to reach into upper or lower calyces or into the ureter for stone fragments.

Adequate local anesthesia can be obtained with several agents injected both in the skin and along the tract. Care should be taken to ensure thorough infiltration of the fascia and particularly of the renal capsule. The patient under local anesthesia may have some discomfort during intrarenal manipulation and distention of the pelvis with irrigant. Different types of anesthesia can be employed for different portions of the procedure.

TECHNIQUES

Nephroscopic Access

OPERATIVE NEPHROSTOMY. Access can be gained to the upper urinary tract by way of a nephrostomy tract, which has been placed either surgically or by percutaneous techniques. The first nephroscopy reported was performed through a preexisting nephrostomy tract. When a nephrostomy tube is placed surgically and there is some consideration for subsequent endoscopic manipulation or inspection of the collecting system, an attempt should be made to place the nephrostomy catheter in a straight tract rather than a sharply angulated one, which might be difficult to traverse with a rigid endoscope postoperatively. In addition, a sufficiently large catheter should be used to maintain a tract adequate for endoscopy. The catheter should be of size 18 to 20 Fr. or larger to allow passage of a rigid nephroscope with little or no dilation. An open-end catheter, such as a Council catheter or a Foley catheter with the tip punctured or cut off, should be used to allow passage of a wire when the catheter is removed. The wire can then serve as a guide for placement of another catheter or the endoscope.

PERCUTANEOUS NEPHROSTOMY. Percutaneous nephrostomy was described as early as 1955[14]. It has only more recently been accepted as a safe, easy access to the upper urinary collecting system[19]. In general, a needle is first placed into the intrarenal collecting system through which a guidewire can be passed down the ureter to remain and to direct dilators into the kidney. A catheter can then be passed over the wire to drain the intrarenal collecting system and provide access.

The kidney and intrarenal collecting system can be located with ultrasound or fluoroscopy, or both. Ultrasound will accurately locate the kidney and collecting system as well as calculi. It minimizes radiation exposure but may not accurately indicate the configuration of the intrarenal collecting system. Fluoroscopy can be used to locate the calyces and renal pelvis after administration of contrast excreted within the urine. Although fluoroscopy then gives only a two-dimensional representation of the kidney, a third dimension can be indicated by changing the plane of the patient relative to the fluoroscope. A fine needle can be introduced directly into the intrarenal collecting system to aspirate urine and inject contrast directly into the collecting system to provide radiographic opacification. A combination of ultrasonic guidance for the initial location and puncture of the kidney followed by injection of contrast and fluoroscopic guidance has proved very satisfactory.

After the intrarenal collecting system has been entered, a guidewire must be passed to maintain access. Various techniques are available, such as placement of a second larger needle that will accept a guidewire or advancement of a sheath of the needle if a coaxial arrangement has been used. The guidewire should be advanced down the ureter as far as possible to provide excess wire within the collecting system and ensure stability.

Dilation can then be started with passage of 6 or 8 Fr. fascial dilators and continued to 8 to 12 Fr. The dilation must be performed under fluoroscopic guidance to determine the placement of the dilators and indicate their position within the renal pelvis in order to avoid perforation of the pelvis or disruption of the ureteropelvic junction. If further dilation is desired at that time, then a second guidewire should be passed to provide both a working and a safety guidewire within the renal collecting system. The safety, or reserve, guidewire is clamped to the side of the working area and remains only to serve as a secondary safety wire in case the working wire is inadvertently removed from the kidney. Dilation can then be continued over the working wire with fascial dilators of increasing size or a dilating balloon. Although it may not be necessary to dilate the tract to a size larger than 26 Fr. when using the rigid percutaneous nephroscope, which has a caliber of 24 Fr., dilation to larger sizes may be indicated when use of a larger sheath is anticipated.

The entire nephrostomy and dilation can be accomplished with local anesthesia and sedation; alternatively, some choose to use local anesthesia when placing a nephrostomy catheter and to complete the dilation with a general anesthesia. Nephrostomy and dilation can be performed on the same day as nephroscopy and stone manipulation or precede the latter by some hours or days. There is always some acute intrarenal bleeding, which may obscure visualization of small calculi. Placement of the nephrostomy tube and subsequent endoscopy several hours or a few days later will allow establishment of fibrosis of the nephrostomy tract and provide a field relatively clear of clots and active bleeding. Any leakage of the irrigant or contrast will then usually be confined to the tract unless there is perforation of the collecting system.

Perforation of the pelvis during nephrostomy or dilation usually heals readily within 1 to 2 days without serious sequelae if the urinary collecting system is adequately drained. In cases of perforation we choose not to proceed with stone manipulation or endoscopy acutely because of the possibility of leakage of large volumes of irrigant into the retroperitoneum. Stone manipulation can be undertaken as a second procedure after allowing a few days for the perforation to seal.

After the tract has been dilated, an open-end catheter is placed to drain the collecting system, tamponade the bleeding, and maintain the percutaneous tract. We prefer a catheter of size 18 to 20 Fr. or larger to maintain the tract at its dilated diameter. The catheter is placed over a guidewire into the intrarenal collecting system, and its position is confirmed radiographically. Contrast injected through the catheter should fill and empty from all calyces. The tube can be secured to the skin with sutures. Inflation of the retaining balloon will help maintain the position but may obstruct a portion of the collecting system.

Introduction of the Nephroscope. Endoscopic inspection of the renal collecting system can be performed through a percutaneous nephrostomy tract with the rigid or flexible nephroscope or some other instrument that will pass through the tract, such as a panendoscope or urethroscope. Instruments without prominent beaks will pass through the tract most readily.

In order to pass the endoscope through the nephrostomy tract into the kidney, the nephrostomy catheter must first be removed. A flexible tip angiographic guidewire should be passed through the catheter into the urinary collecting system before the catheter is removed. This wire will provide access into the kidney if the tract becomes interrupted, if the endoscope is inadvertently dislodged from the kidney, or if bleeding obscures the lumen of the tract. Two guidewires should be placed so that one can be held in reserve as a safety guidewire while the other is used as the working guidewire. This step is essential if the tract must be dilated further or the nephroscope passed. In order to pass the rigid nephroscope, which has a caliber of 24 Fr., the tract should be at least 22 Fr. in size or should be dilated as necessary.

The nephroscope can be passed over the working guidewire along the tract into the kidney. The sheath of the rigid nephroscope with the obturator in place is placed over the working wire and passed into the tract and into the renal pelvis. This maneuver should be observed under the fluoroscope to be certain of the position of the instrument. As the tip enters the renal pelvis, the obturator can be removed. The guidewire can be removed as well, but if the position of the instrument is at all questionable, then it is safer to leave the wire in place and pass it through the working channel of the operative nephroscope as it is inserted into the sheath. The renal pelvis can then be inspected directly through the endoscope and the final position determined.

The working guidewire can subsequently be removed but the safety wire should be held in reserve in its position along the nephrostomy tract but outside the sheath of the nephroscope. It must extend into the renal collecting system, preferably into the bladder or distal ureter.

It is usually difficult to place the rigid percutaneous nephroscope under direct vision through the percutaneous tract because of the configuration of the tip. Because there is no beak or rounding of the end of the sheath to allow atraumatic passage, placement over a guidewire with the obturator is preferred. Another endoscope, such as a urethroscope or a panendoscope, usually has a less traumatic tip and can be passed under direct vision. Neither of these two instruments should be passed in a blind fashion with only tactile control since both can easily perforate the wall of even a well-established tract. Either visual or fluoroscopic control should be used.

The flexible nephroscope can also be passed over a guidewire into the kidney. The working guidewire, which has been previously placed into the kidney, is inserted into the working channel at the tip of the nephroscope, and the instrument is passed along this wire through the tract and into the kidney. This passage can be followed fluoroscopically or under direct vision through the instrument.

Alternatively, in a tract that is well established and has a size greater than 15 Fr., the flexible instrument can be passed under direct vision to follow the guidewire along the tract and into the kidney. When passing the instrument under direct vision, the well-established tract forms a firm cylindrical lumen, which may change in appearance to a darker, more vascular bed as the nephroscope passes into the kidney. The urothelium is then recognized as the collecting system is entered. It may appear essentially normal or, more frequently, inflamed, erythematous, and edematous. It is very difficult and possibly dangerous to attempt to pass the instrument under direct vision alone in a new or recently dilated tract. The lumen may be obscured by blood and there is the risk of leakage of irrigant into the retroperitoneal tissues since the tract has not yet formed a seal along the surface of the lumen. In a fresh tract we prefer to pass the flexible nephroscope through a working sheath.

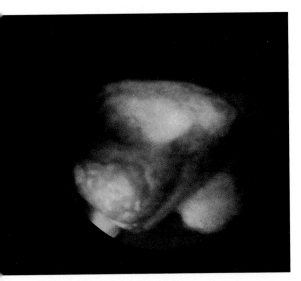

Figure 17-7. *A struvite calculus is located in the renal pelvis (rigid percutaneous nephroscopic view).*

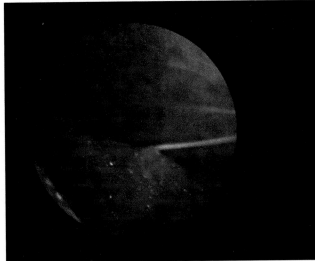

Figure 17-9. *The nephroscope has been dislodged from the renal collecting system and renal parenchyma, and shows perirenal adipose and connective tissue. The characteristic glistening surface of the fatty tissue and the bands of connective tissue are never seen within the lumen of the urinary collecting system.*

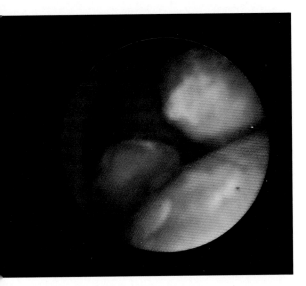

Figure 17-8. *Three struvite (magnesium ammonium phosphate) calculi are located within a dilated calyx and are viewed with a flexible nephroscope placed through a percutaneous nephrostomy tract.*

Inspection of the Intrarenal Collecting System. The accessible portion of the intrarenal collecting system should be inspected as the endoscope enters the kidney. Any calculi, infundibula, or ureter through which calculi or fragments may pass should be located (Figs. 17-7, 17-8). The safety guidewire can be located and followed through the renal pelvis and into the ureter. Treatment of calculi should be started as early as possible after identification of the dangerous areas within the collecting system. If the nephroscope is withdrawn from the kidney into the perinephric tissue, the characteristic fibrous bands and glistening fat can be recognized (Fig. 17-9).

The unoperated kidney is remarkably mobile. The rigid nephroscope will usually pass into infundibula located more than 90 degrees from the nephrostomy tract. Many other calyces can be entered by passing the flexible nephroscope through either the rigid sheath or the percutaneous tract alone. Calculi in these locations can then be grasped or fragmented with the electrohydraulic lithotriptor. It is often more difficult with the flexible instrument, which has a much smaller working channel, limited irrigation capacity, and the limitations as well as the advantages of flexibility.

Table 17-1. Complications of Percutaneous Nephrolithotomy

Series	Year	Patients (total no.)	Complication (no. patients)				
			Inadequate Nephrostomy Tract	Sepsis	Hemorrhage	Residual Calculi	Operation Required
Alken et al. [12]	1981	19	0	0	2	1	0
Wickham et al. [21]	1983	50	8	3	4	12	11
Segura et al. [20]	1983	194	13	1	2	6*	10
Marberger et al. [17]	1983	84	8	NS	3	9	9

*After repeated therapy.
NS = not stated.

Percutaneous Lithotripsy. The techniques of percutaneous nephrostomy and nephroscopy have been combined with the endoscopic fragmentation of stones to alter the treatment of upper urinary calculi radically. Calculi small enough to be trapped in a stone basket or grasper and withdrawn through the nephrostomy tract can be removed intact. The average or moderate size (1–3 cm in diameter) calculus can be fragmented entirely with the ultrasonic lithotriptor. Larger calculi up to and including massive staghorn calculi can be disintegrated and removed in several pieces [13]. Both the ultrasonic and the electrohydraulic lithotriptors have been used in individually selected cases for fragmentation of renal calculi.

In 1975, Raney and Handler [18] reported the fragmentation and removal of renal calculi with the electrohydraulic lithotriptor and a cystoscope passed through a nephrostomy tract. In 1977, Kurth, Hohenfellner, and Altwein [16] reported the removal of a staghorn calculus from a solitary kidney using an ultrasonic lithotriptor inserted through a preexisting nephrostomy tract. Alken's group [12] described the use of this approach with a percutaneous nephrostomy tract. More recently, several series of percutaneous nephrolithotomy have been reported (Table 17-1).

Calculi must first be located with the rigid nephroscope and then disintegrated. The ultrasonic probe is passed through the working channel of the operative percutaneous nephroscope and advanced to touch the calculus under direct vision. Suction is applied from a standard surgical aspirator pump to the sonotrode to remove fragments during disintegration of the calculus and to cool the instrument. The probe is then applied to the stone to fragment and disintegrate it. A small stone can often be broken into a few fragments, which can be removed through the working sheath with the grasping forceps. It is often easier to grasp smaller fragments that will fit through the sheath than to fragment them further with the sonotrode. This method also minimizes the chance of losing fragments to calyces or the ureter.

Fragmentation is begun by applying the tip of the sonotrode to the calculus with simultaneous irrigation through the instrument and suction through the lumen of the sonotrode (Fig. 17-10). The tip is thus tightly applied to the calculus. If possible, an irregular point in the surface of the stone should be chosen for fragmentation. As holes are drilled into a soft calculus by the sonotrode, fragmentation may occur early, or it may be necessary to place several holes into the calculus at different angles to break it. It is advantageous when possible to apply the sonotrode to several peripheral areas of the stone to reduce the size rather than to fragment it.

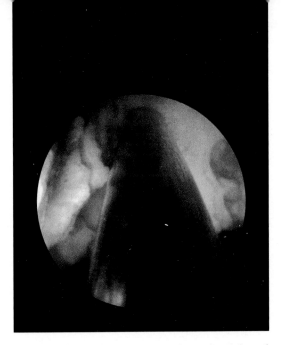

Figure 17-10. *The ultrasonic transducer placed through the rigid nephroscope enters the center of the field and is applied to the calculus. Partial disintegration of the calculus leaves the defects demonstrated superiorly and inferiorly.*

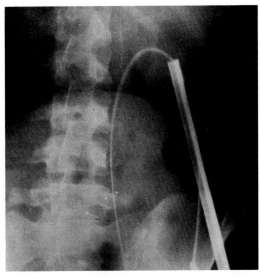

Figure 17-11. *A radiogram made after ultrasonic removal of a renal calculus demonstrates the absence of residual fragments. The rigid nephroscope, ultrasonic probe, and safety guidewire are present.*

The ureter can be secured further from migrating fragments by filling the lumen with an instrument. The wire passing into the ureter affords minimal obstruction against migratory fragments. Occasionally the percutaneous tract is large enough to allow passage of an open-end catheter over the safety guidewire, but more often it will not accept both the sheath and a catheter. Therefore, a ureteral catheter should be passed in a retrograde fashion. Even with a patient in the prone position, a flexible nephroscope can be passed transurethrally into the bladder to function as a flexible cystoscope. As the ureteral orifice is visualized, a guidewire can be passed into the orifice and proximally within the ureter and left in place as the instrument is removed. An open-end ureteral catheter can then be passed over the guidewire into the ureter under fluoroscopic control. This catheter will serve to obstruct the lumen and prevent migration of fragments into the ureter. A balloon catheter can be used to obstruct the lumen most securely. It can be passed in an antegrade or retrograde fashion.

When the calculi have been removed, as determined by visual endoscopic inspection and fluoroscopy, a plain radiogram of the renal area is taken to identify any residual fragments (Fig. 17-11). If all of the pieces have been removed, then a guidewire is replaced through the nephroscope into the collecting system, preferably into the ureter. The nephroscope is removed, leaving the guidewire in place, and a nephrostomy catheter is subsequently passed over the guidewire. The position is determined fluoroscopically. The final view is taken with contrast placed through the nephrostomy tube to be certain that the tube drains all portions of the kidney. The tube is then sutured to the skin and left in place for an additional 24 or 48 hours or until hematuria clears. Another plain radiogram or tomogram of the abdomen should be taken to detect any residual fragments.

We also prefer to inspect the intrarenal collecting system with a flexible nephroscope at the time of nephrostomy tube removal. Often very small (<1 mm in diameter) fragments can be detected at this point, although they are not seen radiographically. These can usually be removed from the collecting system with wire grasping forceps or flushed from the pelvis with irrigation fluid. This procedure can be performed without any anesthesia in an outpatient setting and allows one to be certain of complete stone removal.

Electrohydraulic Lithotripsy. The technique for electrohydraulic lithotripsy within the intrarenal collecting system is similar to that used for bladder calculi. The electrohydraulic lithotriptor probe is passed through the instrument and the tip placed near the calculus. It should not be in direct contact with the calculus. The instrument is then activated and the spark applied repetitively as necessary to fragment the calculus. The instrument should be placed in a low power setting, which is increased until a spark develops.

There are several potential problems with electrohydraulic lithotripsy within the kidney. As noted in Chapter 12, the irrigant used for electrohydraulic lithotripsy must be poorly conductive and, therefore, dilute (1/6–1/7 normal) saline is used. This solution is hypotonic and should not be employed when there is a perforation of the pelvis or extravasation outside the kidney. Absorption of this fluid may result in hemolysis, hyperkalemia, and hyponatremia.

Fragmentation with the electrohydraulic lithotriptor cannot be controlled and the fragments must be removed individually. No instrument is available for simultaneous aspiration of the fragments. Thus, there is a constant risk of losing fragments to other portions of the intrarenal collecting system and to the ureter. In contrast, the advantages of this technique are its speed and power in the fragmentation of large and dense calculi. It should be used with care in selected individuals when necessary.

RESULTS OF PERCUTANEOUS NEPHROLITHOTOMY. Percutaneous nephrolithotomy, particularly with the use of the ultrasonic lithotriptor, has been highly successful for removal of calculi with minimal morbidity. Among the series available, successful stone removal has ranged from 80 to 90 percent. Overall, residual calculi have been present in 8 percent of patients and an open surgical procedure was required in 8.6 percent (Table 17-1).

The major difficulty with the technique has been an inadequate nephrostomy tract. Placement of a second tract to provide access to the calculus or a decision to proceed with other treatment may be necessary. It must be stressed that accurate placement of the nephrostomy tract as close as possible to the calculus is the first step in a successful procedure.

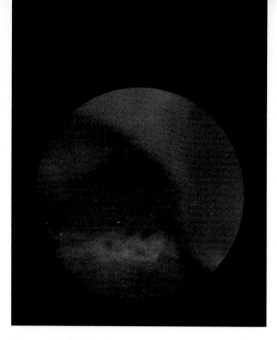

Figure 17-12. *The field of vision of the nephroscope placed operatively within the renal pelvis in this 21-year-old male with a 1-year history of gross hematuria demonstrates the flow of bloody urine from a lower infundibulum.*

Other complications of percutaneous procedures have been hemorrhage and sepsis. Serious bleeding can occur during the initial puncture of the kidney and collecting system or, more often, the dilation of the tract. It also can occur with removal of the nephrostomy tube. The bleeding can arise either from vessels within the muscular layers or from the kidney itself. Usually, the bleeding is easily controlled by placing either a dilator into the tract for several minutes or a large catheter into the tract. Rarely, it is also necessary to inflate the balloon of a catheter within the tract of the kidney to tamponade the bleeding. Continued active bleeding should be localized with angiography and embolized as necessary. Nephrectomy should be considered only as a very last resort for life-threatening hemorrhage. Some bleeding with formation of clots, both in the renal pelvis and in the nephrostomy tube, should be expected in this procedure. Hemorrhage requiring transfusion has occurred in 3 percent of patients.

Figure 17-13. *Inspection within the infundibulum shown in Fig. 17-12 reveals an irregular papillary tip with active bleeding. This appearance is consistent with papillary necrosis, which also was diagnosed from the pathology specimen.*

Sepsis has not been reported as a major complication, but its development may have been avoided in some series by specific exclusion of patients with infectious stones. The risk of sepsis can be minimized by using antibiotics perioperatively and, in patients with infected calculi, preoperatively. In addition, we prefer to stage the nephrostomy-dilation and the endoscopic manipulation as two separate procedures when there is a risk of infection. In this way the kidney can be drained of any infected urine and a tract established to contain contaminated irrigation fluid before the additional pressure of endoscopic inspection and manipulation is added.

Hospital stay has been reported as 5 days in one series and 8.3 in another. Patients usually tolerate the procedure well with only mild discomfort. The patients can usually return to full activity within a very short period after removal of the nephrostomy tube and discharge from the hospital. In general, complications have been mild and relatively rare.

Nephroscopy in Kidneys With Urothelial Tumors. Nephroscopy, operative or percutaneous, should be avoided when there is a suspicion of a urothelial tumor, which, judging from the data, presents too high a risk of spillage of tumor and implantation along the nephrostomy tract. Recurrences have been noted after operative pyeloscopy in kidneys with urothelial tumors [8]. No series is available for percutaneous procedures. Therefore, we consider the presence of a filling defect that is suspicious for urothelial tumor to be a contraindication to percutaneous nephroscopy. A diagnosis should be made by other techniques such as ureteropyeloscopy and brushing prior to any percutaneous procedure.

Nephroscopy for Hematuria. Endoscopic inspection of the intrarenal collecting system has been highly successful in locating a source of bleeding in patients with chronic unilateral hematuria (Figs. 17-12, 17-13) [2]. This procedure should be limited to patients in whom there is no other evidence and minimal suspicion of a malignant source. Since the introduction of ureteropyeloscopy, we have advocated that procedure as the major endoscopic technique in evaluation of chronic unilateral hematuria (see Chaps. 15, 16).

REFERENCES

Operative Nephroscopy

1. Gittes, R. F. Operative nephroscopy. *Trans. Am. Assoc. G. U. Surg.* 67:49, 1975.
2. Gittes, R. F., and Varody, S. Nephroscopy in chronic unilateral hematuria. *J. Urol.* 126:297, 1981.
3. Hertel, E. Intraoperative nephroscopy. *Urology* 4:13, 1974.
4. Leadbetter, W. F. Instrumental visualization of the renal pelvis at operation as an aid to diagnosis: Presentation of a new instrument. *J. Urol.* 63:1006, 1950.
5. McAninch, J. W., and Fay, R. Flexible nephroscope in calculous surgery. *J. Urol.* 128:5, 1982.
6. Rupel, E., and Brown, R. Nephroscopy with removal of stone following nephrostomy for obstructive calculous anuria. *J. Urol.* 46:177, 1941.
7. Takayasu, H., et al. Our new pyelonephroscope for observation of the upper urinary tract. *Endoscopy* 4:105, 1972.
8. Tomera, K. M., Leary, F. J., and Zinche, H. Pyeloscopy in urothelial tumors. *J. Urol.* 127:1088, 1982.
9. Trattner, H. R. Instrumental visualization of the renal pelvis and its communications: Proposal of a new method. Preliminary report. *J. Urol.* 60:817, 1948.
10. Vatz, A., Berci, G., Shore, J. M., Kudish, H., and Nemoy, N. Operative nephroscopy. *J. Urol.* 107:355, 1972.
11. Zingg, E. J., and Futterlieb, A. Nephroscopy in stone surgery. *Br. J. Urol.* 52:333, 1980.

Percutaneous Nephroscopy

12. Alken, P., Hutschenreiter, G., Günther, R., and Marberger, M. Percutaneous stone manipulation. *J. Urol.* 125:463, 1981.
13. Clayman, R. V., et al. Percutaneous nephrolithotomy, an approach to branched and staghorn renal calculi. *J. A. M. A,* 250:73, 1983.
14. Goodwin, W. E., Casey, W. C., and Woolf, W. Percutaneous trocar (needle) nephrostomy in hydronephrosis. *J. A. M. A.* 157:891, 1955.
15. Kato, H., Suzuki, T., Ito, A., Tanaka, M., and Urahashi, S. Changes in optic glass-fibers due to X-ray irradiation. *Chest* 76:672, 1979.
16. Kurth, K. H., Hohenfellner, R., and Altwein, J. E. Ultrasound litholapaxy of a staghorn calculus. *J. Urol.* 117:242, 1977.
17. Marberger, M. Disintegration of renal and ureteral calculi with ultrasound. *Urol. Clin. North Am.* 10:729, 1983.
18. Raney, A. M., and Handler, J. Electrohydraulic nephrolithotripsy. *Urology* 6:439, 1975.
19. Schilling, A., Goettinger, H., Marx, F. J., Schueller, J., and Bauer, H. W. New technique for percutaneous nephropyelostomy. *J. Urol.* 125:475, 1981.
20. Segura, J. W., Patterson, D. E., LeRoy, A. J., May, G. R., and Smith, L. H. Percutaneous lithotripsy. *J. Urol.* 130:1051, 1983.
21. Wickham, J. E. A., Kellet, M. J., and Miller, R. A. Elective percutaneous nephrolithotomy in 50 patients: An analysis of the technique, results and complications. *J. Urol.* 129:904, 1983.

18
PEDIATRIC CYSTOURETHROSCOPY

R. Lawrence Kroovand

Cystourethroscopy is an established and essential tool for adult urologic evaluation. With the high quality of uroradiographic technique and the types of pediatric urologic problems encountered, the indications for pediatric cystoscopy are less clear. Certainly cystoscopy should be done when required; when recommending cystoscopy for a pediatric patient, however, the urologist must balance the risk of anesthesia and the potential complications of the procedure against the sometimes questionable diagnostic and therapeutic benefits to the child. Prior to any endoscopic evaluation of the urinary tract in a child, an intravenous pyelogram (IVP) and voiding cystourethrogram (VCUG) should be done to define the anatomic and functional status of the urinary tract. The use of expression cystourethrography or methylene blue cystography under anesthesia is unphysiologic and inaccurate and has little place in modern pediatric urologic evaluation[11]. Similarly, the substitution of a retrograde pyelogram for an IVP is to be discouraged.

INDICATIONS. The most common indication for cystoscopy in the pediatric patient has been urinary tract infection. It is well documented that children with uncomplicated urinary infections and normal x-rays (IVP, VCUG) generally do not have pyelonephritis[5,7,9,12]. Endoscopic examination in these children is most often normal, or any "abnormal" findings are incidental and do not alter treatment or outcome; in this situation, therefore, cystoscopy appears unnecessary. Cystoscopic examination in children with multiple recurrent infections, especially in those with voiding dysfunction, may document cystitis follicularis or cystitis cystica and reinforce the need for long-term antibiotic treatment.

Children with symptoms of voiding dysfunction (frequency, urgency, day wetting, or nocturnal enuresis) and without documented urinary infections usually have normal physical examinations, urinalyses, and x-rays (IVP, VCUG). Here, again, cystoscopy is usually normal or the abnormal findings are incidental and do not alter treatment or outcome.

The indications for cystoscopy in children with vesicoureteral reflux and urinary infections remain controversial. Because the lesser grades of reflux (2A/4 or 2/5 or less) are infrequently associated with renal scarring or renal growth failure and usually resolve spontaneously, cystoscopic examination in such children seems unwarranted. For children with more severe grades of reflux (2B/4, 3/5) and in those with renal scarring or long-term persistent reflux, cystoscopy may provide the anatomic data on which to base the decision to operate rather than pursue nonoperative management. Here, cystoscopy at the time of planned surgical correction usually provides sufficient indication for or against operative intervention and avoids a separate anesthetic exposure.

Routine cystoscopy for children with hematuria also appears unwarranted since the most common cause for gross or microscopic hematuria in the child is glomerulonephritis, not the bladder tumors so common in adults [3]. We have found, as have others, that most significant bladder and upper urinary lesions producing hematuria in children are radiographically evident [7,12]. Thus, in children with hematuria, if the IVP and VCUG are normal, cystoscopy is almost always normal. Cystoscopy in children with radiographically evident lesions is confirmatory for biopsy, and its function is possibly therapeutic rather than diagnostic. Exceptions to this rule are found after cyclophosphamide therapy [4] and in boys with anterior (bulbar) urethritis who have the characteristic symptom complex of bloody spotting on the shorts or terminal hematuria with or without dysuria and with no pyuria and a negative urine culture. Cystoscopy in boys with the anterior urethritis symptom complex will confirm the anterior urethritis (Fig. 18-1) but is rarely indicated due to the pathognomonic signs and symptoms; additionally, cystoscopy in this situation may cause later stricture formation.

Urinary calculi are uncommon in children [10] and are managed as they are in adults. They may pass or may require manipulation of either retrograde technique or open surgical removal.

Because of the increased accuracy of uroradiographic technique, cystoscopy for observation or for retrograde ureteropyelography is rarely indicated in the pediatric population, as is observation cystoscopy. When retrograde studies are necessary, they should be done under fluoroscopic monitoring.

Figure 18-1. *Anterior (bulbar) urethritis in an 11-year-old boy.*

The role of cystoscopy in the evaluation of congenital anomalies, such as severe hypospadias, ambiguous genitalia, persistent urogenital sinus, and cloacal malformations, is unquestioned. The precise definition of the anatomic abnormalities in such children is invaluable preoperative information that facilitates surgical planning and may reduce the extent of dissection during surgical repair (Fig. 18-2).

The essentials of a pediatric cystoscopic set include interchangeable telescopes (direct vision and forward oblique) and sheaths of assorted sizes to permit both observation (examination) and operative manipulation. I have found that the purely observation or observation-irrigation instruments are neither necessary nor useful because of limited application and the declining indications for observation cystoscopy.

TECHNIQUE. Cystoscopic technique in the infant and child is similar to that in the adult and, therefore, will not be presented in detail. There are, however, certain precautions relevant to pediatric endoscopic technique, which will be discussed. The proper assessment and interpretation of cystoscopic observations often require considerable experience to recognize the subtle and varied congenital anomalies seen in pediatric urology, especially those of the male urethra.

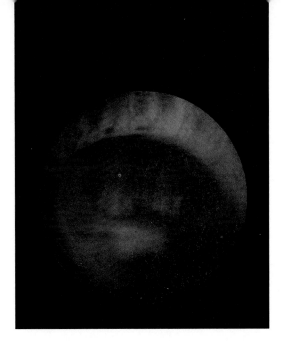

Figure 18-2. *Entrance of the vagina into the urethra of a 2-year-old girl with adrenogenital syndrome.*

Cystoscopy in the child requires general anesthesia and, therefore, should be done in a well-equipped room within an operating or anesthesia suite. The child should be examined in the lithotomy position, although in small infants and young girls an exaggerated frog-leg position is also acceptable. The legs should be carefully taped in position to prevent accidental injury during the procedure. A thorough surgical preparation is essential prior to cystoscopy, and sterile technique is maintained throughout the procedure. The urologist should scrub preoperatively and wear a mask, surgical cap, sterile gown, and gloves.

Instrumentation. Particular care during instrumentation is required to avoid urethral injury. Consistent gentle technique is mandatory. In children urethral instrumentation may present difficulties and, in male children, be followed by stricture. There is a normal range of urethral caliber for each age group, but my preference is to use the smallest diameter instrument appropriate for the examination. In the male child the range of urethral size is limited[1]. The narrowest portion of the male urethra is the external urethral meatus; frequently a simple crush meatotomy is required prior to passage of the instrument. The urethra of a male neonate usually will admit an 8 or 10 Fr. instrument and that of midchildhood a 13 to 14 Fr. instrument without difficulty. Occasionally the penile urethra is too small to permit passage of even the smallest (8 Fr.) infant cystoscope. In such instances a perineal urethrotomy can be done, permitting easy access to the larger diameter bulbar urethra for endoscopic examination and manipulation for treatment of posterior urethral valves or for retrograde ureteropyelography. Because of the accuracy of uroradiographic evaluation, I do not feel that a perineal urethrotomy is warranted for observation cystoscopy.

I do not recommend routine urethral calibration or dilation of the urethra prior to endoscopy, especially in male children, as these procedures may result in iatrogenic injury to the delicate urethral tissues. Rather, I prefer to introduce the instrument into the meatus with the obturator in place; the telescope is then inserted and the urethra examined by direct visual observation during passage of the instrument. This not only minimizes trauma but, more importantly, permits observation of the entire urethra prior to any instrumentation and possible iatrogenic change.

For the female infant and child, the choices for instrument size are broader due to the elasticity and distensibility of the female urethra[6]. The value of urethral dilation in girls with urinary infection and/or voiding dysfunction is questionable[8]. It does not appear to alter the frequency of recurrent infections and rarely enhances resolution of the symptoms of voiding dysfunction.

In the female, the sheath, with obturator in place, may be introduced directly into the bladder and the telescope then inserted. Prior to formal endoscopic evaluation of the bladder in either sex, a urine specimen is usually obtained for urinalysis and, if indicated, culture and sensitivity.

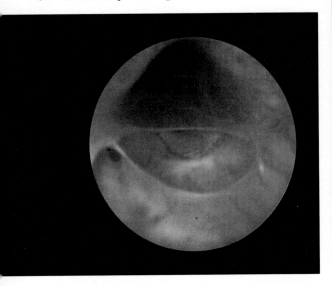

Figure 18-3. *Entrance of Cowper's ducts* (lower lateral) *into the bulbar urethra. The characteristic bulbar urethral diverticulum is present* (lower center).

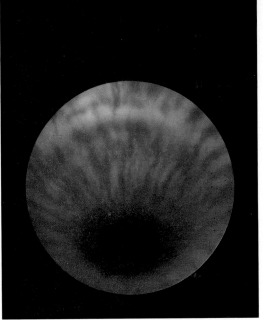

Figure 18-4. *Normal increased prominence of the longitudinal vascular pattern of the male urethra at the urogenital diaphragm.*

Endoscopic Solutions. Irrigating solutions, warmed to body temperature, may be composed of either water or saline. Because of the reduced risks for intravascular absorption or intraperitoneal perforation during endoscopic surgery in infants and children, sterile water is an appropriate medium for such surgery.

The lumen of the pediatric cystoscope, especially the infant cystoscope, allows a reduced rate of irrigating solution flow as compared to that of an adult instrument. The endoscopist, therefore, must be more patient in distending the urethra and bladder. The irrigating solution should not be elevated higher than 1 m above the symphysis pubis. Care should be taken not to overdistend the bladder as this may cause bladder mucosal tears or, in extreme cases, bladder rupture. Approximate bladder capacity in ounces can be calculated using the following formula[2]:

Bladder capacity (oz) = Age (yr) ± 2

This volume should rarely be exceeded.

Normal Endoscopic Findings. The prepubertal male urethra is pale, pink, and of uniform caliber except at the penoscrotal angle and at the urogenital diaphragm where physiologic narrowing and sphincter spasm, respectively, may be misinterpreted as urethral stricture. The entrance of Cowper's ducts deep in the bulbar urethra occasionally may be visualized (Fig. 18-3). The longitudinal vascular pattern normally seen in the penile and bulbar urethra becomes more prominent at the urogenital diaphragm (Fig. 18-4) and should not be misinterpreted as inflammation. The prostatic urethra, verumontanum, and bladder neck are, similarly, more vascular than the remainder of the urethra (Fig. 18-5). A prominent utriculus masculinus may occasionally be seen in boys with severe hypospadias (Fig. 18-6).

The bladder neck in both sexes is supple and easily negotiated, but may bleed easily in response to minimal trauma because of its prominent submucosal vasculature (see Fig. 18-5). In children with long-standing urinary outlet obstruction (urethral valves, sphincter vesical dyssynergia, or urethral stricture), the bladder neck may appear more prominent than normal and possibly obstructive. Generally, such is not the case. These visual obstructions will resolve after relief of the outlet obstruction; surgical correction of bladder neck obstruction is infrequently necessary.

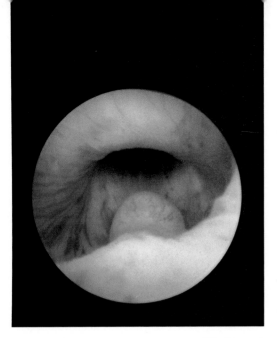

Figure 18-5. *Normal verumontanum and bladder neck.*

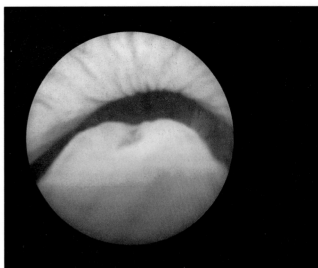

Figure 18-6. *Large prostatic utricle in a 1-year-old boy with perineoscrotal hypospadias.*

The trigone is normally smooth, with ureteral orifices visible within one or two visual fields of the midtrigone. In the postpubertal girl the trigone may be somewhat irregular due to estrogen effect on the trigonal tissues. These findings should not be mistaken for inflammatory or neoplastic changes.

Because position of the ureteral orifices and length of the submucosal tunnel with the bladder distended are important guidelines in predicting resolution of vesicoureteral reflux, great care should be taken in making these observations. The visual perception of the ureteral orifice varies, depending on the type of telescope used (direct vision or forward oblique). Each endoscopist should develop a routine best suited to his or her needs. The endoscopic photographs accompanying this chapter were taken through a direct vision telescope.

Submucosal tunnel length can be estimated or more accurately measured using a small ureteral catheter. Exact dimensions of the submucosal tunnel vary with age and are not absolute for any age. The shape (cone, stadium, horseshoe, golf hole) and position of the ureteral orifices should be observed during bladder filling and recorded with the bladder empty and full (Fig. 18-7). Orifice position and configuration appear to be more consistent determinations than measurement of submucosal tunnel length and, therefore, seem more important parameters in predicting resolution of vesicoureteral reflux.

The normal ureteral orifice (Fig. 18-8) is "volcano" or "cone" shaped and located in the *A* position on the trigone with a generous submucosal tunnel. The orifice maintains its shape and does not migrate laterally during bladder filling. The "stadium" orifice (Fig. 18-9) is located more laterally on the trigone (*B*), is oval in shape, and may migrate laterally during bladder filling; the submucosal tunnel here is shorter than with the normal orifice. The "horseshoe" orifice (Fig. 18-10) has lost its medial rim and some of its attachment to the trigonal muscle along with further shortening of the submucosal tunnel; this orifice is commonly in the *B* or *C* position and migrates farther laterally with bladder filling. The "golf hole" orifice (Fig. 18-11) is located quite laterally on the trigone (*D*) and has little or no submucosal tunnel or trigonal attachment. The gaping appearance may become more apparent with bladder filling. Ureteral orifices located within a bladder diverticulum are frequently difficult to visualize (Fig. 18-12). Ectopic orifices are located distally from the normal trigonal position. Careful examination of the bladder neck and urethra is necessary to locate these ectopic ureteral orifices (Fig. 18-13). In the male, ectopic ureteral orifices, anticipated from preendoscopy urograms, may be encountered in the prostatic urethra proximal to the verumontanum, at the bladder neck, or on the distal trigone (Fig. 18-13). In the female, ectopic ureteral orifices may also be found in the urethra, perineum, or vagina.

CHILDREN'S HOSPITAL OF MICHIGAN

CYSTOSCOPIC EXAMINATION

DATE

PATIENT NO.

PATIENT NAME

MEDICAL RECORD NO.

BIRTH DATE   SEX

PHYSICIAN

HISTORY _____

_____

PHYSICAL FINDINGS _____

IVP _____

CYSTOGRAM _____
URINALYSIS
  BLADDER _____ (R)_____ (L)_____
URINE CULTURE
  BLADDER _____ (R)_____ (L)_____

INSTRUMENT SIZE _____ LENS _____ BLADDER RESIDUAL _____
URETHRA
  MEATUS _____ LENGTH _____ MUCOSA _____

    CALIBRATION FR. ____ DILATATION FR. ____ MEATOTOMY ____ URETHROTOMY ____ OTHER ____
BLADDER
  BLADDER NECK _____ TRIGONE _____ CAPACITY _____

  MUCOSA _____ TRABECULATION _____

URETERAL ORIFICES

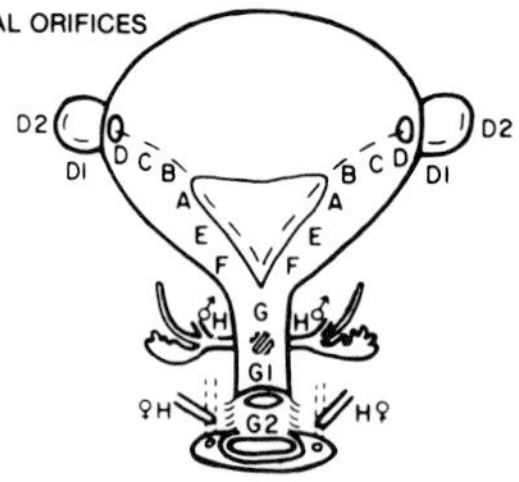

RETROGRADE STUDIES (R)_____ (L)_____

PERISTALSIS   (R)_____ (L)_____

OTHER OBSERVATIONS & CONCLUSIONS _____

_____

_____

PLAN _____

_____

_____

SURGEON _____

FORM OR 3

	Rt. Orifice Posn								(✔)		Lt. Orifice Posn							
H	G	F	E	D	C	B	A	Shape	A	B	C	D	E	F	G	H
								Golf Hole								
								Horseshoe								
								Stadium								
								Normal								
								Size								
								Small(S) Med.(M) Large(L)								
								Patulous(P) NonPat(NP)								
								Submucosal Tunnel m.m.								

▨ If ureteric orifice is duplicated, describe U.O. corresponding with cranial renal segment in shaded part of appropriate column.

★ Paraureteral   R. Present ☐   Not Present ☐
Diverticulum   L. Present ☐   Not Present ☐

If present, denote site of U.O. in relation to diverticulum as shown on diagram D, D1, D2 when possible in D column/s.

White, MEDICAL RECORD — Canary, SURGEON — Pink, RESIDENT — Gold, DEPT.

DO NOT WRITE IN THIS MARGIN

Figure 18-7. *Cystoscopy record for recording endoscopic findings. This should become a permanent part of the patient's record.*

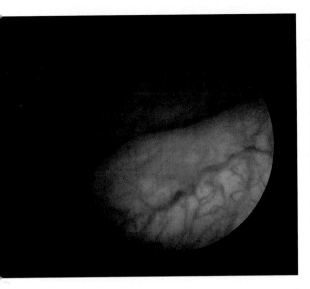

Figure 18-8. *Normal cone- or volcano-shaped ureteral orifice.*

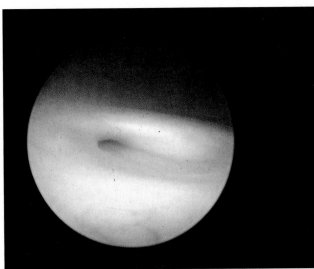

Figure 18-10. *Horseshoe-shaped ureteral orifice; the orifice has lost its medial rim.*

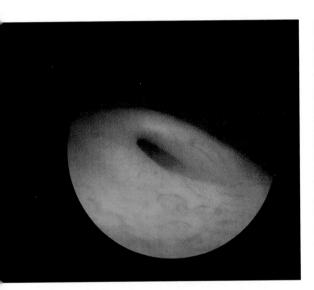

Figure 18-9. *Stadium-shaped ureteral orifice.*

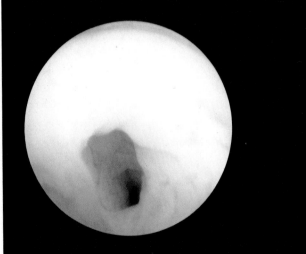

Figure 18-11. *Golf hole-shaped ureteral orifice; there is no submucosal tunnel.*

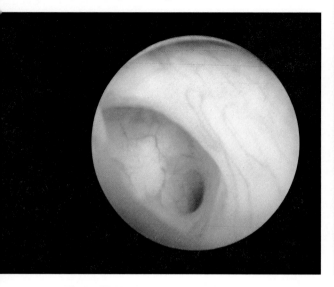

Figure 18-12. *Ureteral orifice located within bladder diverticulum.*

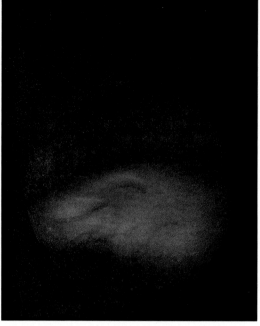

Figure 18-14. *Total ureteral duplication. The upper and more lateral ureteral orifice drains the lower renal segment; the lower and more medial ureteral orifice drains the upper renal segment.*

In addition to the position and shape of the ureteral orifice and the length of the submucosal tunnel, observations should be made for the presence of ureteral duplication (Fig. 18-14) or ectopia, bladder trabeculation, diverticulum, bleeding point, tumor, stone, and foreign body. Bladder capacity should be measured and all data recorded on a cystoscopy report, which becomes a permanent part of the patient record (see Fig. 18-7).

In girls, I perform vaginoscopy using a direct viewing telescope to detect any vaginal abnormalities (e.g., foreign bodies, discharge) that may contribute to urinary symptoms or previously undiagnosed anomalies. In the prepubertal girl, the vagina is relatively long and narrow with the cervix seen as a small, pale structure frequently hidden in the mucosal folds of the vaginal fornix and, therefore, easily missed (Fig. 18-15). The vagina may be distended by gently occluding the vaginal orifice with a finger; overdistention should be avoided because retrograde passage of irrigant into the peritoneum may cause peritonitis.

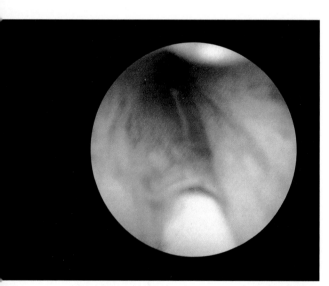

Figure 18-13. *Ectopic ureteral orifice located in the proximal urethra near the bladder neck; the ectopic orifice has been catheterized.*

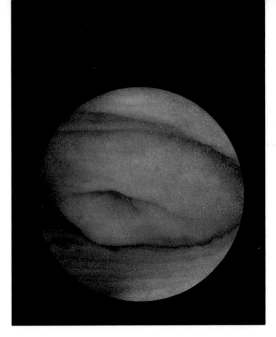

Figure 18-15. *Vaginoscopy. A normal prepubertal cervix located in the folds of the vaginal fornix is shown.*

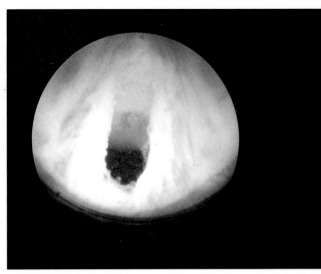

Figure 18-16. *Posterior urethral valves.*

ENDOSCOPIC SURGERY. Operative cystoscopy is easily done using the various pediatric instruments available. Posterior urethral valves (Fig. 18-16) are easily recognized on a voiding cystourethrogram and may be carefully incised using either a pediatric resectoscope or a cystoscope with a 3 or 4 Fr. ureteral catheter converted into an electrode by a wire stylet. Care should be exercised to incise only the valve leaflets and not to injure the external sphincter or verumontanum; residual obstruction may be treated electively. Similarly, anterior urethral valves and urethral diverticula, when small, may be incised transurethrally; larger lesions usually require open revision.

Transurethral incision of ureteroceles is of limited long-term value because it trades obstruction for reflux into a dilated and poorly draining segment of the urinary tract and is generally unwise. Transurethral incision of an ectopic ureterocele in the septic infant, however, may be lifesaving; formal reconstruction may be done later, electively. Large ectopic ureteroceles may collapse during cystoscopic examination or even evert through the detrusor hiatus, simulating a bladder diverticulum (Fig. 18-17). Simple ureteroceles are usually asymptomatic and are rarely diagnosed in children.

Bladder neck obstruction has become an unusual diagnosis in childhood. Most such obstructions are more apparent than real and will resolve after relief of the urinary outlet obstruction. Transurethral resection of such obstructions is rarely indicated and may lead to retrograde ejaculation in boys or to vesicovaginal fistula in girls.

Urinary calculi in children are managed in a manner similar to those in the adult. Urethral size in the male limits the size of the instruments used; however, 4 and 5 Fr. stone retrievers are available for use through a 10 Fr. sheath. Similarly, miniature biopsy forceps may be used to retrieve small objects from the urethra or bladder; larger objects often require open retrieval.

COMPLICATIONS. In a discussion of pediatric endoscopy, it is appropriate to conclude with a brief section on those complications relating to pediatric cystoscopy. Most complications can be avoided or minimized through gentle technique and by keeping the procedure as brief as possible, especially in the male. The use of a suitable teaching attachment minimizes the need for multiple examiners to manipulate the cystoscope and, therefore, reduces iatrogenic trauma. Adherence to meticulous sterile technique is essential and minimizes the risk of postoperative infection. Sepsis is more common after prolonged or vigorous instrumentation, especially in an anomalous or infected urinary system with poor emptying characteristics.

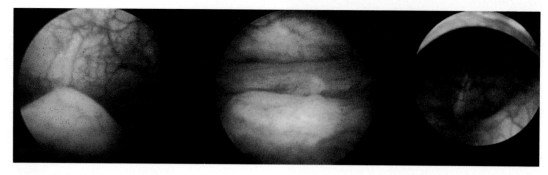

Figure 18-17. *Ectopic ureterocele (left to right). With bladder filling, the ureterocele flattens and everts outside the bladder muscle, simulating a bladder diverticulum.*

Incontinence after transurethral incision of urethral valves and bladder perforation or vesicovaginal fistula after transurethral resection of the bladder neck in girls are well-known complications and should easily be avoided by adherence to careful technique. A too tightly fitting sheath or rough instrumentation may lacerate, perforate, or produce false passages in the male urethra. When removing the cystoscope from the male child, the instrument should be withdrawn in a gentle curve to avoid urethral injury as the cystoscope passes the suspensory ligament of the penis. Difficult endoscopic examinations dictate careful follow-up to detect late stricture formation (see Fig. 18-14). In young or physically small boys, transient postoperative urinary retention due to dysuria or edema may occur and necessitate brief indwelling catheterization. Finally, an infrequently encountered but potentially dangerous complication of pediatric cystoscopy is hypothermia, which may result from using irrigating solutions at room temperature. The use of warm irrigating solutions and careful monitoring of body temperature should prevent this complication.

REFERENCES

1. Allen, J.S., Summers, J.L., and Wilkerson, S.E. Meatal calibration in newborn boys. *J. Urol.* 107:498, 1972.
2. Berger, R.M., et al. Bladder capacity (ounces) equals age (years) plus 2 predicts normal bladder capacity and aids in diagnosis of abnormal voiding patterns. *J. Urol.* 129:347, 1983.
3. Chan, J.C.M. Hematuria and proteinuria in the pediatric patient. Diagnostic approach. *Urology* 11:205, 1978.
4. Droller, M.J., Saral, R., and Santos, G. Prevention of cyclophosphamide-induced hemorrhagic cystitis. *Urology* 20:256, 1982.
5. Dunn, M., Smith, J.B., and Abrams, P.H. Endoscopic examination in children. *Br. J. Urol.* 50:586, 1978.
6. Immergut, M.A., and Wahman, G.E. The urethral caliber of female children with recurrent urinary tract infections. *J. Urol.* 99:189, 1968.
7. Johnson, D.K., Kroovand, R.L., and Perlmutter, A.D. The changing role of cystoscopy in the pediatric patient. *J. Urol.* 123:232, 1980.
8. Kaplan, G.W., Sammons T.A., and King, L.R. A blind comparison of dilation, urethrotomy and medication alone in treatment of urinary tract infections in girls. *J. Urol.* 109:917, 1973.
9. Kroovand, R.L. Pediatric Endoscopy. In P. Kelalis, L. King, and B. Belman (Eds.), *Clinical Pediatric Urology* (2nd ed). Philadelphia: Saunders. In press, 1984.
10. Reiner, R.J., Kroovand, R.L., and Perlmutter, A.D. Unusual aspects of urinary calculi in children *J. Urol.* 121:480, 1979.
11. Timmons, J.W., Watts, F.B., and Perlmutter, A.D. A comparison of awake and anesthesia cystography. *Birth Def.* 13(5): 1977.
12. Walther, P.C., and Kaplan, G.S. Cystoscopy in children: Indications for its use in common urologic problems. *J. Urol.* 122:717, 1979.

19
UROLOGIC ENDOSCOPIC PHOTOGRAPHY

Jeffry L. Huffman

Demetrius H. Bagley

Edward S. Lyon

Historically, urologic endoscopic photography languished for decades following the development of the cystoscope, largely as a consequence of inadequate instrumentation. The small size of the urologic instruments, slow film speeds, and low levels of illumination resulted in poor quality photographic images. Subsequent improvements, including the development of cameras with built-in exposure metering, optically superior telescopes, high-speed fine grain color films, and external photographic light sources connected to the telescope by efficient light-carrying cables and to the camera for automatic light sensing and emission adjustments, have made urologic endoscopic photography a reality.

For the urologist, endoscopic photography provides a means of documentation of pathological processes. Lesions that are identified endoscopically in the urethra, bladder, and upper urinary tract can be permanently recorded in individual patients. The urologist can also use the photographs for recording and teaching normal urologic anatomy, pathology, and the various urologic procedures, including ureteropyeloscopy, operative nephroscopy, and percutaneous nephroscopy.

INSTRUMENTATION

Illumination for Photography. It is essential to the technique of endoscopic photography to provide enough light within the urinary tract and to the camera to obtain properly exposed photographs. The light is initially provided by a light source unit in the form of an electronic flash generator or a continuous high-intensity light. It is then transmitted to the telescope by means of a fiberoptic or fluid-filled light bundle. Once it has passed through the telescope to illuminate the object, the light must return through the objective lens of the telescope to the camera lens and adaptor in order to reach the film. Therefore, proper illumination for urologic endoscopic photography depends not only on the light-supplying unit, or flash generator, but also on the light-carrying bundle, telescope, camera lens, and film. It is for this reason that in discussing proper illumination for endoscopic photography every part of the system must be evaluated individually for its efficiency in light generation or transmission.

Each major instrument manufacturer produces light sources that can be used for routine endoscopy and for photography. Both manual electronic flash units and automatic flash exposure systems are available. The manual flash units have settings for different flash intensities, and the automatic systems are used in conjunction with automatic exposure cameras to determine precisely the correct flash intensity for proper exposure.

Table 19-1. Specifications of Photographic Units

Manufacturer	Photographic Unit	Flash Exposure Mode	Observation Lamp Intensity (watts)	Recommended Camera[a]
ACMI	Xenon light source — model 1210	Manual	300	Olympus OM-1, OM-2n, or OM-4
Olympus	Cold light supply — model CLE-F	Automatic and manual	150	Olympus OM-1, OM-2n, or OM-4; EC-3 Polaroid; SC16-3R Auto 16 mm
	Xenon cold light supply (flexible instrumentation) — model CLV	Automatic and manual	300	Olympus OM-1, OM-2n, or OM-4; SC16-3R Auto 16 mm; EC-3 Polaroid
Pentax	Xenon light source — model LX-75F	Automatic and manual	75	Pentax MF; Olympus OM-1, OM-2n, or OM-4
Karl Storz	Computer flash unit and cold light fountain — model 600 CA	Automatic and manual	150	Olympus OM-2n or OM-4[b]
Wolf	Endo-Computer flash — model 5007	Automatic and manual	100	Olympus OM-2n or OM-4[b]

[a]The Pentax MF automatic camera for endoscopic photography can be used in conjunction with any of the light sources listed.
[b]Other cameras that have through-the-lens photosensing capabilities and are adaptable to the individual systems may be used.

Although an electronic flash unit is more commonly used, a high-intensity light source also provides enough light continuously to enable photographs to be taken without a flash generator. This system is occasionally useful in photographing well-illuminated regions, such as the urethra: often the exposure time required for still photography is so long, however, that it is difficult to prevent movement of the endoscopic instrument and camera.

The light generated by either system is transmitted to the object being photographed by a light cable and a telescope. The most efficient system is the one with the least loss of light by this transmission. Therefore, the integral bundle system in which the fiberoptic bundle is permanently attached to the telescope is most satisfactory for photography. Other systems that require a connection between the light cable and telescope are acceptable, but there is considerable loss of light at the connection and less illumination of the object.

Further variations in the light-carrying bundle may also enable better illumination. A fluid-filled bundle transmits light more efficiently than a standard fiberoptic bundle and may improve photography. Also, a fiberoptic bundle from one manufacturer actually focuses the transmitted light on the smaller light-carrying core of the telescope through a condensor lens. The standard fiberoptic bundle has uniform illumination and only the portion striking the telescope bundle will be transmitted to the object being photographed.

Superior telescopes also enhance endoscopic photography. Lenses that are optically efficient in transmitting light provide the best illumination of the object. The H. H. Hopkins rod-lens system for rigid endoscopes revolutionized telescope construction. This system, routinely used today, increases light transmission 80-fold through the telescope in comparison with previous telescope designs.

The diameter of the telescope lens also influences illumination. The standard cystoscope lens is 4 mm in diameter. Photographic telescope lenses, 5 mm in diameter, provide better illumination and are available for cystourethroscopy. Smaller telescopes, such as those used for ureteropyeloscopy, have lenses that are only 2.7 mm in diameter. Because these lenses provide less illumination, photography through a small telescope can be difficult, although the addition of an integral fiberoptic bundle does produce satisfactory photographs.

Camera. Several types of cameras are acceptable for urologic endoscopic photography (Table 19-1). The type we have found most useful is a 35-mm single lens reflex camera. This type of camera is small and light enough to attach directly to the endoscope. It also allows the urologist to see directly the object being photographed and to move the instrument and perform procedures with the camera in place. In addition, it can be used for other medical and personal purposes and is not limited to endoscopic photography.

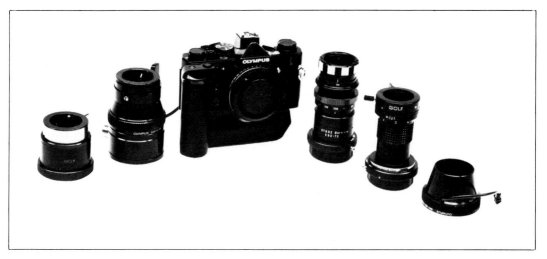

Figure 19-1. *The Olympus OM-2n camera is shown with a power winder. Five endoscopic adaptors are also shown. From left to right are the ACMI adaptor without focusing, the Olympus variable focus (SM-EFR), the Storz variable focus zoom lens, the Wolf variable focus, and the Olympus SM-2S adaptor for the flexible endoscope.*

To be acceptable for adaptation to urologic endoscopic photography, a camera should have (1) readily interchangeable focusing screens, (2) interchangeable lenses with adaptability to the endoscope, (3) capability of synchronization with a flash generator, and, ideally, (4) through-the-lens (TTL) light-sensing automatic flash control. Automatic film advance is not mandatory but its benefits far outweigh its cost. To be used in conjunction with the Karl Storz or Richard Wolf automatic exposure systems, the camera must have a through-the-lens light-sensing device to control the electronic flash and synchronization capabilities with the flash generator. For the Olympus automatic exposure system, either the Olympus OM-1, OM-2n, or OM-4 camera may be used.

We have used the Olympus OM-2 and OM-2n cameras with power winders, which satisfy all of these requirements (Fig. 19-1). Cameras from other manufacturers are also acceptable if they have the capabilities listed above. For example, an automatic camera manufactured by Pentax is suitable for use with any light source presently available. It has a half-frame format, which doubles the number of exposures; however, it is a fixed focus system.

FOCUSING SCREEN. Either the Olympus clear endoscopic viewing screen (1–9) or the cross-hairs, clear field focusing screen (1–12) is used. The 1–9 clear screen is used in conjunction with a standard camera lens with the focus set at infinity to allow clear identification of the object even at low light levels at which other screens may become too dark to allow the urologist to see well. The 1–12 screen is used with special lenses adapted for endoscopic photography in a variable focus system and allows one to focus on the object sharply.

LENSES. A standard photographic lens used in conjunction with a specific adaptor can be attached to the individual endoscope eyepiece. The longer the focal length, the larger the image on the film, but the less light per unit area for film exposure. Therefore, a 100-mm lens requires more exposure time for the same object than a 50-mm lens but does produce an adequate-sized image on the film with most cystoscopic telescopes.

A standard lens should have its aperture (f-stop) set wide open (or at the lowest f-stop) to avoid constricting the field of view. Unlike conventional photographic situations in which aperture variation influences film exposure and depth of focus, the parallel light rays emanating from the endoscope completely defeat diaphragm use in both exposure control and depth of field selection.

Specially designed lenses are available for urologic endoscopic photography and are highly desirable for the more than casual endoscopic photographer. These lenses are variable focus and available in a variety of focal lengths: Wolf, 105 mm; Olympus, 100 mm; and Storz, 70–140 mm (zoom) (Fig. 19-1). They will be described in more detail below.

Table 19-2. Camera and Photographic Unit Settings Using Olympus OM-2n Camera With ASA 200 Daylight Color Film

Camera Settings	ACMI (model 1210) Manual	Olympus (CLE-F)		Olympus CLV (flexible endoscope)[b]		Pentax LX-75F (flexible endoscope)[h]		Karl Storz 600 CA		Wolf 5007	
		Automatic[a]	Manual	Automatic[b]	Manual	Automatic[h]	Manual	Automatic	Manual	Automatic	Manual
Exposure mode	Manual	Manual[a]	Manual	Automatic[b]	Manual	Automatic[h]	Manual	Automatic	Manual	Automatic	Manual
Shutter speed	1/15 sec	1/4 sec	1/4 sec	1/4 sec	1/4 sec	1/4 sec	1/4 sec	1/15 sec	1/15 sec	1/15 sec	1/15 sec
ASA setting	NA	NA[a]	NA	NA[b]	NA	NA[h]	NA[h]	800[c]	NA	800[d]	NA
Synchronization terminal and setting	X	FP	FP	X	X	FP	FP	X[f]	X	X[g]	X
Flash intensity setting on photographic unit	1–3[e]	3[a]	Full and 1–6[e]	3[b]	1–5	1[h]	1–3[e]	3	1–3[e]	4	1–4[e]

[a]Applicable only with SM-EFR Olympus adaptor and Olympus telescopes. ASA setting entered on CLE-F unit, not camera.

[b]Applicable only with Olympus adaptors for flexible fiberscopes (SM-2S or SM-4S). ASA setting entered on CLV unit, not camera.

[c]Varies with focal length of lens (800 used when Storz zoom lens set at 70 mm). (See text for explanation.)

[d]Varies with focal length of lens and type of telescope (refer to manufacturer's chart).

[e]Varies depending on amount of flash required (greater distance from telescope requires higher setting).

[f]Special synchronization cord attaches to through-the-lens auto connector Type 4 in hot shoe socket.

[g]Special synchronization cord attaches to Accessory Shoe 4 in hot shoe socket.

[h]Applicable only with Pentax MF camera for endoscopic photography and Pentax flexible endoscopes. ASA setting entered on LX-75F unit, not camera. Exposure index set on 1 using PA-M105 adaptor and ASA 200 film.

NA = not applicable.

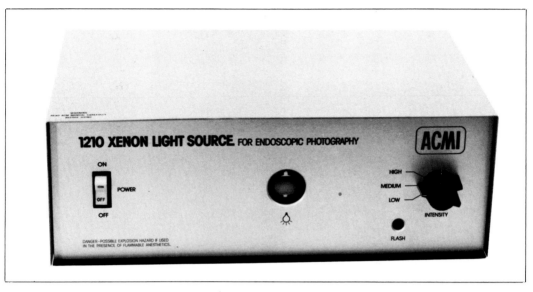

Figure 19-2. *ACMI xenon light source—Model 1210.*

SYNCHRONIZATION CORDS. The electronic flash generated by the light source must be timed to occur entirely when the camera shutter is open. For this, the proper setting must be made on the camera and synchronization cords are needed to synchronize shutter release with flash generation. Each instrument manufacturer has different synchronization cords to attach the Olympus camera to its individual flash generators. These will be discussed individually below.

AUTOMATIC FILM ADVANCE. Although not an absolute necessity, an automatic film advance allows the endoscopist to take photographs without having to advance the film manually. Manual winding often entails readjusting instrument position and focus prior to taking another exposure. The battery-operated electronic winder will automatically advance the film to the next exposure after the shutter release is activated.

FILM. For color slides, daylight type film ASA 200 has proved satisfactory when using a light source with electronic flash. Color matching the film to the light source is important for proper colors in the projected image. Since 400 ASA film has more grain to its appearance than 200 ASA film, we usually use 200 ASA film unless the extra film speed is required. This film is developed in a standard fashion, although for added speed (increased ASA rating) special processing to double the effective film speed may be requested at many laboratories for a slight additional cost.

CHOOSING A PHOTOGRAPHIC SYSTEM. In deciding which system to use for endoscopic photography, several factors should be considered. If a urologist is starting with no instrumentation and desires consistently excellent photographs, one of the automatic exposure systems would be most satisfactory. These are relatively expensive and often are not interchangeable with equipment from different manufacturers. Nevertheless, they do routinely produce high-quality photographs and are very reliable. The manual flash generators are less expensive and often can be used in conjunction with instruments from different companies. Each manufacturer has a manual flash unit; these units will be discussed in detail below. Although more exposures often are required to obtain one high-quality photograph, selected final photographs usually are comparable to those obtained with the automatic systems.

Each major instrument manufacturer has a top-of-the-line photographic system available commercially. These systems, including their specifications, will be discussed individually below (Tables 19-1, 19-2).

ACMI Xenon Light Source for Endoscopic Photography (model 1210)—Manual Exposure. The ACMI photographic unit contains a high-output xenon lamp, which, for exposure, is boosted in intensity to correspond with shutter opening (Fig. 19-2). There are three different intensity selections for photographic use.

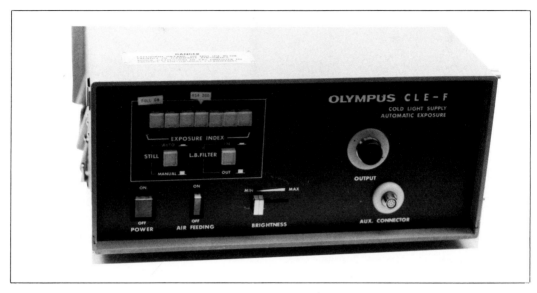

Figure 19-3. *Olympus CLE-F cold light supply.*

This unit is a manual exposure system. It can be used with most 35-mm cameras with an ACMI synchronization cord. The cord connects to the light source and to the camera synchronization terminal set at "X." One should increase the intensity as the distance to the location of the object in the urinary tract increases. The shutter speed should be set at 1/15 second (see Fig. 7-18).

A standard photographic lens can be used in conjunction with a screw-on telescope eyepiece connector. Also, many of the variable focus lenses from other manufacturers are acceptable.

Olympus CLE-F Cold Light Supply—Automatic and Manual Exposure. When the Olympus CLE-F system is used for automatic flash exposure, the Olympus telescopes and fiberoptic light cable must also be employed (Fig. 19-3). A specially designed SM-EFR lens (100 mm) includes a photosensing device that automatically adjusts the light output of the Olympus electronic flash unit in much the same way as the OM-2 camera with the Storz and Wolf flash units. The CLE-F unit contains a synchronization cable that connects the lens to the synchronization terminal on the Olympus OM-1 or OM-2n camera (set at focal plane, FP). A second synchronization cable connects the lens to the auxiliary connector terminal on the light-generating unit.

For automatic exposure, the CLE-F unit is set on "auto" and the exposure index selector (Full and 1–6) is set to correspond to the speed (ASA) rating of film being used. The camera is set on its manual exposure mode since the light sensor in the SM-EFR adaptor controls the automatic flash exposure. The shutter speed is set on 1/4 second and the synchronization terminal of the camera is set on FP (see Fig. 7-12).

For manual or nonautomatic exposure, the CLE-F unit is set on "manual" and the exposure index selector is varied according to the level of flash intensity required. Once again, the camera is set on its manual exposure mode, 1/4-second shutter speed, and FP synchronization.

The Olympus CLV xenon cold light supply is the preferred unit for endoscopic photography, using an Olympus flexible endoscope. Although the CLE-F unit is also acceptable, the CLV unit has a high-intensity xenon flashtube that provides the increased light needed for photography through the flexible instrumentation. When used in conjunction with the Olympus OM-2, OM-2n, OM-4, or SC-16 cameras, it allows for automatic flash exposure. Each Olympus flexible instrument contains a photosensing device that automatically adjusts the light output of the CLV unit.

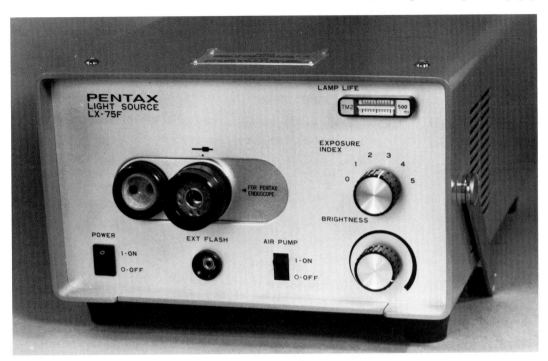

Figure 19-4. *Pentax xenon light source—Model LX-75F.*

For automatic exposure, either the Olympus SM-2S or SM-4S adaptor must be used to connect the flexible fiberscope to the Olympus camera. These adaptors have a synchronization cord that connects to the synchronization terminal on the Olympus camera (set on X). The exposure mode of the camera is set on manual and the shutter speed at 1/4 second. The exposure index selector on the CLV unit is then varied according to the ASA rating of the film being used.

Pentax Light Source LX-75F—Automatic and Manual Exposure. The Pentax light source model LX-75F has a xenon flashtube for endoscopic photography (Fig. 19-4). This system is designed to be used with their flexible endoscope, their model MF endoscopic camera, and the Pentax PA-M55, PA-M75, or PA-M105 adaptors. The camera is of half-frame format, which doubles the number of exposures per roll of film. It has a built-in photosensor for automatic exposure and can be used with most standard light sources. There is no provision for changing viewing screens, however, and thus it is a fixed focus system.

For automatic exposure, using the entire Pentax system and ASA 200 film, the camera is set on 1/4-second shutter speed and the exposure index on the light source is maintained at 1 (if the PA-M105 adaptor is used). The ASA setting on the camera is adjusted to correspond to the film speed used, and the flash synchronization is set on FP (see Fig. 7-21).

A photosensor in the flexible endoscope adjusts the output of xenon flash from the LX-75F unit. Using this system, therefore, the camera is maintained at 1/4-second shutter speed and its automatic exposure capabilities are not utilized. The exposure index on the light source does need adjustment depending on the ASA rating of the film and the focal length of the lens used. If ASA 200 film is used, the index should be set on 5 for the 55-mm lens adaptor (PA-M55), 3 for the 75-mm lens adaptor (PA-M75), and 1 for the 105-mm lens adaptor (PA-M105).

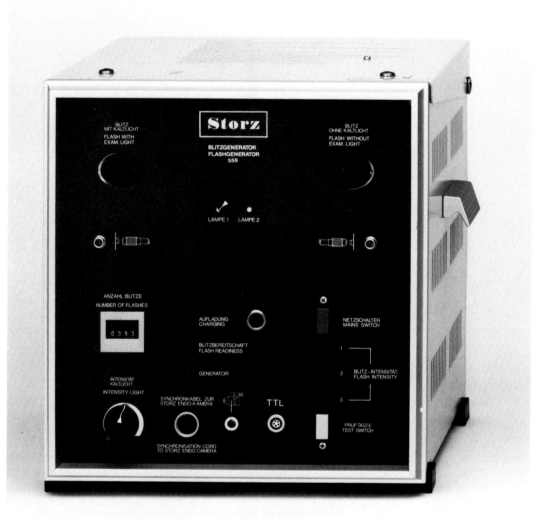

Figure 19-5. *Karl Storz computer flash unit and cold light fountain — Model 600 CA.*

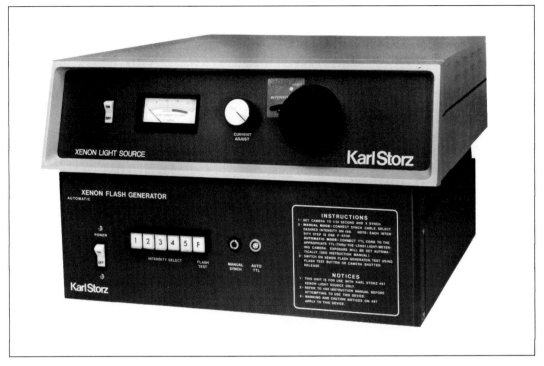

Figure 19-6. *Karl Storz xenon light source and flash generator—Model 617.*

Karl Storz Computer Flash Unit and Cold Light Fountain 600 CA—Automatic and Manual Exposure. The Karl Storz computer flash unit contains two observation lamps and one flashtube (Fig. 19-5). The cold light fountain has an intensity of 150 watts for observation and the flashtube has 3 different outputs for manual exposure.

This system can be used with the Olympus OM-2n or OM-4 camera for automatic through-the-lens exposure or with other cameras for manual flash exposure. These cameras contain photosensors that measure the light quantity passing through the lens to the film and automatically switch off the flash impulse at the precise moment for proper exposure. For automatic exposure, a synchronization cord fits into the hot shoe of the Olympus OM-2n or OM-4 camera and also into the synchronizing port of the light source. The camera is set on automatic exposure and the flash intensity on the light source at 3.

The camera ASA setting is varied according to the type of film used and the focal length of the lens. These settings are available in table form from the manufacturer. For automatic exposure using 200 ASA film and the lens at 70 mm, for example, the camera ASA should be set at 800. The 70-mm focal length gives a small image on the film and the camera actually overexposes the photograph. "Underexposing," by setting the ASA at 800, compensates for this small image and results in proper exposure (see Fig. 11-2).

For manual exposure, the synchronization cable is attached to the camera synchronization terminal (set at X) and to the light source at a separate synchronization port. The camera is set on manual exposure with a shutter speed of 1/15 second. The flash intensities are varied according to the level of flash required.

Either the automatic or manual Storz system can be used in conjunction with the variable focus 70- to 140-mm zoom lens specially designed for adaptability to urologic telescopes. This lens allows variable magnification and, at higher focal lengths, produces an image that almost entirely covers the film.

Karl Storz is also currently testing a newer model, the 617, which utilizes a xenon flashtube and has automatic flash exposure control as well (Fig. 19-6).

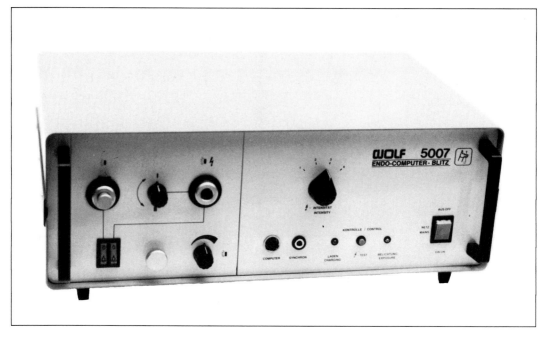

Figure 19-7. *Richard Wolf Endo-Computer flash — Model 5007.*

Wolf Endo-Computer Flash (model 5007) — Automatic and Manual Exposure. The Wolf automatic flash unit contains two observation light sources and one flash generator (Fig. 19-7). The observation lamp has an intensity of 100 watts and the electron flashtube has 4 different outputs when used for manual flash exposure.

Once again, this unit is used with the Olympus OM-2n or OM-4 camera for automatic exposure. A synchronization cord attaches to the hot shoe of the camera and to the synchronization terminal of the light source. This enables the TTL automatic exposure system of the camera to function in the same fashion as described previously for the Storz system. The flash intensity of the light source is set at 4 and the camera exposure mode is set on automatic (see Fig. 7-8).

For manual flash exposure, a different synchronization cord, which inserts into the camera body alongside the lens and then into a separate synchronization port on the light source, is required. Using this system, the synchronization terminal on the Olympus camera should be at X, the exposure mode on manual, and the shutter speed at 1/15 second.

The Wolf focusing lens has a 105-mm focal length and can be adapted to other telescopes. Depending on the type of telescope and type of film used, the setting of the Olympus camera must be varied. For example, if a standard 5-degree telescope is used with ASA 200 film with the automatic exposure system, the camera should be set on an ASA of 800 to compensate for the small area of image on the film. These settings are listed in table form available from the manufacturer.

TECHNIQUE. Once a system has been selected, it is important prior to beginning the procedure that the photographic equipment be checked and set up properly (Table 19-3). It is essential that the camera settings be accurate and the film properly loaded into the camera. The synchronization cord should be attached to the camera and flash generator and the correct synchronization setting should be selected.

Extra time should be allowed for the procedure in order to take photographs and also to finish the procedure. To obtain satisfactory photographs, time is needed to ensure sharp focus, clear irrigation, and proper centering of the object.

Table 19-3. Checklist for Endoscopic Photography

1. Film
   a. Correct ASA rating?
   b. Color daylight film?
   c. Properly loaded in camera?
2. Camera
   a. Correct exposure mode setting (auto or manual)?
   b. Correct shutter speed and f-stop?
   c. Correct ASA setting for film type used?
   d. Proper synchronization setting for electronic flash (X or FP)?
3. Light source
   a. Correct exposure mode and flash setting?
   b. Proper connection for synchronization cord and light cable?

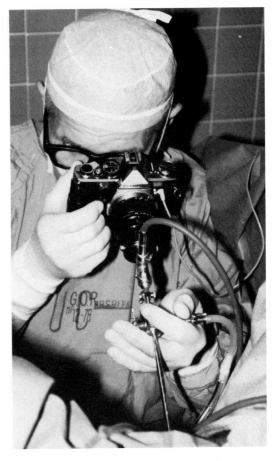

Figure 19-8. *The urologist wears two sets of gloves and holds the camera attached to the endoscope. The endoscopic field is seen through the camera. A power winder permits operation of the camera with one hand.*

The sterility of the photographic procedure can be a problem. At our institution, the urologist performing the procedure wears two sets of gloves and, after finishing photography, removes one set to finish the procedure. The actual photographic process is done by one person. The urologist can control the camera with one hand while stabilizing the endoscope with the other (Fig. 19-8).

Photography of the Urethra. In taking pictures of the urethra, the cystoscope is actually advanced with the camera in place. The pictures are taken while urethroscopy is being performed and irrigation maintained so that the urethral lumen does not collapse around the telescope.

The flash intensity, if using a manual system, should be set at a low or medium setting because of the close proximity of the lumen and the relatively smaller amount of light needed for good illumination.

Photography of the Bladder. Once inside the bladder, the flash intensity should be set at a maximum setting if a manual system is being used. Thorough irrigation of all debris, blood, and urine from the bladder is performed until the irrigation fluid is absolutely clear. Any amount of blood or debris will cloud the photographs (see Figs. 9-4, 12-9).

As observed with standard flash photography, objects in the foreground appear more illuminated than those in the background, which appear dark. It is, therefore, more desirable to have all objects in the photograph approximately the same distance from the telescope. This serves for uniform illumination and uniform focus.

Should the urologist desire an estimate of the site of a lesion photographed in the bladder (e.g., tumor), an object of known size can be photographed in the same field. For example, a ureteral catheter with centimeter markings can be inserted next to the tumor and an approximate size can be determined (see Fig. 6-14).

Photography of the Ureter and Renal Pelvis. Photography of the ureter and renal pelvis is different from that of the bladder and urethra. It is important while taking pictures in the upper tract to prevent overdistention of the ureter and renal pelvis. Usually, it is necessary to maintain irrigation to keep the lumen distended. Because of the delicate nature of the instruments used in the upper urinary tract, an assistant should always be available to help handle the camera and support the instrument.

Table 19-4. Causes of Unsatisfactory Pictures

1. Poor illumination
    a. Malfunctioning flash generator (picture may appear yellow).
    b. Improper synchronization between shutter release and flash generation.
    c. Worn fiberoptic light bundle with broken light-conducting fibers.
    d. Telescope with poor light transmission.
    e. Excessive distance between end of telescope and object photographed.
    f. Incorrect film type and/or speed.
2. Cloudy or out-of-focus pictures
    a. Excessive blood in irrigation (see Fig. 9-3).
    b. Excessive debris in irrigation (see Fig. 12-9).
    c. Poor focusing of object (if variable focus system is used).
    d. Dried lubricant or debris on camera lens or telescope.
    e. Telescope with improper focus of lenses.
    f. Movement of object.

The telescopes used for ureteroscopy and pyeloscopy are smaller in diameter (2.7 mm) than the standard cystoscopic telescopes. Therefore, adequate illumination for proper exposure is difficult and usually necessitates integral light bundles. This is especially important in the renal pelvis where there is a larger area to be illuminated and proper exposure almost always requires an integral fiberoptic light bundle and high-speed (ASA 400) film.

Another obstacle unique to photography within the kidney is the continuous movement of the kidney with respiration. It is difficult to time the shutter release and to focus on the moving object. Therefore, it is often necessary to have the anesthesiologist temporarily stop the patient's breathing when the photograph is taken.

COMMON PROBLEMS. It is usually possible to obtain very satisfactory photographs using the systems that have been described. Poor results do occur, however, usually because the subjects are not well illuminated or appear out of focus. Some possible causes for these poor results are listed in Table 19-4.

20
ANESTHESIA FOR UROLOGIC ENDOSCOPY

Donald W. Benson

In terms of the number of procedures done by the average urologist, it is probably safe to say that the vast majority are transurethral. Of these, many are performed in an office or clinic without the benefit of regional or general anesthesia. The anesthesiologist is partner only to those transurethral and other endoscopic procedures done in a cystoscopic suite, which is usually part of an operating room system. Depending, of course, on the number of urologists, endoscopy can constitute an important part of the workload of a busy surgical suite and deserves more attention from the anesthesiologist than is usually given.

THE PATIENT POPULATION. Perusal of patients subjected to transurethral and other endoscopic procedures usually demonstrates that they are predominantly males in the older age group, namely 40 years or older. Relatively few young children are patients; as people approach the age of stone formation, namely the 20s or 30s, the number of patients increases. As the process of aging takes over, the frequency increases. The gamut of concomitant disease is the same as that witnessed in any other practice but, again because of the age factor, those diseases related to atherosclerosis, such as coronary and cerebral vascular disease and hypertension, tend to predominate.

PATIENT PREPARATION. Every surgical or anesthetic intervention carries with it a discreet morbidity and possibly mortality rate. There is a strong tendency on the part of us all to consider a quick look with a cystoscope under local anesthesia with a little sedation as a benign procedure. It certainly can be but, at the same time, the potential for a variety of serious complications is always present, and it behooves the attending surgeon and anesthesiologist to observe consistently some common-sense rules of patient preparation.

The patient should be in the best possible physical shape that can reasonably be accomplished. Factors such as uncontrolled hypertension, incipient congestive heart failure, and pulmonary infection should be treated and controlled, provided, of course, that the delay involved does not outweigh the advantage of early surgical intervention. There should be a common-sense approach to this problem. One obviously can never achieve the ideal situation in very sick patients but, whenever possible, physiologic reserve should be built up for the patient's protection.

Many patients these days are treated as outpatients and, in a sense, prepare themselves for the procedure. There should be a clear understanding on the part of the patient, usually facilitated by an understandable printed handout, of the requirements for outpatient surgery. These include such simple measures as no food or drink intake for 8 hours previous to the procedure and a shower or bath in close relationship. The history, physical examination, and necessary laboratory studies should be done prior to the procedure but within a reasonable length of time, usually 7 to 10 days. Immediately before the surgical procedure, a brief history and physical examination should be done to ensure that no intercurrent catastrophe or change has occurred.

All of the above requirements generally hold for the inpatient as well, except that orders concerning food intake, bathing, enemas, and the like can be written for an inpatient and left with a nurse. Premedication is problematic. This decision is a very personal matter for many anesthesiologists and, since the advent of many new techniques and procedures, premedicant drugs are frequently not required. They are of importance in patients who are going to be treated under local anesthesia with sedation, as will be discussed later.

CHOICE OF ANESTHESIA. The choice of anesthesia is, first of all, dictated somewhat by the procedure that is to be undertaken. For example, in procedures in which coughing or uneven breathing cannot be tolerated, such as transureteral endoscopy, general anesthesia is probably the best choice. At the other end of the spectrum, simple short procedures, such as cystoscopy, can be done with little or no sedation and, rarely, even without local anesthesia. A second important factor is patient acceptance. It is the author's opinion that most transurethral procedures should be done under some form of regional or local anesthesia. Unfortunately, patients very often prefer to be unconscious during the procedure and will insist on a general anesthesia despite a probable increase in morbidity. This situation is ameliorated to some degree in transurethral surgery because the age group involved, namely 60- to 80-year-old patients, have a greater equanimity than their younger counterparts and will accept a spinal or an epidural when it is suggested. A third factor is the status of the patient, inpatient or outpatient, and the recovery room facilities available. General anesthesia necessitates a well-managed recovery room with all of its attendant facilities whereas, for the most part, regional anesthesia requires much less care from the anesthesiologist's point of view in the recovery period. Lastly, there are indications and contraindications specifically related to the patient's condition that also dictate the type of anesthesia. A surgeon's preference should not be ignored in this consideration, but it cannot be an overriding requirement.

Regional Anesthesia. Regional anesthesia is the anesthesia of choice whenever possible in transurethral surgery. No clinical studies support this obvious bias, but few anesthesiologists or urologists would disagree[4]. There are some very real advantages, which include:

1. Minimal disruption of body homeostasis by the anesthetic technique and drugs
2. Patient awareness of the procedure and the possibility of patient cooperation, such as holding the breath during x-ray or appreciating shoulder and abdominal pain when there is a perforation with extravasation
3. Ideal surgical conditions with no enhancement of bleeding, as may occur with some of the general anesthetic agents
4. Rapid recovery, which allows early ambulation and food and water intake

There are, of course, disadvantages, which include:

1. The everpresent specter of postspinal headache, which can occur even with a epidural when perforation of the dura occurs
2. Occasional unpleasant experiences during the procedure, such as nausea and vomiting, pain, and awareness

Although regional anesthesia poses other advantages and disadvantages, the above are the major ones and should be considered when addressing the type of anesthesia for a given patient.

SPINAL ANESTHESIA. Spinal anesthesia is by far the easiest form of anesthesia to accomplish and can be used to manage practically every type of transurethral surgery, especially if excellent patient cooperation can be achieved. As mentioned above, one of the major problems associated with spinal anesthesia is headache; it is interesting to note, however, that, again in the older age group, headache is a rare occurence and can be minimized by proper administration. It is not the purpose of this chapter to discuss techniques, but some specific details are worth noting. The sitting position, although not mandatory, is of great help in localizing the spread of the local anesthetic. Many patients, however, have to be anesthetized while lying on their side because they either are unstable or may even have orthostatic hypotension because of premedication or other drugs. Giving 2 cc of a hyperbaric solution, such as 100 mg of lidocaine in 7.5% glucose in water, to the average adult in the sitting position and allowing the patient to sit for approximately 2 minutes before lying down will produce a level of about T10 with some upward spread over time almost routinely. The T10 level is desirable because the pelvic viscera are innervated from T10 downward. Furthermore, the level should be high enough so that hip joint pain from the lithotomy position, especially in patients with arthritic changes, is controlled at the same time. If the spinal is injected with the patient lying on the side, the head should be tilted up so that the spinal column is slanted upward by about 10 degrees to minimize the upward spread.

The drugs most commonly used are lidocaine and tetracaine. Tetracaine is considered to last approximately 50 percent longer than lidocaine ($1–1\frac{1}{2}$ hr) and, of course, the spinal anesthetic should last as long as the procedure. In the author's hands, tetracaine has a 10- to 15-percent failure rate, so lidocaine is used far more frequently despite its somewhat shorter action. Tetracaine can be adjusted to last approximately $2\frac{1}{2}$ to 3 hours, especially if a very small amount of epinephrine, roughly 0.1 ml of 1 : 1,000 solution, is mixed with the spinal drug. Lidocaine can be extended to $1\frac{1}{2}$ to 2 hours with the same procedure, although it does not seem to be quite as reliable in this respect. As one becomes familiar with these drugs, one's choice is probably based more on experience than on any other indication.

Spinal headache is probably the most common complication of this type of anesthesia. It has been reasonably well demonstrated that the use of a 25- or 26-gauge needle carefully inserted will reduce the incidence of headache to a very low figure. It is unfortunate, however, that many of the individuals who need this type of anesthesia very often have some of the most difficult access because of arthritic changes and require the use of a 22-gauge spinal needle, which makes a larger hole and thus results in the spinal leak thought to cause the spinal headache. Postspinal headache is managed, for the most part, by providing symptomatic relief for the day so that the usual headache persists. Other therapeutic modalities such as blood patching are discussed in detail elsewhere[1,6]. Headache is not a feared complication, however, and should not stand in the way of utilization of this technique.

EPIDURAL ANESTHESIA. Epidural anesthesia is a reasonable technique to consider for transurethral work. Its use does, however, carry a slightly higher complication rate than spinal anesthesia and requires somewhat greater skill. Its greatest virtue is that it does not pose the specter of a spinal headache. It should be pointed out, however, that if the large needle used causes a dural puncture it makes a very large leak, which more often than not will result in a severe headache. In the older age group, epidural anesthesia tends to be somewhat spotty on occasion and also carries with it occasional systemic reaction to the local agent.

Epidural anesthesia can be induced through either the caudal or the lumbar approach. The caudal approach may be more difficult because variations in the caudal hiatus make entrance and recognition thereof somewhat difficult. Generally speaking, it is easier to use the lumbar route, again with the patient sitting or, if necessary, lying on the side. Entrance into the epidural space is detected by a variety of methods, such as loss of resistance or aspiration of a hanging drop on the end of the needle. Once the space is recognized, the anesthetic solution is injected, either through the needle directly or, if a catheter is expected to be left in place for a long procedure or postoperative analgesia, through a catheter. The volume of solution used is the major determinant of the level of anesthesia achieved. In general, it takes approximately 20 cc in the sitting position to achieve good solid perineal anesthesia and a level of T10 in the average individual. Very tall people and very short people, however, need more and less, respectively. It is not uncommon to have inadequate perineal anesthesia, especially when the anesthetic is injected with the patient lying on the side. The use of a larger volume, such as 25 or 30 cc, causes a greater spread in the needed downward direction, of course, but also spreads in a cephalad manner.

The concentration of the solution dictates the degree of muscle paralysis. Very low concentrations, such as 0.5% lidocaine or 0.25% bupivacaine, produce reasonably good sensory anesthesia. With 1 to 1.5% lidocaine and 0.75% bupivacaine, one can achieve good motor paralysis. It is important to make a safe compromise, however, since, as was suggested earlier, the incidence of reaction is higher in epidural anesthesia than in spinal anesthesia simply because of the quantity of drug necessary. For example, 20 cc of 2% lidocaine equals 400 mg, an amount that is very close to the toxic limit usually attributed to lidocaine.

There are some distinct advantages to the epidural approach. One is that it is possible to use bupivacaine, which has not yet been released for spinal anesthesia. Bupivacaine lasts two to three times longer than lidocaine and, in general, both easily encompasses the surgical time and provides some hours of postoperative analgesia. Another advantage to the epidural approach is that an indwelling catheter can be used and anesthesia extended for a very protracted period of time by adding alioquots of the local agent as the initial doses lose effectiveness. Using the catheter also permits the level of anesthesia to be raised should surgical intervention into the abdomen become necessary. Another advantage of the catheter is the administration of narcotics into the epidural space for the control of pain for the first 24 to 48 hours[3]. A dose of 2 to 6 mg of morphine in approximately 10 cc of saline provides several hours of pain relief equal to or greater than intramuscular injections of morphine. Morphine carries with it the occasional undesirable response of severe respiratory depression and sometimes nausea and itching. It does have a place, however, and should be considered in the overall anesthetic management of these patients.

CONTINUOUS SPINAL ANESTHESIA. For the sake of completeness, continuous spinal anesthesia should be mentioned. Very few patients require the duration of either continuous epidural or continuous spinal anesthesia but, from the standpoint of manageability and minimal possibility of systemic reaction, continuous spinal is superior to continuous epidural anesthesia. It has lost favor, however, because of the increased incidence of spinal headache. Again, it should be pointed out that, in individuals above 60 years of age, the likelihood of spinal headache, even in the presence of an indwelling catheter, is reasonably remote.

HYPOTENSION. The most commonly encountered complication of both spinal and epidural anesthesia is acute hypotension. When anesthesia is limited to the lower half of the body, hypotension is generally not too severe; if anesthesia extends upward to include the sympathetics to the upper body and the arms, however, rather severe hypotension can occur. This complication is the result of a loss in systemic resistance, which, if high enough, leads to a decrease in venous return, a slowing of the heart, and thus a decrease in cardiac output.

For the most part, drops in blood pressure that are not severe are best left alone. A judgment will have to be made, based on the state of the circulation of the patient, as to whether or not adequate perfusion of organs is being achieved at the level of blood pressure that has occurred. Fixed resistances in carotid arteries, coronary arteries, and renal vessels need higher blood pressures, and severe drops result in inadequate perfusion. In general, it can be said that the average individual tolerates comfortably and without harm a 30 percent drop in systolic blood pressure. Although adequate infusion of crystalloids can generally prevent the blood pressure from falling below this level, overload is not desirable and it is wise to reverse the hypotension in a pharmacologic manner. The author generally uses 50 mg of ephedrine mixed with the local anesthesia used for placement of the spinal or epidural. This ensures a slow release of a drug with both a modest inotropic and chronotropic effect as well as a peripheral vasopressor effect. Inasmuch as the cause of the blood pressure fall is largely related to peripheral vasodilation, carefully titrated doses of an alpha-agonist such as phenylephrine (0.5–1 mg) are in order.

General Anesthesia. The choice of agents for general anesthesia is less important than the technique employed for endoscopic procedures. The direct and indirect effects of breathing, coughing, and straining on the bladder, ureters, and kidneys are obvious. A sudden squeezing down of the bladder produced by a cough might easily result in a perforation. Analogous situations can be described for the ureters and the kidneys as well, which obviously implies the use of relaxation and controlled ventilation for most of the procedures done under general anesthesia. This is not meant to rule out the use of short-acting barbiturates and nitrous oxide with a mask in short procedures in which the scope of the surgery is predetermined and certain, for example, simple cystoscopies. Endoscopic efforts to remove kidney stones and stones lodged in the ureters are often very time consuming, and the requirement for constant smooth ventilation becomes very important. Thus, endotracheal anesthesia with proper relaxation is probably the method of choice.

It is very difficult to make a case for specific agents. Choice of an anesthetic largely depends on the skill of the anesthesiologist with the agents under consideration. Indications for or against specific agents are certainly conceivable, however. Liver disease, for example, tends to rule out halogenated hydrocarbons. This would indicate some other technique such as a narcotic relaxant method. Many anesthesiologists prefer, in the presence of known heart disease, to use a narcotic technique. It must be borne in mind that the greatest risk by far in protracted endoscopic work that does not involve cutting and bleeding is the anesthetic. The technique that offers the safest anesthetic and is the most useful for the surgical procedure should be the choice.

HIGH-FREQUENCY VENTILATION. The introduction of high-frequency ventilation into clinical use suggests an excellent application to anesthesia for endoscopic work, especially those procedures requiring entrance into the ureters and into the kidneys with rigid scopes. The field has not yet been clearly defined, but presently two major forms for producing high-frequency ventilation are evident — namely, the jet and the oscillation techniques [2,8]. In the jet method, short puffs of air are introduced into the endotracheal tube through a small nozzle at a frequency of approximately 100 to 200 times per minute. The volume of each jet varies according to the pressure and time that flow is allowed. Each jet causes an entrainment of gases from an enclosed anesthetic system. Rather than the usual in-and-out alveolar ventilation, this method uses an increased conduction convection into the airway to supply oxygen and remove carbon dioxide.

The oscillation method is somewhat similar but it supplies a continuous flow instead of an intermittent jet of gas into the airway, and the column of gas in the airway is vibrated at very high frequencies, usually between 10 and 15 Hz. Again, there is a reliance on an efficient mixing process to provide for improved gas exchange.

An important advantage of either of these techniques for urologic endoscopic work is that diaphragm motions, which might possibly interfere with the capture of stones in the kidney, for example, are reduced to a minimum. Only a faint vibration is transmitted to the kidney or ureter. Both of these techniques are currently in the experimental stage despite the fact that they have been recognized for many years. The reader is referred to current journals and review articles for detailed descriptions of these techniques.

Local Techniques and Sedation. Of all the methods utilized for endoscopic work, the simple application of a local anesthetic to the urethra and bladder probably accounts for more procedures than all the other techniques combined. The methods for producing anesthesia and sedation are as varied as the individuals using them, and it would be presumptuous to suggest a best way. A few important factors should be considered, however.

Local anesthetics are generally used in very high concentrations. Lidocaine, for example, is often supplied in a liquid or jelly form in a concentration of 4 to 5%. It is possible to produce quite good local anesthesia in the urethra (especially that of the male, which is probably most painful), provided that the agent is put in place and then given adequate time to work. The mucous membranes of the tract must absorb the agent to provide the anesthesia, and this is not accomplished immediately.

Special note should be made of the fact that it is quite possible to produce a local anesthetic reaction with this technique. If, for example, the urethra or the neck of the bladder is traumatized and entry into the circulation is possible, this highly concentrated local anesthetic can enter the circulation and, with a boluslike effect, produce a systemic reaction. The author has seen such an episode on at least two occasions, which required control of agitation and support of the blood pressure. While this complication is certainly rare, those using these techniques should be aware of its possibility and be prepared to manage the reaction.

While some patients who have been followed for bladder tumors, for example, and have received frequent cystoscopy can tolerate the procedures with little or no sedation and often even without any local anesthesia, most individuals have considerable discomfort and anxiety. Sedation is certainly an important adjunct to local anesthesia. While it can be accomplished in numerous ways, sedation, in general, should include a drug that reduces anxiety, such as diazepam or one of its congeners, and a narcotic for obtunding the pain and discomfort. There are those who would argue that the narcotic is not necessary, and this may well be true for certain patients; however, good pharmacology would dictate a combination of the two as a sounder approach to sedation.

Dosages should be adjusted to the size, general physical condition, and anxiety level of the patient. If too little sedation is given, the patient may be uncomfortable and, because of modest disorientation, very uncooperative. On the other hand, the author has been called more than once in a great rush to the cystoscopy room to resuscitate an individual who had received an overdose of a drug for sedation. It is a mistake to standardize dosages. It is far more appropriate to give small amounts of sedative drugs intramuscularly preoperatively and then to give supplementation intravenously as needed.

A word should be added about the use of barbiturates for sedation. In the elderly, these drugs can be very disturbing. Older patients, usually in the age group of 65 years and over, become very confused and disoriented, and thus very uncooperative. Narcotics and several of the newer sedative drugs are less likely to provoke this type of response. The state of sedation to aim for should be one wherein the patient is calm, somewhat sleepy, but at all times aware of the situation and cooperative.

Anesthesia for the Flank Approach. Throughout this discussion, the transurethral approach to the bladder, ureter, and kidney has been emphasized. It must be remembered, of course, that the kidney pelvis can be approached through the flank using endoscopic techniques. Simple local infiltration of the tract to the kidney will manage the major discomfort caused by the insertion of the instrument. Once the instrument is inserted, pain varies widely from patient to patient. Any of the three techniques — local, regional, or general anesthesia — will work well for the procedure. The position is an uncomfortable one and movement of the endoscope in a variety of directions can sometimes be painful regardless of excellent local anesthesia. General endotracheal anesthesia is the author's first choice for this procedure. Epidural and spinal anesthesia work quite well and, as usual, local infiltration with sedation suffices in the hands of the skilled operator. It is very likely that, as the skills as well as the instrumentation needed for stone removal improve, the discomfort produced will be minimal, causing local anesthesia to become the predominate technique of choice.

WATER INTOXICATION. No discussion of anesthesia for urologic endoscopy would be complete without mention of the syndrome caused by water intoxication (see Chap. 9). The anesthesiologist is usually the first to notice the symptoms and usually initiates the therapy; such early recognition of the syndrome is yet another reason for regional anesthesia for these procedures. The patient usually demonstrates some confusion along with hypotension and sometimes tachycardia, which progresses to complaints of tightness in the chest, difficulty in breathing, and even the wheezes of pulmonary edema. The first treatment is to initiate the diuresis, usually with a loop blocker such as furosemide or ethacrynic acid. Positive airway pressure with high oxygen concentrations decreases the dyspnea that is present in the awake patient as well as helps to ameliorate some of the pulmonary edema that might occur. In the patient undergoing general anesthesia, a rise in airway pressure from a fall in pulmonary compliance as pulmonary edema commences is one of the first signs. The application of positive-end expiratory pressure in these patients is of great help in reversing the pulmonary edema.

The incidence of water intoxication is not nearly as common as awareness of the problem, and the use of preventive measures has increased on the part of both surgeon and anesthesiologist. Also, the use of fluids that are osmotically equivalent has reduced the red cell laking that so commonly occurred in the past with water intoxication. As described above and in Chapter 9, the anesthesiologist's role in water intoxication involves recognition and treatment of the problem.

PRIAPISM. Priapism during transurethral endoscopy, while not always painful to the anesthetized patient, is certainly discomfiting for the surgeon. It is usually reflexive in origin and ordinarily occurs only under general anesthesia, not under spinal or epidural anesthesia. The fact that many modes of therapy have been suggested probably means that none of them work very well. In the author's hands, modest hypotension has provided the best results. This usually has been achieved by deepening halothane anesthesia. On one occasion, when this technique did not work, sodium nitroprusside was titrated intravenously to provide hypotension, which resulted in a successful subsidence of the priapism. Gale[5] reported on the use of ketamine to prevent priapism, and Ravindran, Dryden, and Sumerville[7] have recently reported on the use of ketamine and physostigmine for control of priapism. None of these experiences occurred in endoscopic procedures. The author recently had an episode, however, in which an erection was about to preclude further cystoscopic endeavors, and the treatment of ketamine 0.5 mg per kilogram, followed in about 5 minutes by 1 mg physostigmine IV, as suggested by Ravindran's series, caused a rapid detumescence. The patient at the time was under general anesthesia consisting of nitrous oxide, oxygen, and enflurane. The detumescence maintained itself to the end of the procedure and allowed the procedure to be completed.

A good level of general anesthesia adequate to depress reflex activity will probably prevent most priapism during manipulation. Once it occurs, such treatment as described above with ketamine and physostigmine is worth trying as well as efforts directed toward vasodilation, which usually include hypotension produced by either the general anesthetic agent or a direct-acting vasodilator.

MONITORING. All patients need some form of observation at all times whether undergoing local anesthesia or the most complicated form of general anesthesia. For the urologist working alone in a cystoscopy room in the dark, the maintenance of some form of vocal contact with the patient throughout the procedure is probably adequate. If the patient has a number of problems, such as cardiovascular instability or respiratory difficulties, however, it is prudent that an anesthesiologist observe constantly. The euphemism of standby anesthesia has pervaded both the surgical and anesthesiologic ranks, who too often regard such monitoring as a necessity without giving it the consistent care and thoughtfulness that is required. There is a definite art in properly sedating patients and maintaining them physiologically through any local procedure.

The electrocardiogram can be attached to a patient under local, regional, or general anesthesia, and is an extremely valuable adjunct. The endoscopist can position the oscilloscope in such a way that the electrocardiogram can be seen; such observation is, of course, vital for the anesthesiologist when monitoring the patient or giving the anesthesia. For protracted cases, especially those in which large volumes of fluid are washed in and out of the bladder (e.g., transurethral resections), the monitoring of temperature is extremely important. Elderly people tolerate hypothermia poorly, and it can produce a variety of ill effects such as arrhythmias and relative overdoses of anesthetics. Warming of solutions used usually prevents this type of complication.

Other types of invasive monitoring, such as intraarterial and pulmonary artery lines, ought to be used where indicated. Management of the very ill patient who needs an endoscopic procedure is undoubtedly easier if all of the monitoring parameters are available for administration of the appropriate therapy.

CONCLUSIONS. It is obvious from this discussion that the author's preference for anesthesia for endoscopic procedures is a regional technique, mainly that of spinal followed by epidural anesthesia. There is an important place for local anesthesia with the proper sedation, a method that should be well understood by both the urologist and the anesthesiologist. General anesthesia can be used in all instances and is especially important for the control of ventilation and the provision of optimal conditions for the newer endoscopic procedures requiring rigid endoscopy of the ureters and the kidneys.

REFERENCES

1. Abouleish, E. Epidural blood patch for treatment of chronic postlumbar puncture cephalgia. *Anesthesiology* 49:291, 1978.
2. Borg, V., Ericksson, I.A., and Sjostrand, V.H. High frequency positive pressure ventilation (HFPPV): A review based upon its use during bronchoscopy and microlaryngeal surgery under general anesthesia. *Anesth. Analg. (Cleveland)* 59:594, 1980.
3. Bromage, P.R., Camporesi, E., and Chestnut, D. Epidural narcotics for postoperative analgesia. *Anesth. Analg. (Cleveland)* 59:473, 1980.
4. Dripps, R.D., and Vandam, L.D. Long-term followup of patients who have received 10,098 spinal anesthetics. *J.A.M.A.* 156:1486, 1954.
5. Gale, A.S. Ketamine prevention of penile turgescence. *J.A.M.A.* 219:1629, 1972.
6. Gormley, J.B. Treatment of postspinal headache. *Anesthesiology* 21:565, 1960.
7. Ravindran, R.S., Dryden, G.E., and Somerville, G.M. Treatment of priapism with ketamine and physostigmine. *Anesth. Analg. (Cleveland)* 61:705, 1982.
8. Sjostrand, V.H., and Ericksson, I.A. High rates and low volumes in mechanical ventilation—not just a matter of ventilatory frequency. *Anesth. Analg. (Cleveland)* 59:567, 1980.

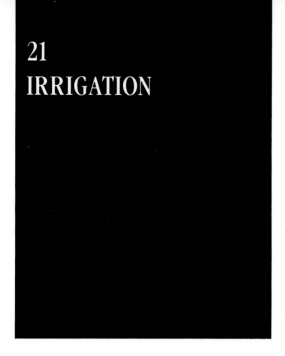

21
IRRIGATION

Demetrius H. Bagley

Jeffry L. Huffman

Edward S. Lyon

Irrigation through an endoscope is essential to distend the lumen of the structure being examined. Each portion of the urinary collecting system has a *lumen,* which is a potential space that can be distended by introducing a fluid under pressure. The intraluminal surface is then moved away from the objective lens into the viewing range. A liquid or gas can be used; in urologic systems, a liquid is usually chosen. The fluid must be clear so that it will not obscure the field of view and should be nonirritating, or at least minimally irritating, to the urothelium. Passage of irrigant through the instrument also washes debris and blood from the lens and dilutes blood within the lumen.

Table 21-1. Irrigating Solutions

1. Nonconductive
   a. Water
   b. Glycine (aminoacetic acid) 1.5%
   c. Sorbitol 3.0%
   d. Mannitol 5.0%
2. Conductive
   a. Saline (sodium chloride) 0.9% or 0.45%
   b. Lactated Ringer's

CHOICE OF IRRIGANT. Liquid irrigants have their own particular advantages, and specific solutions can be designed to maximize different features (Table 21-1). The decision to use water, a hypotonic solution, an isoosmotic nonconductive solution, or an isoosmotic conductive or electrolyte solution is based on several factors. The procedure to be performed usually dictates the type of solution that should be used. If there is minimal chance of fluid absorption, as with simple diagnostic cystoscopy, then any of the commonly available irrigating solutions can be used satisfactorily. If, on the other hand, the possibility of fluid absorption is significant, as with transurethral resection of the prostate, then an isoosmotic or otherwise nonhemolyzing solution should be used. With special procedures such as nephroscopy and ureteroscopy, there is an even greater possibility of direct intravenous absorption of the irrigant through pyelovenous backflow; therefore, an irrigant suitable for intravenous administration such as saline or Ringer's solution should be employed. A similar risk of absorption during visual internal urethrotomy would dictate the use of a nonhemolytic or isoosmotic solution.

Water. Sterile water has some specific advantages that can recommend its use. Since it is hypotonic, it rapidly lyses red blood cells and renders vision in the presence of bleeding slightly clearer. It also offers some theoretic advantage in the resection of bladder tumors since tumor cells dispersed within the irrigant may also be lysed. This advantage remains theoretic as no benefit in terms of lower rates of tumor growth has been demonstrated in animal systems. Since water is nonconductive, it is also a reasonable choice if an electrocautery is to be used and there is little risk of absorption of the irrigant. These conditions are met with cystoscopic biopsy of small papillary tumors and subsequent fulguration of the base. Water is not recommended as an irrigant for transurethral resection of the prostate[5].

Some institutions have designed systems for sterile water production from a central water supply, and thus have large volumes of irrigant available at low cost. This supply can be a major consideration in the choice of irrigant when physiologic factors do not contraindicate its use. Thus, water may become the first choice as an irrigant for cystoscopy when such a source is available. The sterility of these systems may be difficult to maintain, and they should be monitored carefully.

Saline. In the spectrum of irrigating fluids, normal (0.9%) saline can be considered on the end opposite from water. It is an isotonic, electrolytic solution that is compatible with biologic tissues. It is well tolerated by the urothelium and can be administered intravenously in large quantities to patients who can tolerate the load of sodium. It is, therefore, the irrigating solution of choice for procedures in which absorption is likely. It can be used for ureteroscopy and for nephroscopy performed for diagnosis or stone removal[3,8]. Ureteroscopy for electroresection or coagulation of urothelial tumors can be performed with isotonic nonconductive solutions for only short periods.

Hypotonic (1/6 or 1/7 normal) saline is used for electrohydraulic lithotripsy (see Chap. 12). When used in the bladder, it presents no unusual problem, but it can be absorbed from the kidney. Therefore, when the electrohydraulic lithotriptor is employed to fragment renal or ureteral calculi, the dilute saline irrigant should be employed for only short periods and under very low pressure. The endoscopist must remain alert to the possibility of absorption of this hemolytic solution.

Ringer's Solution. Another physiologic electrolytic solution that can be used as an irrigant is lactated Ringer's solution. It contains potassium chloride and sodium lactate in addition to sodium chloride. It is tolerated slightly better by the urothelium than saline but offers no other advantages. It can be used for diagnostic endoscopy when there is risk of absorption. Ringer's lactate, like other electrolytic solutions, cannot be used for electrosurgical procedures since it will disperse the current ineffectively.

Nonhemolytic, Nonconductive Solutions. The value of nonhemolytic, nonconductive irrigation solutions in transurethral resection of the prostate was discovered once the procedure's complications were recognized. Absorption of hypotonic solutions resulted in hyponatremia and in hemolysis with hyperkalemia and renal damage. The use of isotonic solutions can minimize these effects, while nonconductive solutions are essential for electrosurgery. The search for the ideal solution has resulted in several commercially available solutions, each with its own advantages.

Glycine. Glycine (aminoacetic acid) is widely used as a 1.5% solution. It was recommended by Nesbit and Glickman in 1948[7]. This solution with an osmolarity of 200 mOsm per liter is slightly hypotonic but has been employed with relatively few direct complications[5]. It is nonhemolytic and nonelectrolytic or very weakly ionized. When glycine enters the systemic circulation, it is converted to serine and glyoxylic acid. Encephalopathy has been reported in patients who underwent transurethral prostatic resection with glycine irrigation and were found in the postoperative period to have elevated blood ammonia levels[2]. Other possible adverse reactions include nausea, lightheadedness, and, when large volumes of fluid are absorbed, cardiovascular overload.

Sorbitol. Sorbitol is available in a 3% solution. Designated as D-glucitol, it is a reduced form of dextrose. The solution is nonhemolytic, nonconductive, and clear. When absorbed intravascularly, it is either metabolized to carbon dioxide and water or excreted by the kidneys. Hyperglycemia may develop in patients with diabetes when absorbed sorbitol is metabolized. This solution is also slightly hypotonic.

Other Irrigants. *Glucose* as a 2.5 or 5% solution is a satisfactory irrigant but exhibits major problems [5]. It forms a very sticky syrup as it dries, making instruments and gloves difficult to handle. It also interferes with glucose determinations in diabetic patients and may lead to hyperglycemia if absorbed.

Urea has been used in a 1% solution but, because it may cause hemolysis and has an unpleasant odor, there is little to recommend it.

Mannitol has been used as a 5% solution. It often tends to crystallize and form a film on surfaces of instruments, however, thus interfering with the action of the resectoscope.

IRRIGATION PRESSURE. The delivery pressure of any irrigating solution is extremely important for the absorption of that solution and the resulting complications. As discussed in Chapter 9, absorption of fluid during prostatic resection increases sharply with pressures greater than 60 cm of water, which can develop when the irrigating bottle or bag is hung 60 cm above the bladder. Absorption can be decreased markedly by lowering the pressure to 30 or 40 cm [1]. Pressure within the bladder and urethra can also be lowered by maintaining a continuous flow, low-pressure system, either with a suprapubic trocar draining the bladder or with a continuous flow resectoscope. Pressure can be monitored clinically by observing the filling of the bladder. If the bladder is only partially filled and the back wall can be seen to be partially collapsed with either a resectoscope in the prostatic urethra or a cystourethroscope within the urethra or the bladder, then the intravesical pressure is within a reasonable range. An even greater monitor of safety can be maintained when a procedure is performed in an alert, awake patient. The patient with a neurologically intact bladder will then develop discomfort if the intravesical pressure reaches an unacceptable level.

Excessive irrigating pressures must be avoided during procedures in which the pressure is transmitted directly to the kidney, such as ureteroscopy and nephroscopy. Absorption of irrigant can occur by pyelovenous, sinus, or lymphatic backflow, just as it does, and can be demonstrated, with retrograde pyelography (see Fig. 13-8A, B). As noted previously, an isotonic, physiologic solution should be used as an irrigant for these procedures.

TEMPERATURE OF IRRIGATING FLUID. The optimal temperature of fluid for irrigation has been the point of several studies and much discussion. The preferred temperature for irrigation solutions that are used for simple cystoscopy is probably body temperature or certainly no less than room temperature to avoid any possible alterations of the patient's body temperature. Fluid at body temperature should definitely be used for percutaneous nephroscopy and for ureteroscopy since body temperature can quickly be changed by irrigation with cold fluids and the rapid heat exchange possible in the interior of the kidney. Because of the large volumes of irrigant employed, fluid temperature is particularly important in percutaneous nephroscopy and stone removal.

There is more controversy regarding the temperature of irrigant for transurethral resection of the prostate. Cold ($2°C$) irrigant has been reported to have an impressive beneficial effect on intraoperative hemostasis, thought to be the result of vasoconstriction induced by the cold irrigant [9]. Other studies have indicated that such cold irrigant inhibits platelet aggregation [4] and actually promotes intraoperative bleeding. All studies have reported an impressive lowering of the patient's body temperature when cold irrigant was employed. At this time the lack of evidence strongly supporting the use of cold irrigant for transurethral resection of the prostate can lead one to conclude that it is preferable to use irrigating solution at room or body temperature during the procedure.

IRRIGATION DELIVERY SYSTEM. Irrigating solutions are available in 1- and 3-liter containers that can be connected by tubing directly to the endoscopic instrument. Two or more containers can be joined with Y-connectors to provide an even larger reservoir of fluid. The final connecting tubing should include a bubble trap (Fig. 21-1). The 1-liter containers of irrigant are often adequate for cystoscopy. Several of the larger containers are used during transurethral resection of the prostate with either the standard or the continuous flow resectoscope. The pressure of the irrigant can be monitored easily by the height at which the reservoir is placed relative to the instrument. Care should be taken to move the fluid reservoir as the operating table is raised or lowered.

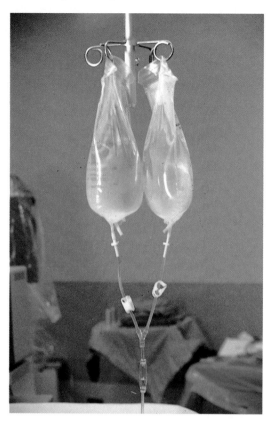

Figure 21-1. *Collapsible plastic bags of irrigant drain through a Y-connector tube and bubble trap to a single tube attached to the endoscope.*

Bubbles. Bubbles passing with the irrigant into the instrument and the endoscopic field of view can be both annoying and, because they distort the view, dangerous. Several techniques can be of help in avoiding bubbles. The irrigant should be allowed to flow through the instrument before the instrument is passed into the orifice. Thus, the air within the instrument is washed from the lumen before it is trapped within the urethra, ureter, or nephrostomy tract. When the irrigating solution container is changed, care should be taken to avoid entry of air into the system. The tubing to the reservoir that is being changed should be clamped to prevent drainage of the fluid with subsequent influx of air. An intermediate reservoir should be used as a bubble trap to prevent any air from entering the system at the highest point and travelling to the level of the endoscope. Bubbles are usually much less of a problem in continuous flow endoscopy since the instruments used generally sweep the air bubbles along with the irrigant into the outflow system.

If bubbles do enter the field of view, the instrument or the patient may be tilted to allow the bubbles to flow away from the instrument to a higher point in the system. Two maneuvers for removal of bubbles from the sheath in front of the lens are (1) to turn the entire endoscope over to allow trapped bubbles under the beak of the instrument to escape and (2) to depress the operator's end of the scope so that the patient's end is higher and bubbles are encouraged to escape from the open tip of the sheath.

Bubbles can be particularly troublesome in the urethra during visual internal urethrotomy since they remain trapped at the objective lens of the instrument throughout the procedure. They can be eliminated by opening the outflow stopcock or by removing the telescope and subsequently replacing it while the fluid is flowing.

Bubbles may also be incapacitating during ureteroscopy. A small bubble can fill the lumen of the ureter and characteristically pass to the highest level in the ureter, which in the supine patient is the portion of the midureter that crosses the psoas muscle. It may not be possible to change a patient's position, which may have been set to optimize the gravitational effects on the calculus or the kidney. The bubbles occasionally can be removed by aspiration with a catheter passed through the ureteroscope into the field. Ironically, the loss of vision caused by a collection of small bubbles can sometimes be effectively cleared by introducing 1 or 2 ml of air or carbon dioxide into the side port of the ureteroscope, thus creating a single large bubble through which vision is good. It is much more important to avoid strenuously the introduction of air into the irrigation system during this procedure.

CARBON DIOXIDE AS AN IRRIGANT. Carbon dioxide has been used relatively little as an irrigant in urologic endoscopy. It has been used with excellent results in both laparoscopy and, in the field of gynecology, urethroscopy, however. In a urologic study comparing carbon dioxide cystoscopy with standard cystoscopy using water, visualization was judged somewhat better with the gas instrument [6]. In the presence of macroscopic hematuria, visualization was markedly better with carbon dioxide. Even minor active bleeding obscured vision when the blood was diluted by water used as an irrigant.

Visibility was significantly improved when carbon dioxide was used since the blood, instead of dispersing within the irrigating fluid, remained localized at the source within the bladder or clotted along the vesical wall. Carbon dioxide is generally safe since it is nonexplosive and is so highly soluble in water that the risk of gas emboli is minimal. It has special benefits for office use since it can be stored readily in cylinders, is often available for urodynamic equipment, and is very convenient and neat to use without the spills associated with liquid irrigants. The use of carbon dioxide as a urologic irrigant is uncommon at this time but may find an important role in urologic endoscopy.

REFERENCES

1. Hagstrom, R. S., and Shaw, J. A. Low pressure irrigation for transurethral prostatic resection. *J. Urol.* 83 : 724, 1960.
2. Hoekstra, P. T., Kahnoski, R., McCamish, M. A., Bergen, W., and Heetderks, D. R. Transurethral resection syndrome — a new perspective: Encephalopathy with associated hyperammonemia. *J. Urol.* 130 : 704, 1983.
3. Huffman, J. L., Bagley, D. H., and Lyon, E. S. Extending cystoscopic techniques into the ureter and renal pelvis: Experience with ureteroscopy and pyeloscopy. *J. A. M. A.* 250 : 2002, 1983.
4. Kattlove, H., and Alexander, B. Effect of cold on bleeding. *Lancet* 2 : 1359, 1970.
5. Madsen, P. O., and Madsen, R. E. Clinical and experimental evaluation of different irrigating fluids for transurethral surgery. *Invest. Urol.* 3 : 122, 1965.
6. Matthews, P. N., Woodhouse, C. R. J., and Hendry, W. F. Carbon dioxide versus water for cystoscopy: A comparative study. Presented at the 78th Annual Meeting of the American Urological Association, Las Vegas, April, 1983.
7. Nesbit, R. M., and Glickman, S. I. The use of glycine solution as an irrigating medium during transurethral resection. *J. Urol.* 59 : 1212, 1948.
8. Schultz, R. E., et al. Percutaneous ultrasonic lithotripsy: Choice of irrigant. *J. Urol.* 130 : 858, 1983.
9. Serrao, A., Mallik, M. K., Jones, P. A., Hendry, W. F., and Wickham, J. E. A. Hypothermic prostatic resection. *Br. J. Urol.* 48 : 685, 1976.

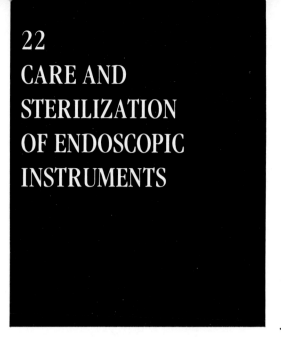

22
CARE AND STERILIZATION OF ENDOSCOPIC INSTRUMENTS

Demetrius H. Bagley

Edward S. Lyon

Jeffry L. Huffman

Urologic endoscopes are expensive instruments that are used in invasive procedures. They must be carefully maintained to preserve their useful life and to avoid transmission of infectious diseases. Rigid endoscopes are generally durable but may be damaged by relatively minor physical shocks or by improper sterilization techniques. Flexible endoscopes are even more fragile and may require specific sterilization techniques. The utmost care is essential for all endoscopes but is crucial for the long, thin ureteropyeloscopes and flexible instruments. Appropriate cleaning and sterilization of endoscopes before and after passage into a patient's body is necessary to prevent the transmission of infectious organisms between patient and medical personnel.

TYPES OF CLEANING

Mechanical Cleaning. Mechanical cleaning is the most important step in the care of endoscopic instruments. Maintenance of the instruments in working order depends largely on thorough mechanical cleansing to remove all particulate matter. Blood and other proteinaceous debris must be removed immediately to prevent pitting of the metal surfaces and to avoid its accumulation in crevices on the instrument, such as the locking mechanism or the point at which the stopcock attaches to the sheath of a cystoscope. Proper cleansing of the telescope is essential to avoid the buildup of opaque debris on the light-transmitting surfaces and subsequent discoloration. The seals must also be preserved to prevent the entry of moisture into the telescopes.

The most important role of mechanical cleaning is to remove bacteria-laden particles. The chance of transmitting an infection can be related to the size of the inoculum of organisms. By removing contaminated debris, a large inoculum can be avoided. Any infectious organisms remaining on the instruments can be rendered inactive by disinfection or sterilization.

Manual Cleaning. Endoscopic instruments can be cleaned thoroughly by handwashing. Sheaths and all submersible instruments should be placed into soapy water, which is flushed through the interior of the sheath and irrigation ports. Adherent debris including tissue, blood, and the accumulated dry irrigant is manually removed and scrubbed from the surface of the instrument. A soft brush or cotton gauze can be employed to reach into less accessible corners. The lumen is further cleaned with a long narrow brush or a pledget of cotton drawn throughout its length. The instrument should be thoroughly rinsed, first in clean running water and then in distilled water, and thoroughly dried. A jet of compressed air can be passed through the lumen to hasten drying. Abrasive washing instruments and cleaners should be avoided because they can roughen the surface of even a stainless steel instrument.

Instruments that cannot be submersed for cleaning should be thoroughly wiped with a cloth wetted with a detergent solution. They are then rinsed with another soft cloth wetted only with water. Care must be taken not to use excess water, which can leak into the critical portions of these instruments (this restraint is especially important with flexible fiberoptic instruments). After washing and rinsing, the entire instrument should be dried with a clean drying cloth.

A detergent should be employed in the cleaning process. In general, moderately alkaline, low-sudsing detergents are satisfactory. The selection of detergent, however, should be guided by the instrument manufacturer's specific recommendations. Ordinary soap should be avoided because of the possible formation of insoluble alkaline films that can coat the instrument.

The exposed ocular and objective lenses of the telescopes are cleaned with a swab moistened with alcohol. This swab will clear the surface of any adherent debris and precipitate. Do not use any metal instruments, even small forceps, for the swab or for cleaning the lens since these may scratch the delicate lens or coating.

Ultrasonic Cleaning. Ultrasonic cleaning of standard operative surgical instruments is routinely employed in most hospitals. It is satisfactory for most surgical instruments but the many different endoscopes are extremely delicate and can be cleaned more safely individually by hand. Ultrasonic cleaning can be used for the metal working instruments, such as biopsy forceps or graspers. It can ensure more thorough cleaning of the many irregularities in these instruments.

DISINFECTION AND STERILIZATION. Transmission of disease by endoscopes is avoided by removing microorganisms from the instruments or by rendering bacteria nonviable. Different organisms have different sensitivities to the physical or chemical modalities employed and, therefore, various levels of disinfection or even sterility can be achieved. Although many common bacteria can be killed by several different techniques, spores, tubercle bacilli, and viruses may require more severe conditions.

The life cycle of a contained population of microorganisms follows that of a general growth curve. After the initial inoculation of viable cells into a liquid medium, a stationary or lag phase ensues, during which there is no increase in the number of organisms. It is followed by logarithmic or exponential growth. During this period, there is a maximum and constant rate of cell multiplication. The next phase is stationary, during which the rates of multiplication and of death of the organisms are in balance. With the progressive increase in the death rate, the population enters a death phase with a decline in population. Initially, the organisms die exponentially but, as the majority of cells die, there may be a small population remaining with a very slow death rate, and some organisms may survive for long periods of time.

It is difficult to define absolute death in a population of microorganisms. One accepted criterion is the inability of the organism to reproduce when placed in an optimal environment. This environment is crucial in determining the viability of the organism. After sublethal injury, organisms may fail to reproduce in certain environments while they may multiply immediately or after a lag phase in other more beneficial environments.

The criteria sought for levels of disinfection of sterility for surgical instruments are based on known effectiveness of various techniques to eradicate known pathogenic organisms. Essential to these criteria of correction is the assumption that the sterilizing machines are accurate and working to the defined limits. Moreover, considering the risks of failure of these machines, techniques for checking the performance must be employed with each cycle.

Risk Categories. Medical and surgical instruments and other equipment can be divided into three categories, based on the risk of infection during their use. These groups were described by Spaulding and co-workers[4] as critical, semicritical, and noncritical.

Critical items are those that carry with them a great risk of imparting infection if they are contaminated. They are introduced directly into normally sterile areas of the body and, therefore, must be sterile. The second category of equipment, termed *semicritical,* includes those items that come in contact with the intact epithelial surfaces but do not ordinarily penetrate beyond the body's physical defenses. Endoscopes generally fall into this group. Sterilization has been considered desirable but not essential. These instruments should at least undergo processing that will destroy ordinary bacteria, spores, tubercle bacilli, and small nonlipid viruses — thorough cleaning and high-level disinfection have often been considered adequate. The third category includes *noncritical* items, which are those that either do not contact the patient directly or touch only unbroken skin. These categories are particularly useful in determining the effort necessary to render materials free of microbial activity since different materials tolerate the rigors of various cleansing processes to varied extents.

Disinfection. *Sterilization* has been defined as the use of procedures to destroy all microbial life within the system, including the highly resistant bacterial spores. *Disinfection,* in comparison, eliminates most recognized pathogenic microorganisms but not necessarily all microbial forms, including possibly spores. Thus, disinfection processes reduce the level of contamination but do not include that margin of overkill inherent in sterilization processes. Disinfection can be achieved by *germicides,* which are chemicals possessing various antimicrobial activities. Although these chemicals generally lack the capacity to kill spores routinely, they can usually remove ordinary vegetative forms of bacteria and, in some cases, can act against the tubercle bacilli, fungi, and nonlipid viruses. An *antiseptic* is defined as a germicide used on skin or living tissue to inhibit or kill microorganisms, while a *disinfectant* is a germicide used exclusively for killing microorganisms on nonliving objects.

Disinfection has also been categorized into three levels: high, intermediate, and low[4]. Since many materials are damaged by the high temperatures achieved in steam autoclaves, they must be sterilized chemically. Consequently, an essential feature of *high-level* disinfection is its achievement of chemical sterilization, which necessarily includes activity of the process against spores, fungi, and viruses. Several disinfectants possess sporicidal activity, an indication of high-level disinfection. These agents include aqueous 2%, glutaraldehyde, 8% formaldehyde solution in 70% alcohol, 6 to 10% stabilized hydrogen peroxide, and ethylene oxide gas. Other agents may also be effective with prolonged exposure.

Intermediate-level disinfectants can inactivate the tubercle bacillus but may not kill large numbers of bacterial endospores. Examples of these agents include 0.5% iodine, 70 to 90% ethanol, and isopropanol. Their effects against viruses may vary widely.

Low-level disinfectants can remove common vegetative bacteria but may be ineffective against bacterial endospores, tubercle bacilli, or small nonlipid viruses. Their activity may vary depending on the concentrations of their ingredients. Examples of these disinfectants include quaternary ammonium compounds, mercurials, and lower levels of iodophores and phenolic compounds.

The selection of disinfectant level can be related to the category of the material regarding the critical nature of antimicrobial treatment. Critical items require sterilization while noncritical equipment may be subjected to other levels of disinfection. Semicritical items may be controversial.

Endoscopic equipment is placed into normally sterile areas of the body but usually comes in contact with intact epithelial surfaces; therefore, it is included in the semicritical or critical categories. Optimally, endoscopes should be submitted to a procedure of cleaning and sterilization. In situations in which this is impractical, they should receive at least thorough mechanical cleaning and high-level disinfection[1,2]. The risk of physical damage to the endoscope, particularly to the flexible fiberoptic endoscope, must be considered in choosing a disinfection regimen[1]. The most widely used high-level disinfectants for endoscopic equipment include ethylene oxide– and 2% glutaraldehyde–based germicides.

Sterilization. As noted in the preceding section, *sterilization* is defined as the absolute destruction of all forms of life. Agents responsible for this process can be grouped as physical or chemical and, further, as liquid, gaseous, or electromagnetic. The severe conditions imposed for sterilization may damage the primary object being sterilized. An endoscope is particularly susceptible to injury because of the many different materials composing the instrument. It cannot be carelessly exposed to wide variations in temperature, humidity, and chemical activity without severe structural damage.

HEAT, MOIST OR DRY. The classic agent for microbial destruction is heat. Dry heat, in comparison to moist heat, is relatively slow and requires fairly high temperatures for sterilization. It is effective, however, in penetrating all kinds of material, including oils and closed containers, which may not be permeable to humidity. Although a temperature of 170°C (340°F) may require only 60 minutes exposure for sterilization, reduction of the temperature to 121°C (250°F) will require overnight exposure. The addition of humidity to heat provides more rapid, effective antibacterial activity. Saturated steam at 121°C may require only minutes to provide extremely strong probability of sterilization.

Sterilization by steam under pressure is one of the least expensive and most common forms of sterilization employed clinically. It must be avoided for equipment that can be damaged by heat and moisture. This description is almost universally true for urologic endoscopes and, therefore, steam sterilization can be used in only a few specific instances. It can be employed for metal working instruments such as biopsy forceps and metal sheaths during emergency situations—for instance, the dropping of the instrument to the floor. It must always be avoided for flexible fiberoptic instruments and it should also be avoided for all endoscopic telescopes. The manufacturers admit that even in those few cases where steam sterilization is permissible, it will shorten the life of the endoscope considerably.

ETHYLENE OXIDE. Ethylene oxide is the most widely used gaseous sterilizing agent. It is used often in hospitals in the United States to sterilize items that cannot be treated in the steam autoclave. Ethylene oxide is a reactive molecule with the following chemical structure:

Its alkylation of nucleic acids results in its bactericidal and sporicidal activity. The effectiveness of ethylene oxide against spores has been related to the relative humidity with the maximal effect at 33 percent. Ethylene oxide inactivates all viruses against which it has been tested.[3] Temperature and exposure time are also important and are standardized to eradicate known microbiologic standards.

After an effective sterilizing cycle, the agent must be removed for safe use of the instrument. Several factors including the material, packaging, and parameters of the sterilizing cycle itself can affect the removal of residual agent. Ethylene oxide has been indicated as a carcinogen in some studies and is a severe local irritant. It must be employed only with the greatest care and with strict attention to aeration. The manufacturer can provide information on the optimal features of sterilization and aeration. It should be noted that optimal cycles for flexible endoscopes may vary widely between manufacturers.

OTHER TECHNIQUES. Gamma-irradiation has been used primarily for sterilization in commercial applications. Although it is an economic and reliable sterilizing agent, it may irreversibly damage some materials. It is not practical for hospital sterilization.

Direct application of ultraviolet radiation can kill microbial agents including bacteria, yeasts, and viruses. This destruction is the result of alteration of the DNA with cross-linking of adjacent thymidine residues and possibly other units as well. The ultraviolet light must penetrate the substance to be sterilized and, therefore, its application for medical and surgical instruments is limited.

STORAGE OF UROLOGIC ENDOSCOPES. Urologic endoscopes should be carefully stored in a planned fashion for several purposes. The intent should be to protect the instruments themselves, to maintain their cleanliness or sterility, and to ensure their ready accessibility for the endoscopist.

Each instrument should be stored in a separate padded container. The individual parts of the endoscope, such as the sheath and the obturator, should be dissembled and wrapped separately but stored together. Interchangeable telescopes should also be stored separately so that they can be used with other endoscopes. As an example, the forward-viewing telescope may fit either a cystoscope, a visual urethrotome, or a resectoscope. By storing that telescope separately, other unnecessary sheaths will not have to be removed from storage when the telescope is used with a single instrument. If a telescope fits only a single endoscope, such as that for the ureteroscope or percutaneous nephroscope, then storage of that telescope with the endoscope may be preferable.

The instrument should be placed in a rigid container and should lie well padded with towels, gauze, or foam. The exact type of container will vary according to the specific instrument and the techniques employed for disinfection or sterilization of the endoscope. A permeable or perforated tray is employed when the instrument is gas sterilized. Other less rigorous containers can be employed when the instrument is to be removed for disinfection in a germicidal solution immediately before use. In that case, the container itself is not subjected to the sterilization process. The tray or case must accommodate the instrument without touching the instrument's sides or necessitating sharp coiling of a flexible instrument.

Instruments must be packaged to maintain cleanliness or sterility. All instruments should be stored in covered containers for protection from environmental contamination. Sterilized instruments should be wrapped to maintain sterility. A double-wrap technique is often employed to ensure sterility as the instrument is unwrapped and passed to the operator in a sterile field. Plastic films are preferred packaging materials for gas sterilization since instruments wrapped in this way remain sterile longer than those packaged in paper or muslin.

Urologic endoscopes and the associated working instruments should be stored in a readily accessible system. Because operating room personnel relatively unfamiliar with the different urologic endoscopes may occasionally staff the urologic suites in many institutions, it is well worth the initial effort needed to establish an accessible storage system. Similar instruments can be grouped together, and the most commonly used instruments can be stored in the most prominent position. A list of instruments and their locations can sometimes prove to be the most important feature in the endoscopy suite during an emergency procedure when unfamiliar personnel are staffing the room. It cannot be overemphasized that instruments must be available and in working order to be of value to the urologist.

REFERENCES

1. Bond, W. W. Favero, M. S., Mackel, D. C., and Mallison, G. F. Sterilization or disinfection of flexible fiberoptic endoscopes. *A. O. R. N. J.* 30 : 350, 1979.
2. Center for Disease Control. *Guidelines for the Prevention and Control of Nosocomial Infections.* Atlanta: Center for Disease Control, 1981.
3. Sidwell, R. W., Dixon, G. J., Westbrook, L., and Pulmodege, E. A. Procedure for the evaluation of the virucidal effectiveness of an ethylene oxide gas sterilizer. *Appl. Microbiol.* 17 : 790, 1969.
4. Spaulding, E. H., Cundy, K. R., and Turner, F. J. Chemical Disinfection of Medical and Surgical Materials. In C. A. Lawrence and S. S. Block (Eds.), *Disinfection, Sterilization and Preservation* (1st ed.) Philadelphia: Lea & Febiger. Pp. 654–684, 1968.

SUGGESTED READINGS

Block, S. S. (Ed.) *Disinfection, Sterilization and Preservation* (3rd ed.). Philadelphia: Lea & Febiger, 1983.

Perkins, J. J. *Principles and Methods of Sterilization in Health Sciences* (2nd ed.). Springfield, Ill.: Charles C. Thomas, 1969.

INDEX

INDEX